AF814902

METHODS IN MOLECULAR BIOLOGY

Series Editor
John M. Walker
School of Life and Medical Sciences
University of Hertfordshire
Hatfield, Hertfordshire, AL10 9AB, UK

For further volumes:
http://www.springer.com/series/7651

Vaccine Adjuvants

Methods and Protocols

Edited by

Christopher B. Fox

Infectious Disease Research Institute, Seattle, WA, USA; Department of Global Health, University of Washington, Seattle, WA, USA

Humana Press

Editor
Christopher B. Fox
Infectious Disease Research Institute
Seattle, WA, USA

Department of Global Health
University of Washington
Seattle, WA, USA

ISSN 1064-3745 ISSN 1940-6029 (electronic)
Methods in Molecular Biology
ISBN 978-1-4939-6443-7 ISBN 978-1-4939-6445-1 (eBook)
DOI 10.1007/978-1-4939-6445-1

Library of Congress Control Number: 2016951959

© Springer Science+Business Media New York 2017
This work is subject to copyright. All rights are reserved by the Publisher, whether the whole or part of the material is concerned, specifically the rights of translation, reprinting, reuse of illustrations, recitation, broadcasting, reproduction on microfilms or in any other physical way, and transmission or information storage and retrieval, electronic adaptation, computer software, or by similar or dissimilar methodology now known or hereafter developed.
The use of general descriptive names, registered names, trademarks, service marks, etc. in this publication does not imply, even in the absence of a specific statement, that such names are exempt from the relevant protective laws and regulations and therefore free for general use.
The publisher, the authors and the editors are safe to assume that the advice and information in this book are believed to be true and accurate at the date of publication. Neither the publisher nor the authors or the editors give a warranty, express or implied, with respect to the material contained herein or for any errors or omissions that may have been made.

Printed on acid-free paper

This Humana Press imprint is published by Springer Nature
The registered company is Springer Science+Business Media LLC New York

Preface

"So far, the results have been very, very exciting... But now we got involved into practical application" --Edgar Ribi [1]

Vaccine adjuvants have an interesting and empirical history, which led immunologist Charles Janeway to refer to them as the "immunologist's dirty little secret." Nevertheless, pioneering work led by Edgar Ribi elucidated structure-function relationships of adjuvant components while emphasizing practical application and manufacturing aspects, leading to the development of the TLR4 ligand MPL® that is now contained in approved human vaccines. In recent years, progress in vaccine adjuvant technology has accelerated to an exciting pace, including FDA approval of adjuvant-containing vaccines such as Cervarix® (2009) and Fluad® (2015), and positive phase III clinical results of adjuvanted vaccines for malaria, shingles, and hepatitis B. In addition to these significant clinical advances, earlier stage progress in adjuvant development including use of synthetic raw materials, novel formulation and characterization approaches, elucidation of mechanisms of action, and technology transfer to developing country institutions is likewise highly encouraging. Moreover, the critical role of adjuvants with regard to global pandemic preparedness is being realized. Given these considerations, there is a clear need for up-to-date information on the practical methods and protocols important for successful adjuvant synthesis, formulation, and evaluation from the experts in the field.

The complex factors involved in the design, synthesis, formulation, physicochemical and bioactivity characterization, and clinical development of vaccine adjuvants are often underestimated, in part because adjuvant access and formulation know-how have historically not been widely available. This collection seeks to elucidate the practical methods necessary for successful adjuvant development, with a particular focus on the synthesis, formulation, manufacturing, and characterization aspects involved. It is anticipated that readers will be empowered to develop effective and stable vaccine adjuvants with product potential through application or adaptation of these techniques. While in some cases there is necessarily some overlap, my intent has been to avoid duplication of material covered in previous books from the Springer Protocols series, including the excellent volumes edited by Derek T. O'Hagan (*Vaccine Adjuvants: Preparation Methods and Research Protocols*, Methods in Molecular Medicine, 2000) and by Gwyn Davies (*Vaccine Adjuvants: Methods and Protocols*, Methods in Molecular Biology, 2010). The reader is referred to these previous books for further information on vaccine adjuvants.

The present volume begins with two review chapters, one focused on an overview of adjuvants in general and the other a specific case study on the development of the CpG adjuvant 1018. Chapters 2–8 concern the in silico design, chemical synthesis, biosynthesis, and/or purification from natural raw materials of specific adjuvant molecules. Chapters 9–15 involve adjuvant formulation approaches, including liposomes, oil-in-water emulsions, aluminum salts, block copolymer gels, biodegradable polymeric particles, and lyophilized cakes. The analytical characterization of adjuvant formulations and adjuvant-containing vaccines is treated in Chapters 16–21, involving particle sizing, vibrational spectroscopy, antigen-specific fluorescent and gel-based techniques, methods to separate antigens from adjuvants prior to analysis, and stressed stability approaches. Finally, chapters 22–26 involve the biological characterization of vaccine adjuvant activity, including in vitro and in vivo approaches, including modern bioinformatic tools, to measure innate and adaptive immune responses. Given the expansiveness of current adjuvant research and development, it was not possible to include every topic of interest. Nevertheless, a wide range of molecular and particulate adjuvants has been represented in the chapters included here.

It is my sincere pleasure to introduce the reader to this volume on vaccine adjuvants. I hope he or she will find it to be as informative and useful as I have, and that the methods described here by expert hands-on authors will facilitate vaccine adjuvant product development efforts. I have long been impressed with the practical approach and helpful notes featured in the Springer *Methods in Molecular Biology* series. By focusing this volume on the pragmatic aspects of vaccine adjuvants, my goal is to help them become more accessible, manufacturable, and better characterized. Ongoing efforts along these lines should help in removing the "dirty little secret" sobriquet from adjuvants, and in the tradition of Edgar Ribi, turn exciting results into practical applications.

Seattle, WA, USA ***Christopher B. Fox***

Reference

1. NIH Oral History Interview (1985) Hamilton, Montana, USA

Contents

Preface . . . . *v*
Contributors . . . . *ix*

1 Overview of Vaccine Adjuvants: Introduction, History, and Current Status . . . 1
Ruchi R. Shah, Kimberly J. Hassett, and Luis A. Brito

2 Development of the CpG Adjuvant 1018: A Case Study 15
John D. Campbell

3 Syntheses of Human TLR8-Specific Small-Molecule Agonists 29
Mallesh Beesu, Hari Prasad Kokatla, and Sunil A. David

4 Semisynthesis of Analogues of the Saponin Immunoadjuvant QS-21 45
Alberto Fernández-Tejada, William E. Walkowicz, Derek S. Tan, and David Y. Gin

5 QS-21 Adjuvant: Laboratory-Scale Purification Method and Formulation Into Liposomes 73
Livia Brunner, Christophe Barnier-Quer, and Nicolas Collin

6 Purification of an Immunoadjuvant Saponin Fraction from *Quillaja brasiliensis* Leaves by Reversed-Phase Silica Gel Chromatography 87
Anna C.A. Yendo, Fernanda de Costa, Carla Kauffmann, Juliane D. Fleck, Grace Gosmann, and Arthur G. Fett-Neto

7 Biosynthetic Approaches to Squalene Production: The Case of Yeast 95
Martin Valachovič and Ivan Hapala

8 In Silico Adjuvant Design and Validation 107
Matthew N. Davies, Helene Pere, Iris Bosschem, Freddy Haesebrouck, Bram Flahou, Eric Tartour, Darren R. Flower, David F. Tough, and Jagadeesh Bayry

9 Manufacturing Methods for Liposome Adjuvants 127
Yvonne Perrie, Elisabeth Kastner, Swapnil Khadke, Carla B. Roces, and Peter Stone

10 Synthesis of Lymph Node-Targeting Adjuvants 145
Melissa C. Hanson and Darrell J. Irvine

11 Preparing an Adjuvanted Thermoresponsive Gel Formulation for Sublingual Vaccination 153
Manjari Lal, Jessica White, and Changcheng Zhu

12 Manufacture of Oil-in-Water Emulsion Adjuvants 165
Jean Haensler

13 Methods to Prepare Aluminum Salt-Adjuvanted Vaccines 181
Sachin G. Thakkar and Zhengrong Cui

14 Production of Adjuvant-Loaded Biodegradable Particles for Use in Cancer Vaccines 201
Cristina Maria de Barros, Emad Ibrahim Wafa, Khanidtha Chitphet, Kawther Ahmed, Sean M. Geary, and Aliasger K. Salem

15 Lyophilization of Adjuvanted Vaccines: Methods for Formulation of a Thermostable Freeze-Dried Product. 215
Michelle Y. Chan, Timothy S. Dutill, and Ryan M. Kramer

16 Stressed Stability Techniques for Adjuvant Formulations 227
Manvi Hasija, Anthony Sheung, Nausheen Rahman, and Salvador F. Ausar

17 Particle Sizing of Nanoparticle Adjuvant Formulations by Dynamic Light Scattering (DLS) and Nanoparticle Tracking Analysis (NTA). 239
Michelle Y. Chan, Quinton M. Dowling, Sandra J. Sivananthan, and Ryan M. Kramer

18 Quantification of Multiple Components of Complex Aluminum-Based Adjuvant Mixtures by Using Fourier Transform Infrared Spectroscopy and Partial Least Squares Modeling. 253
Quinton M. Dowling and Ryan M. Kramer

19 Determination of Protein Content in Alhydrogel®-Based Vaccines by *O*-Phthalaldehyde Assay 263
Kelly M. Rausch and Daming Zhu

20 Staining and Transfer Techniques for SDS-PAGE Gels to Minimize Oil-in-Water Emulsion Adjuvant Interference 273
Alicia M. Schwartz, Michelle Y. Chan, Dawn M. Fedor, Sandra J. Sivananthan, and Ryan M. Kramer

21 Interactions Between Antigens and Nanoemulsion Adjuvants: Separation and Characterization Techniques 285
Michelle Y. Chan, Dawn M. Fedor, Tony Phan, Lucien Barnes V, and Ryan M. Kramer

22 Screening Vaccine Formulations in Fresh Human Whole Blood. 295
Jalil Hakimi, Sepideh Aboutorabian, Frederick To, Salvador F. Ausar, Nausheen Rahman, and Roger H. Brookes

23 Analysis of the Innate Response to Adjuvants: Characterization of the Draining Lymph Node by Fluorescence-Activated Cell Sorting 305
Anthony L. Desbien

24 Assessment of Antigen-Specific Cellular Immunogenicity Using Intracellular Cytokine Staining, ELISpot, and Culture Supernatants 313
Elyse A. Beebe and Mark T. Orr

25 Eliciting Epitope-Specific CD8 T Cell Response by Immunization with Microbial Protein Antigens Formulated with α-Galactosylceramide: Theory, Practice, and Protocols. 321
Pavlo Gilchuk, Frances C. Knight, John T. Wilson, and Sebastian Joyce

26 Molecular Methods and Bioinformatic Tools for Adjuvant Characterization by High-Throughput Sequencing 353
Steven R. Wiley and Vanitha S. Raman

Index *369*

Contributors

SEPIDEH ABOUTORABIAN • *Bioprocess Research and Development, Sanofi Pasteur, Toronto, ON, Canada*
KAWTHER AHMED • *Division of Pharmaceutics and Translational Therapeutics, College of Pharmacy, University of Iowa, Iowa City, IA, USA*
SALVADOR F. AUSAR • *Bioprocess Research and Development, Sanofi Pasteur, Toronto, ON, Canada*
CHRISTOPHE BARNIER-QUER • *Vaccine Formulation Laboratory, Department of Biochemistry, University of Lausanne, Epalinges, Switzerland*
CRISTINA MARIA DE BARROS • *Division of Pharmaceutics and Translational Therapeutics, College of Pharmacy, University of Iowa, Iowa City, IA, USA*
JAGADEESH BAYRY • *Institut National de la Santé et de la Recherche Médicale, Paris, France; Equipe-Immunopathology and Therapeutic Immunointervention, Centre de Recherche des Cordeliers, Paris, France; Sorbonne Universités, Paris, France; Université Paris Descartes, Sorbonne Paris Cité, Paris, France*
ELYSE A. BEEBE • *Infectious Disease Research Institute, Seattle, WA, USA*
MALLESH BEESU • *Department of Medicinal Chemistry, University of Minnesota, Minneapolis, MN, USA*
IRIS BOSSCHEM • *Department of Pathology, Bacteriology and Avian Diseases, Faculty of Veterinary Medicine, Ghent University, Merelbeke, Belgium*
LUIS A. BRITO • *Moderna Therapeutics, Cambridge, MA, USA*
ROGER H. BROOKES • *Bioprocess Research and Development, Sanofi Pasteur, Toronto, ON, Canada*
LIVIA BRUNNER • *Vaccine Formulation Laboratory, Department of Biochemistry, University of Lausanne, Epalinges, Switzerland*
JOHN D. CAMPBELL • *Dynavax Technologies Corporation, Berkeley, CA, USA*
MICHELLE Y. CHAN • *IDRI, Seattle, WA, USA*
KHANIDTHA CHITPHET • *Division of Pharmaceutics and Translational Therapeutics, College of Pharmacy, University of Iowa, Iowa City, IA, USA*
NICOLAS COLLIN • *Vaccine Formulation Laboratory, Department of Biochemistry, University of Lausanne, Epalinges, Switzerland*
FERNANDA DE COSTA • *Plant Physiology Laboratory, Center for Biotechnology and Department of Botany, Federal University of Rio Grande do Sul (UFRGS), Porto Alegre, RS, Brazil*
ZHENGRONG CUI • *Pharmaceutics Division, College of Pharmacy, The University of Texas at Austin, Austin, TX, USA; Dell Pediatric Research Institute, The University of Texas at Austin, Austin, TX, USA*
SUNIL A. DAVID • *Department of Medicinal Chemistry, University of Minnesota, Minneapolis, MN, USA*
MATTHEW N. DAVIES • *Translational Oncogenomics Laboratory, Centre for Evolution and Cancer, Division of Molecular Pathology, The Institute of Cancer Research, London, UK*
ANTHONY L. DESBIEN • *Aduro Biotech, Inc., Berkeley, CA, USA*

QUINTON M. DOWLING • *IDRI, Seattle, WA, USA*
TIMOTHY S. DUTILL • *Lyophilization Technology, Inc., Ivyland, PA, USA*
DAWN M. FEDOR • *IDRI, Seattle, WA, USA*
ALBERTO FERNÁNDEZ-TEJADA • *Chemical Biology Program, Memorial Sloan Kettering Cancer Center, New York, NY, USA; Chemistry Research Laboratory, Department of Chemistry, University of Oxford, Oxford, UK*
ARTHUR G. FETT-NETO • *Plant Physiology Laboratory, Center for Biotechnology and Department of Botany, Federal University of Rio Grande do Sul (UFRGS), Porto Alegre, RS, Brazil*
BRAM FLAHOU • *Department of Pathology, Bacteriology and Avian Diseases, Faculty of Veterinary Medicine, Ghent University, Merelbeke, Belgium*
JULIANE D. FLECK • *Molecular Microbiology Laboratory, Feevale University, Novo Hamburgo, RS, Brazil*
DARREN R. FLOWER • *School of Life and Health Sciences, University of Aston, Birmingham, UK*
SEAN M. GEARY • *Division of Pharmaceutics and Translational Therapeutics, College of Pharmacy, University of Iowa, Iowa City, IA, USA*
PAVLO GILCHUK • *Veterans Administration, Tennessee Valley Healthcare System, US Department of Veterans Affairs, Nashville, TN, USA; Department of Pathology, Microbiology and Immunology, School of Medicine, Vanderbilt University, Nashville, TN, USA*
DAVID Y. GIN • *Chemical Biology Program, Memorial Sloan Kettering Cancer Center, New York, NY, USA; Tri-Institutional Research Program, Memorial Sloan Kettering Cancer Center, New York, NY, USA*
GRACE GOSMANN • *Phytochemistry Laboratory, Faculty of Pharmacy, UFRGS, Porto Alegre, RS, Brazil*
JEAN HAENSLER • *Sanofi Pasteur R&D, Marcy l'Etoile, France*
FREDDY HAESEBROUCK • *Department of Pathology, Bacteriology and Avian Diseases, Faculty of Veterinary Medicine, Ghent University, Merelbeke, Belgium*
JALIL HAKIMI • *Bioprocess Research and Development, Sanofi Pasteur, Toronto, ON, Canada*
MELISSA C. HANSON • *Department of Cell Biology and Infection, Institut Pasteur, Paris, France*
IVAN HAPALA • *Institute of Animal Biochemistry and Genetics, Slovak Academy of Sciences, Ivanka pri Dunaji, Slovakia*
MANVI HASIJA • *Bioprocess Research and Development, Sanofi Pasteur, Toronto, ON, Canada*
KIMBERLY J. HASSETT • *Valera, Cambridge, MA, USA*
DARRELL J. IRVINE • *Department of Biological Engineering, Massachusetts Institute of Technology, Cambridge, MA, USA; Department of Materials Science & Engineering, Massachusetts Institute of Technology, Cambridge, MA, USA; David H. Koch Institute for Integrative Cancer Research, Massachusetts Institute of Technology, Cambridge, MA, USA; The Ragon Institute of MGH, MIT, and Harvard, Cambridge, MA, USA; Howard Hughes Medical Institute, Chevy Chase, MD, USA*
SEBASTIAN JOYCE • *Veterans Administration, Tennessee Valley Healthcare System, US Department of Veterans Affairs, Nashville, TN, USA; Department of Pathology, Microbiology and Immunology, School of Medicine, Vanderbilt University, Nashville, TN, USA*

Elisabeth Kastner • *School of Life and Health Sciences, Aston University, Birmingham, UK*
Carla Kauffmann • *Faculty of Pharmacy, Univates University Center, Lajeado, RS, Brazil*
Swapnil Khadke • *Aston Pharmacy School, School of Life and Health Sciences, Aston University, Birmingham, UK*
Frances C. Knight • *Department of Biomedical Engineering, School of Engineering, Vanderbilt University, Nashville, TN, USA*
Hari Prasad Kokatla • *Department of Medicinal Chemistry, University of Minnesota, Minneapolis, MN, USA*
Ryan M. Kramer • *IDRI, Seattle, WA, USA*
Manjari Lal • *PATH, Seattle, WA, USA*
Mark T. Orr • *Infectious Disease Research Institute, Seattle, WA, USA; Department of Global Health, University of Washington, Seattle, WA, USA*
Helene Pere • *INSERM U970 PARCC (Paris Cardiovascular Research Center), Université Paris Descartes, Sorbonne Paris Cité, Paris, France; Hôpital Européen Georges-Pompidou, Service d'Immunologie Biologique, Paris, France*
Yvonne Perrie • *School of Life and Health Sciences, Aston University, Birmingham, UK; Strathclyde Institute of Pharmacy and Biomedical Sciences, University of Strathclyde, Glasgow, UK*
Tony Phan • *IDRI, Seattle, WA, USA*
Nausheen Rahman • *Bioprocess Research and Development, Sanofi Pasteur, Toronto, ON, Canada*
Vanitha S. Raman • *Henry M. Jackson Foundation, Bethesda, MD, USA*
Kelly M. Rausch • *Laboratory of Malaria Immunology and Vaccinology, National Institutes of Allergy and Infectious Disease, National Institutes of Health, Rockville, MD, USA*
Carla B. Roces • *Strathclyde Institute of Pharmacy and Biomedical Sciences, University of Strathclyde, Glasgow, UK*
Aliasger K. Salem • *Division of Pharmaceutics and Translational Therapeutics, College of Pharmacy, University of Iowa, Iowa City, IA, USA*
Alicia M. Schwartz • *IDRI, Seattle, WA, USA*
Ruchi R. Shah • *Northeastern University, Boston, MA, USA*
Anthony Sheung • *Bioprocess Research and Development, Sanofi Pasteur, Toronto, ON, Canada*
Sandra J. Sivananthan • *IDRI, Seattle, WA, USA*
Peter Stone • *Aston Pharmacy School, School of Life and Health Sciences, Aston University, Birmingham, UK*
Derek S. Tan • *Chemical Biology Program, Memorial Sloan Kettering Cancer Center, New York, NY, USA; Tri-Institutional Research Program, Memorial Sloan Kettering Cancer Center, New York, NY, USA*
Eric Tartour • *INSERM U970 PARCC (Paris Cardiovascular Research Center), Université Paris Descartes, Sorbonne Paris Cité, Paris, France; Hôpital Européen Georges-Pompidou, Service d'Immunologie Biologique, Paris, France*
Sachin G. Thakkar • *Pharmaceutics Division, College of Pharmacy, The University of Texas at Austin, Austin, TX, USA*
Frederick To • *Bioprocess Research and Development, Sanofi Pasteur, Toronto, ON, Canada*

DAVID F. TOUGH • *Epinova Discovery Performance Unit, Immuno-inflammation Therapeutic Area, GlaxoSmithKline, Medicines Discovery Centre, Stevenage, UK*
LUCIEN BARNES V • *IDRI, Seattle, WA, USA*
MARTIN VALACHOVIČ • *Institute of Animal Biochemistry and Genetics, Slovak Academy of Sciences, Ivanka pri Dunaji, Slovakia*
EMAD IBRAHIM WAFA • *Division of Pharmaceutics and Translational Therapeutics, College of Pharmacy, University of Iowa, Iowa City, IA, USA*
WILLIAM E. WALKOWICZ • *Chemical Biology Program, Memorial Sloan Kettering Cancer Center, New York, NY, USA*
JESSICA WHITE • *PATH, Seattle, WA, USA*
STEVEN R. WILEY • *Imdaptive Inc., Seattle, WA, USA*
JOHN T. WILSON • *Department of Biomedical Engineering, School of Engineering, Vanderbilt University, Nashville, TN, USA; Department of Chemical & Biomolecular Engineering, School of Engineering, Vanderbilt University, Nashville, TN, USA*
ANNA C.A. YENDO • *Plant Physiology Laboratory, Center for Biotechnology and Department of Botany, Federal University of Rio Grande do Sul (UFRGS), Porto Alegre, RS, Brazil*
CHANGCHENG ZHU • *PATH, Seattle, WA, USA*
DAMING ZHU • *Laboratory of Malaria Immunology and Vaccinology, National Institutes of Allergy and Infectious Disease, National Institutes of Health, Rockville, MD, USA*

Chapter 1

Overview of Vaccine Adjuvants: Introduction, History, and Current Status

Ruchi R. Shah, Kimberly J. Hassett, and Luis A. Brito

Abstract

Adjuvants are included in sub-unit or recombinant vaccines to enhance the potency of poorly immunogenic antigens. Adjuvant discovery is as complex as it is a multidiscplinary intersection of formulation science, immunology, toxicology, and biology. Adjuvants such as alum, which have been in use for the past 90 years, have illustrated that adjuvant research is a methodical process. As science advances, new analytical tools are developed which allows us to delve deeper into the various mechanisms that generates a potent immune response. Additionally, these new techniques help the field learn about our existing vaccines and what makes them safe, and effective, allowing us to leverage that in the next generation of vaccines. Our goal in this chapter is to define the concept, need, and mechanism of adjuvants in the vaccine field while describing its history, present use, and future prospects. More details on individual adjuvants and their formulation, development, mechanism, and use will be covered in depth in the next chapters.

Key words Adjuvant, Alum, Nanoemulsion, Vaccine, Immunopotentiator

1 Introduction

Vaccination has protected the human race from numerous devastating diseases, improved the quality of life, and extended the average lifespan. According to statistics released by National Institute of Health in 2010, vaccines have prevented approximately 2.5 million deaths and countless cases of illness each year [1]. The modern day concept of vaccination was introduced by Edward Jenner in the eighteenth century when he made the connection between the lack of small pox infections and milk maids. Using this observation Jenner took cow pox (which does not cause severe disease in humans) and inoculated individuals. Those individuals were then found to be protected against small pox infection [2]. However, well before Jenner's observation many Asian and African countries had practiced a similar concept of variolation (using infected material to immunize a healthy individual against the same infection) for centuries [2, 3]. This history of vaccination is not only

Christopher B. Fox (ed.), *Vaccine Adjuvants: Methods and Protocols*, Methods in Molecular Biology, vol. 1494, DOI 10.1007/978-1-4939-6445-1_1, © Springer Science+Business Media New York 2017

interesting but also suggestive of the empirical approach that has always been a trademark of vaccine development from inception until today, despite our increasing understanding of the field of vaccinology [4].

Vaccination is a process of mimicking infection in the body leading to the activation of the immune system for the generation of a potent immune response [5, 6]. Once injected, pathogen-associated molecular patterns (PAMPs) present in the vaccine interact with the pattern recognition receptors (PRRs) on the innate immune cells present at the site of injection (SOI) and initiate an immune cascade. This involves upregulation in the production of chemokines and cytokines that subsequently lead to an increase in the number of antigen presenting cells (APCs) at the SOI. The APCs are involved in antigen uptake and subsequent presentation to T-cells that ultimately are responsible for priming CD4+ and CD8+ responses. These T-helper cells also activate the B cells, leading to the production and secretion of antibodies. Activation of both B and T cells is required for a robust immune response. A portion of the total T and B cells transform into memory cells which can mount an adaptive immune response quickly during future infections [6].

As medical science advanced the crude methodology of Jenner was refined leading to an improvement in the safety and efficacy of vaccines. Building directly from Jenner's work, live attenuated and whole killed pathogens are considered the first generation of vaccines. Live attenuated vaccines contain weakened versions of the pathogen, virus or bacteria. These attenuated pathogens can replicate inside the host leading to long lasting immunity. These vaccines are highly effective; yet there is a concern of reversion to its virulent form. For example the vaccine for Venezuelan Equine Encephalitis has to undergo only two-point mutations to return to virulence, limiting its utility to vaccinating high-risk individuals such as lab workers [7]. Whole killed vaccines on the other hand are incapable of replication as they undergo a viral inactivation step such as crosslinking, or viral splitting. Despite the lack of reversion for these types of vaccines, safety is still a concern. In the 1960s a formalin-inactivated vaccine against RSV in a clinical trial killed an infant subject [8]. This tragedy hampered the RSV field, and until recently no vaccine candidates have entered into late-stage clinical trials [9]. Another type of commercially available vaccine is the inactivated toxoid, e.g., tetanus. These traditional vaccines are still in use as they are highly potent; but in certain disease targets there are safety concerns and issues with the manufacturing process and in some non-cultivable microorganisms this traditional approach does not work [10, 11]. The limitations outlined above led to the introduction of subunit and recombinant protein vaccines. Subunit and recombinant proteins are highly purified antigens which require only a part of the pathogen to generate a protective immune response. These antigens improved vaccine development as they proved to be safe with no ability to revert to a virulent form and were easier to manufacture and characterize. Also, these antigens exhibit low potency due to fewer PAMPs in comparison to the conventional attenuated or whole inactivated vaccines. Adjuvants were thus introduced in vaccines to enhance the immunogenicity of these weaker antigens and help in improving the overall potency of poorly immunogenic subunit vaccines [11].

Adjuvants are defined as materials added to vaccines in order to improve the immunological response. Adjuvants have many potential benefits such as reducing the frequency of vaccination, reducing the dose of antigen per vaccine (dose sparing), improving the quality of the immune response, and promoting cross-clade immunity and in certain cases they may improve the stability of the final vaccine formulation [12]. Adjuvants have been used to improve immunogenicity of vaccines in immune-comprised patients (e.g., HIV positive), infants, and elderly patients. Adjuvants such as MF59 and AS04 have even improved the efficacy profile of the vaccine in comparison to non-adjuvanted vaccines or placebo [13, 14]. In this chapter we focus on adjuvants which are added specifically to enhance the immune responses of a poorly immunogenic antigen.

Conventional classification schemes based on origin, disease target, route of administration, type of formulation, mechanism of action, intended use (delivery vs. immune potentiation), etc. may not be directly applied to vaccine adjuvants. One way to classify adjuvants is according to different generations—based on how they interact with the immune system and their composition [15]. Particulate adjuvants like alum, emulsions, liposomes, and microparticles can be considered as the first generation of vaccine adjuvants. This first generation can also be considered as antigen delivery systems which promote the uptake of the co-administered antigen from the SOI [15]. The second generation of vaccine adjuvants may be best described as combinational adjuvants as they are comprised of immune potentiators combined with the first generation of vaccine adjuvants, e.g., AS04 which is included in Cervarix® and consists of alum and a TLR4 agonist [15]. AS04 is a part of the adjuvant systems by GlaxoSmithKline which applies a similar concept of combining delivery systems and immune potentiators into one single system; we will discuss these individually in the following sections.

Currently there are many types of adjuvants available for vaccine use being evaluated throughout various stages of vaccine development. Ultimately the selection of an adjuvant for a vaccine should take many factors into consideration. Safety of an adjuvant is the first criteria and it is dependent on the risk to benefit ratio of the intended vaccine. An adjuvant should be safe, well tolerated, easy to scale up and manufacture, pharmaceutically acceptable (in regard to pH, osmolality, endotoxin levels, etc.) with a reasonable shelf life, compatible with the antigen, and economically feasible [16].

Establishing all these parameters while maintaining the safety of the adjuvanted vaccine is a difficult time-consuming process; therefore currently only a handful of vaccine adjuvants are included in commercial vaccines.

2 Current Adjuvants

Although many well-respected academic and industry groups have excellent adjuvant research programs, very few of their discoveries have successfully translated to components in licensed vaccines. In the USA aluminum salts, AS04 (monophosphoryl lipid A [MPL] with aluminum hydroxide), AS03 (oil-in-water emulsion consisting of squalene, alpha-tocopherol, and Tween 80), and MF59 (oil-in-water emulsion consisting of squalene, polysorbate 80, and sorbitan trioleate) are adjuvants included in licensed vaccines [17, 18]. In addition to adjuvants licensed in the USA, Europe has licensed vaccines containing virosomes [17]. Each vaccine adjuvant has had its own challenges and successes. Experiences from previously studied adjuvants and the pharmaceutical feasibility of adjuvants have impacted and directed the development of the future adjuvants.

2.1 Aluminum-Based Adjuvants

Aluminum salt solutions were originally added to growth medium to help purify tetanus and diphtheria vaccine antigens through precipitation, but it was soon discovered that aluminum precipitated antigens were more immunogenic than the soluble antigens [19]. Aluminum-based adjuvants have been used since the 1920s, making them the adjuvant used for the longest period of time and the most frequently used adjuvant in licensed vaccine products with approximately one-third of licensed vaccines containing alum [20]. As a result alum has an extensive track record of safety in vaccines.

Although potassium aluminum sulfate was originally referred to as alum, aluminum hydroxide and aluminum phosphate are more commonly referred to as alum in the vaccine community. Aluminum hydroxide has a crystalline needle like morphology whereas aluminum phosphate appears as amorphous loose aggregates [21]. Alum has been used as an antigen delivery system where the antigen interacts primarily though electrostatic interactions and ligand exchange. The electrostatic interactions of antigen and alum are a function of pH and type of alum. The point of zero charge (PZC) will determine the charge of alum; for aluminum hydroxide and aluminum phosphate the PZC are approximately 11 and 5, respectively [22]. Based on the formulation pH and the isoelectric point (PI) of the antigen, the appropriate alum adjuvant can be chosen to maximize adjuvant-antigen electrostatic interactions by having oppositely charged antigen and adjuvant [23]. Ligand exchange occurs when hydroxide groups on the alum exchange with phosphate groups present on the antigen. Although association of antigen to alum allows the antigen to remain at the site of injection for longer periods of time, association of antigen to alum may not be critical for immune potentiation [24].

Alum promotes a strong Th2-biased response, also referred to as a humoral immune response. Although the exact mechanism of action for alum is still unknown, proposed mechanisms include depot effect, an inflammatory response which recruits antigen-presenting cells, NALP3 inflammasome activation, release of DNA from cell death causing danger-associated molecule pattern (DAMP) recognition, and enhanced phagocytosis by antigen-presenting cells [15, 25–27]. Despite the success of alum use in many vaccines, it has limitations particularly for use against intracellular pathogens and pathogens that require a strong cellular immune response. In addition, alum is sometimes found to be not potent enough as an adjuvant for some antigens, e.g., influenza vaccines where alum was found to be a poor adjuvant [28, 29].

One approach to overcome the limitations of alum is to use it to co-deliver it with additional adjuvants. Adjuvant system AS04 combines aluminum hydroxide or aluminum phosphate with the immunostimulatory molecule monophosphoryl lipid A (MPL) [30]. Mechanistic studies suggest that alum and MPL do not work synergistically, but alum facilitates the delivery of MPL at the site of injection and increases the duration of cytokines [31]. Monophosphoryl lipid A (MPL) is a modified version of lipopolysaccharide (LPS) that is significantly less toxic but still remains a TLR4 agonist [32]. By including MPL with aluminum hydroxide, both a Th1 and Th2 response can be created [30]. AS04 is currently used in licensed human papillomavirus (Cervarix®) and hepatitis B (Fendrix®) vaccines [30].

Alum-based vaccine formulations have limitations regarding stability. When alum is frozen, alum particles significantly aggregate leading to a decrease in vaccine efficacy when administered [33–36]. To avoid potential freezing, vaccines need to be transported and stored in a very narrow temperature range throughout the cold chain. Although no commercial formulations containing alum are stored frozen or lyophilized, proof-of-concept studies have shown the feasibility of lyophilizing alum formulations [20, 36–38].

2.2 Emulsions

Another approach that has an extensive history of use as vaccine adjuvants are emulsions. The earliest used emulsion designed as a vaccine adjuvant was a mineral oil-based water-in-oil emulsion called Freund's adjuvant. The water-in-oil (w/o) emulsion comes in two forms, complete Freund's adjuvant (CFA) which contains mineral oil, emulsifier, and killed bacteria *M. tuberculosis* and incomplete Freund's adjuvant (IFA) which has the same composition as CFA without the bacteria [39]. Although Freund's adjuvant has a long history of use, it will likely never be included as originally described in human vaccines due to safety concerns; it has been approved for use in certain large animal veterinary vaccines [40]. Toxicity issues were caused by the non-biodegradable oil, high levels of oil in the emulsion (water-in-oil), reproducibility of emulsion, and poor oil and/or emulsifier quality [41–45]. Despite this, CIMAvax EGF, a therapeutic non-small lung cancer vaccine developed and marketed in Cuba contains another mineral oil containing water-in-oil emulsion adjuvant Montanide ISA 51 by Seppic [46].

To create an adjuvant without the tolerability issues associated with FCA or IFA, oil-in-water emulsions prepared with biodegradable/biocompatible oils such as squalene (e.g., MF59) were developed in the 1980s [47]. MF59 is primarily used in influenza vaccines since it can improve immune responses and improve cross-reactivity to a wide array of influenza strains [48]. MF59 has been shown to be safe and well tolerated with millions of doses administered in over 35 countries [49]. MF59 is composed of squalene, Span 85, and Tween 80 in 10 mM sodium citrate buffer at pH 6.5 with an average droplet size of approximately 165 nm [47, 50]. Recently the mechanism of action of MF59 has been extensively studied and although it is still ongoing various theories have been established [51, 52]. MF59 does not create an antigen depot at the site of injection and the antigen and MF59 are cleared independently from the site of injection. An immune competent environment is created at the SOI leading to an influx of APCs and other immune cells. MF59 also upregulates production of cytokines and chemokines which further attracts the immune cells to the SOI. This migration of APCs leads to an increase in uptake of the antigen, especially by neutrophils and monocytes, and translocation to draining lymph nodes where MF59 also helps in priming the immune responses [51, 52].

AS03, a GlaxoSmithKline proprietary adjuvant, has also been used for influenza vaccines where it enhances immune responses similar to MF59 [53]. The difference in composition (squalene, alpha-tocopherol, and Tween80 in phosphate buffered saline) of AS03 leads to a different mechanism than MF59 [54]. Alpha-tocopherol (vitamin E) has been shown to have antioxidant and immunostimulatory properties which have been found to be critical to the adjuvant effect of AS03 [55]. AS03 and antigen must be delivered to the same site for an enhanced immune response to be achieved but emulsion and antigen do not have to be associated to generate the enhanced immune response [55]. Monocytes and granulocyte recruitment at the SOI are responsible for mechanism of action of AS03 [55].

To further enhance the immunogenicity of AS03, adjuvant system AS02 consists of the AS03 emulsion and incorporates the immune potentiators QS-21 and MPL to induce both strong antibody and cellular immune responses [30, 56]. QS-21 is a saponin from the soap bark tree, *Quillaja saponaria*, and has been found to enhance the immune response by producing high antibody titers, improving responses for T cell-independent antigens, and promoting CD8+ T cell responses [57].

Another emulsion that contains a TLR4 agonist is stable emulsion with glucopyranoside lipid adjuvant (GLA-SE). GLA-SE contains squalene, glycerol, phosphatidylcholine, glucopyranoside lipid adjuvant (GLA), and pluronic F68 in ammonium phosphate buffer [58]. A synthetic analogue of MPL, GLA has been shown to be more potent per molecule and less toxic than MPL [59]. The particles formed in stable emulsion are 100 nm in diameter [58]. Formulations containing GLA create a Th1 type of immune response. GLA can also be formulated as an aqueous formulation, in a liposome or adsorbed to alum, where each delivery system yields a slightly different immune response [58]. Additional emulsions have been evaluated as adjuvants including AF03 and WEC50; for a more detailed discussion on emulsion adjuvants the reader is referred to previously published reviews [10, 60].

2.3 Lipid-Based Particles

Liposomes are spherical particles containing a bilayer of phospholipids with an aqueous center [61]. Liposomes can be used to deliver both antigen and immunostimulatory molecules [61]. Components can be encapsulated within, associated with the membrane, or adsorbed on to liposomes [62]. Since liposomes alone do not create a strong immune response, they are often combined with immunostimulatory molecules [63–65]. Cationic liposomes have been found to improve immune responses more than neutral or anionic liposomes since cationic liposomes increase the uptake of entrapped antigen to cells [66]. CAF01, a cationic liposomal adjuvant developed by Statens Serum Institute containing DDA (dimethyldioctadecylammonium) and TDB (trehalose dibehenate), is now being clinically tested as a component of a tuberculosis vaccine [67].

Immunostimulating complexes (ISCOMs) were developed in the 1980s. ISCOMs originally had antigen incorporated with Quil A adjuvant with phospholipids and cholesterol [68]. To facilitate antigen association with the 40 nm ISCOMATRIX particles, it was found that the antigen must be amphiphilic [69]. Due to its poor tolerability Quil A is now replaced with more refined saponin preparations [70]. ISCOMATRIX has a dual role: immunomodulation and antigen delivery [69]. While it modulates the immune response by activation of immune cells and upregulation of cytokines and chemokines, it is hypothesized that it interacts with membranes on the cell surface and endosomes to deliver the antigen into the cytosol [69, 71]. As ISCOMATRIX can efficiently induce CD8+ responses it has been used as the gold standard for CTL immune responses [15].

The most clinically advanced liposomal adjuvant is AS01, a liposome composed of 1,2-dioleoyl-sn-glycero-3-phosphocholine (DOPC), cholesterol, MPL, and QS21. Immediately before injection, AS01 is combined with the antigen. It has been reported that for AS01 to be effective, the adjuvant and antigen must be delivered to the same injection site at the same time which leads to AS01 recruiting antigen-presenting cells to the injection site [72].

2.4 Polymeric Particles

During the 1980s poly(lactide-co-glycolide) (PLG) microparticles began to be evaluated for use as adjuvants [73]. In addition to being biodegradable and bio-compatible, these particles offer the possibility of a single-shot vaccine, thus overcoming the need for booster shots [74]. Since PLG is biodegradable, antigen entrapped within the polymer was able to be released once the particle was introduced into an aqueous environment [75]. Unfortunately, harsh conditions are required to entrap the antigen in PLG which results in a loss of antigen stability [76]. To overcome the loss of antigen stability during incorporation of antigen into the PLG particle, adsorption of antigen on the surface of PLG particles has also been attempted [77]. Since PLG particles induce immune responses only marginally better than alum, further development of this adjuvant has been halted since alum has a long history of use and safety. To increase the immune response generated with PLG particles, immune stimulating molecules have also been entrapped in the microparticle [76, 78]. Polymeric nanoparticles have also been evaluated as adjuvants, but there has been no biological advantage to the use of nanoparticles as opposed to microparticles [79].

3 Future Prospects for Adjuvants

Adjuvant research is an active field due in part to an increased need to improve immune responses of poorly immunogenic antigens, an increased understanding of the molecular mechanism of the innate immune system, improved biophysical analytical techniques for analysis of nanoscale assemblies, and a number of clinical successes in the past 15–20 years. Approval of an adjuvanted influenza vaccine containing MF59 in 1997 in Europe illustrated a path forward for emulsion adjuvants. Emulsions such as AS03, AF03, and SE soon followed a similar path and the field largely focused on the use of squalene as the oil of choice within emulsion adjuvants. Alternate oils have been evaluated further supporting the use of squalene as an adjuvant [80]. Interesting to note is the sizes were not evaluated in that report; we recently identified the size of the oil droplet to be critical to eliciting the appropriate immune response with changes as little as 70 nm impacting immune responses [81]. Recently a series of papers have focused on detailing the mechanism of action of MF59 [52, 82]. This increased mechanistic understanding is useful to benchmark novel adjuvants against a safe well-tolerated class of adjuvants.

A number of adjuvanted clinical candidates have recently gained significant attention. The adjuvant systems developed by

GSK have been advancing through the clinic. Recently scientists at GSK reported >96% efficacy with an $AS01_B$-adjuvanted herpes zoster vaccine in a phase III clinical trial [83]. An AS01-adjuvanted malaria vaccine was recently given a positive recommendation from the EMA [84]. Additionally the AS04 adjuvanted hepatitis B and human papilloma virus vaccines have successfully been in use for a number of years [85]. These examples clearly illustrate how an adjuvant can improve immune responses for vaccines where the mechanism of neutralization is understood in part.

Dynavax's hepatitis B vaccine Hepsilav-B has shown promising results in three phase III trials. Hepsilav-B includes immunostimulatory sequence 1018 which contains unmethylated CpG motifs allowing it to act as a TLR 9 agonist [86]. Several advantages over currently marketed products have been seen in Hepsilav-B including a reduced number of doses required from three doses over 6 months (Engerix-B) to two doses in 1 month to achieve seroprotection, and increased seroconversion in hypo-responsive populations such as obese, smokers, males, and diabetics while maintaining a similar safety profile to approved vaccines [86]. After receiving a rejection on the FDA regulatory filing in 2013 due to insufficient safety data and concerns about adjuvant caused autoimmunity, Dynavax hopes to resubmit the application in 2016 with an increased number of safely immunized patients and positive results from the latest phase III trials [87].

The late-stage failure of the AS15-adjuvanted cancer vaccine is a reminder that a powerful adjuvant alone cannot generate the desired immune response [88, 89]. Deep understanding of biology is needed to generate the appropriate immune response. Although the field of immune-oncology has clearly made significant advances through the use of PD-1 antibodies and CAR-T therapy, the field in general has not yet reached a consensus on how to generate the most potent immune response against cancer cells within the patient. Therapeutic vaccines will rely heavily on adjuvants in order to coax the immune system to break tolerance (in the case of cancer vaccines), generate tolerance (in the case of allergy vaccines), or generate antibodies against poorly immunogenic antigens (e.g., nicotine vaccine).

Early-stage concepts include a recent report from Wu et al. describing a novel small-molecule adjuvant that binds to alum for enhanced responses [90]. Combining an existing well-established adjuvant with a novel immunostimulator leverages the existing safety record of alum while introducing a novel potent adjuvant for improving cellular responses and breadth of response. Recent phase II data for a peptide-based vaccine adjuvanted with the Matrix M2 saponin-based adjuvant was found to be highly effective in reduction of viral shedding for herpes simplex virus [91, 92].

During the 2009 influenza pandemic, a small but significant subset of vaccinated individuals who received AS03-adjuvanted flu vaccine in Europe developed narcolepsy [93, 94]. It was not until recently that Soheil et al. identified homology between an antigen found in the vaccine and a protein found in the human body to lead to narcolepsy [95]. As the adjuvant improved the overall immune response of the vaccine, it likely helped elicit antibodies against this protein in a subset of patients. This example is a reminder that adjuvants need to be combined with well-defined and well-characterized vaccine antigens. Although vaccine adjuvants can improve responses and lead to improved health, particularly for unmet medical needs, an in-depth understanding of the biology and well-characterized antigens is critical for the field to succeed as a whole.

The increased use of recombinant proteins will inevitably lead to a greater use of adjuvants. Not many vaccines will require the "kitchen sink" approach where multiple immune stimulators are combined to create a varied and long-lasting immune response, although recent late-stage trials are illustrating the clear need to combine different classes of adjuvants for improving responses. As our understanding of the immune system improves through the use of antibody repertoire analysis and deep sequencing combined with other recent bio-analytical advances the immune system will be harnessed not only to be used for preventing infectious disease, but for treating autoimmunity and cancer, and there is a high likelihood that vaccine adjuvants will be a central player in those next-generation treatments.

References

1. The decade of vaccines—a plan to extend vaccine benefits to the whole world. December 18, 2012 November 5, 2015]. http://www.niaid.nih.gov/topics/vaccines/Pages/decadeVaccines.aspx
2. Riedel S (2005) Edward Jenner and the history of smallpox and vaccination. Proc (Baylor Univ Med Cent) 18(1):21–25
3. Gross CP, Sepkowitz KA (1998) The myth of the medical breakthrough: smallpox, vaccination, and Jenner reconsidered. Int J Infect Dis 3(1):54–60
4. Hilleman MR (2000) Vaccines in historic evolution and perspective: a narrative of vaccine discoveries. Vaccine 18(15):1436–1447
5. Medzhitov R, Janeway CA Jr (1997) Innate immunity: impact on the adaptive immune response. Curr Opin Immunol 9(1):4–9
6. Pashine A, Valiante NM, Ulmer JB (2005) Targeting the innate immune response with improved vaccine adjuvants. Nat Med 11(4 Suppl):S63–S68
7. Kinney RM et al (1993) Attenuation of Venezuelan equine encephalitis virus strain TC-83 is encoded by the 5'-noncoding region and the E2 envelope glycoprotein. J Virol 67(3):1269–1277
8. Haynes LM (2013) Progress and challenges in RSV prophylaxis and vaccine development. J Infect Dis 208(Suppl 3):S177–S183
9. Kallerup R, Foged C (2015) Classification of vaccines. In: Foged C et al (eds) Subunit vaccine delivery. Springer, New York, pp 15–29
10. Shah R, Brito L, O'Hagan D, Amiji M (2014) Emulsions as vaccine adjuvants. In: Foged C, Rades T, Perrie Y, Hook S (eds) Subunit vaccine delivery. Springer, New York
11. Coffman RL, Sher A, Seder RA (2010) Vaccine adjuvants: putting innate immunity to work. Immunity 33(4):492–503
12. Schijns VE, Lavelle EC (2011) Trends in vaccine adjuvants. Expert Rev Vaccines 10(4):539–550
13. Vesikari T et al (2011) Oil-in-water emulsion adjuvant with influenza vaccine in young children. N Engl J Med 365(15):1406–1416
14. Roteli-Martins CM et al (2012) Sustained immunogenicity and efficacy of the HPV-16/18 AS04-adjuvanted vaccine. Hum Vaccin Immunother 8(3):390–397
15. Brito LA, O'Hagan DT (2014) Designing and building the next generation of improved vaccine adjuvants. J Control Release 190: 563–579

16. Brito LA, Malyala P, O'Hagan DT (2013) Vaccine adjuvant formulations: a pharmaceutical perspective. Semin Immunol 25(2):130–145
17. Rambe DS et al (2015) Safety and mechanism of action of licensed vaccine adjuvants. Int Curr Pharma J 4(8):420–431
18. FDA approves first seasonal influenza vaccine containing an adjuvant. 2015 [cited 2016 3/18/2016]. http://www.fda.gov/NewsEvents/Newsroom/PressAnnouncements/ucm474295.htm
19. Glenny A, Pope CG, Waddington H, Wallace U (1926) Immunological notes XVII to XXIV. J Pathol 29:31–40
20. Hassett KJ et al (2013) Stabilization of a recombinant ricin toxin A subunit vaccine through lyophilization. Eur J Pharm Biopharm 85(2):279–286
21. Romero Méndez IZ et al (2007) Potentiation of the immune response to non-adsorbed antigens by aluminum-containing adjuvants. Vaccine 25(5):825–833
22. al-Shakhshir R et al (1994) Effect of protein adsorption on the surface charge characteristics of aluminium-containing adjuvants. Vaccine 12(5):472–474
23. Seeber SJ, White JL, Hem SL (1991) Predicting the adsorption of proteins by aluminium-containing adjuvants. Vaccine 9(3):201–203
24. Noe SM et al (2010) Mechanism of immunopotentiation by aluminum-containing adjuvants elucidated by the relationship between antigen retention at the inoculation site and the immune response. Vaccine 28(20):3588–3594
25. Marichal T et al (2011) DNA released from dying host cells mediates aluminum adjuvant activity. Nat Med 17(8):996–1002
26. Marrack P, McKee AS, Munks MW (2009) Towards an understanding of the adjuvant action of aluminium. Nat Rev Immunol 9(4):287–293
27. Oleszycka E, Lavelle EC (2014) Immunomodulatory properties of the vaccine adjuvant alum. Curr Opin Immunol 28:1–5
28. Traquina P et al (1996) MF59 adjuvant enhances the antibody response to recombinant hepatitis B surface antigen vaccine in primates. J Infect Dis 174(6):1168–1175
29. Granoff DM et al (1997) MF59 adjuvant enhances antibody responses of infant baboons immunized with Haemophilus influenzae type b and Neisseria meningitidis group C oligosaccharide-CRM197 conjugate vaccine. Infect Immun 65(5):1710–1715
30. Garcon N, Chomez P, Van Mechelen M (2007) GlaxoSmithKline Adjuvant Systems in vaccines: concepts, achievements and perspectives. Expert Rev Vaccines 6(5):723–739
31. Didierlaurent AM et al (2009) AS04, an aluminum salt- and TLR4 agonist-based adjuvant system, induces a transient localized innate immune response leading to enhanced adaptive immunity. J Immunol 183(10):6186–6197
32. Casella CR, Mitchell TC (2008) Putting endotoxin to work for us: monophosphoryl lipid A as a safe and effective vaccine adjuvant. Cell Mol Life Sci 65(20):3231–3240
33. Chen D et al (2009) Characterization of the freeze sensitivity of a hepatitis B vaccine. Hum Vaccin 5(1):26–32
34. Salnikova MS et al (2012) Influence of formulation pH and suspension state on freezing-induced agglomeration of aluminum adjuvants. J Pharm Sci 101(3):1050–1062
35. Braun LJ et al (2009) Development of a freeze-stable formulation for vaccines containing aluminum salt adjuvants. Vaccine 27(1):72–79
36. Hassett KJ et al (2015) Glassy-state stabilization of a dominant negative inhibitor anthrax vaccine containing aluminum hydroxide and glycopyranoside lipid A adjuvants. J Pharm Sci 104(2):627–639
37. Clausi AL et al (2009) Influence of protein conformation and adjuvant aggregation on the effectiveness of aluminum hydroxide adjuvant in a model alkaline phosphatase vaccine. J Pharm Sci 98(1):114–121
38. Clausi A et al (2008) Influence of particle size and antigen binding on effectiveness of aluminum salt adjuvants in a model lysozyme vaccine. J Pharm Sci 97(12):5252–5262
39. Lindblad EB (2000) Freund's adjuvant. In: O'Hagan D (ed) Vaccine adjuvants. Humana Press, Totowa, NJ, pp 49–64
40. Aucouturier J, Dupuis L, Ganne V (2001) Adjuvants designed for veterinary and human vaccines. Vaccine 19(17-19):2666–2672
41. Hilleman MR (1966) Critical appraisal of emulsified oil adjuvants applied to viral vaccines. Prog Med Virol 8:131–182
42. Murray R, Cohen P, Hardegree MC (1972) Mineral oil adjuvants: biological and chemical studies. Ann Allergy 30(3):146–151
43. Stills HF Jr (2005) Adjuvants and antibody production: dispelling the myths associated with Freund's complete and other adjuvants. ILAR J 46(3):280–293
44. Stuewart-Tull DE et al (1976) Immunosuppressive effect in mycobacterial adjuvant emulsions of mineral oils containing low molecular weight hydrocarbons. Int Arch Allergy Appl Immunol 52(1–4):118–128

45. Whitehouse MW et al (1974) Freund's adjuvants: relationship of arthritogenicity and adjuvanticity in rats to vehicle composition. Immunology 27(2):311–330
46. Rodríguez PC, Rodríguez G, González G, Lage A (2010) Clinical development and perspectives of CIMAvax EGF, Cuban vaccine for non-small-cell lung cancer therapy. MEDICC Rev 12(1):17–23
47. O'Hagan DT et al (2013) The history of MF59((R)) adjuvant: a phoenix that arose from the ashes. Expert Rev Vaccines 12(1): 13–30
48. O'Hagan DT et al (2011) MF59 adjuvant: the best insurance against influenza strain diversity. Expert Rev Vaccines 10(4):447–462
49. Schultze V et al (2008) Safety of MF59 adjuvant. Vaccine 26(26):3209–3222
50. Manmohan S (2007) Vaccine adjuvants and delivery systems. Wiley, Hoboken, NJ, pp 115–129
51. O'Hagan DT et al (2012) The mechanism of action of MF59 - an innately attractive adjuvant formulation. Vaccine 30(29):4341–4348
52. Seubert A et al (2008) The adjuvants aluminum hydroxide and MF59 induce monocyte and granulocyte chemoattractants and enhance monocyte differentiation toward dendritic cells. J Immunol 180(8):5402–5412
53. Moris P et al (2011) H5N1 influenza vaccine formulated with AS03A induces strong cross-reactive and polyfunctional CD4 T-cell responses. J Clin Immunol 31(3):443–454
54. Garcon N, Vaughn DW, Didierlaurent AM (2012) Development and evaluation of AS03, an adjuvant system containing alpha-tocopherol and squalene in an oil-in-water emulsion. Expert Rev Vaccines 11(3):349–366
55. Morel S et al (2011) Adjuvant system AS03 containing alpha-tocopherol modulates innate immune response and leads to improved adaptive immunity. Vaccine 29(13):2461–2473
56. Garcon N, Van Mechelen M (2011) Recent clinical experience with vaccines using MPL- and QS-21-containing adjuvant systems. Expert Rev Vaccines 10(4):471–486
57. Kensil CR, Kammer R (1998) QS-21: a water-soluble triterpene glycoside adjuvant. Expert Opin Investig Drugs 7(9):1475–1482
58. Fox CB et al (2013) TLR4 ligand formulation causes distinct effects on antigen-specific cell-mediated and humoral immune responses. Vaccine 31(49):5848–5855
59. Coler RN et al (2011) Development and characterization of synthetic glucopyranosyl lipid adjuvant system as a vaccine adjuvant. PLoS One 6(1):e16333
60. Fox CB (2009) Squalene emulsions for parenteral vaccine and drug delivery. Molecules 14(9):3286–3312
61. Copland MJ et al (2005) Lipid based particulate formulations for the delivery of antigen. Immunol Cell Biol 83(2):97–105
62. Felnerova D et al (2004) Liposomes and virosomes as delivery systems for antigens, nucleic acids and drugs. Curr Opin Biotechnol 15(6):518–529
63. Pichyangkul S et al (2004) Pre-clinical evaluation of the malaria vaccine candidate P. falciparum MSP1(42) formulated with novel adjuvants or with alum. Vaccine 22(29–30): 3831–3840
64. Davidsen J et al (2005) Characterization of cationic liposomes based on dimethyldioctadecylammonium and synthetic cord factor from M. tuberculosis (trehalose 6,6'-dibehenate)-a novel adjuvant inducing both strong CMI and antibody responses. Biochim Biophys Acta 1718(1-2):22–31
65. Banerji B, Alving CR (1979) Lipid A from endotoxin: antigenic activities of purified fractions in liposomes. J Immunol 123(6): 2558–2562
66. Christensen D et al (2007) Cationic liposomes as vaccine adjuvants. Expert Rev Vaccines 6(5):785–796
67. van Dissel JT et al (2014) A novel liposomal adjuvant system, CAF01, promotes long-lived Mycobacterium tuberculosis-specific T-cell responses in human. Vaccine 32(52): 7098–7107
68. Morein B et al (1984) Iscom, a novel structure for antigenic presentation of membrane proteins from enveloped viruses. Nature 308(5958):457–460
69. Drane D et al (2007) ISCOMATRIX adjuvant for prophylactic and therapeutic vaccines. Expert Rev Vaccines 6(5):761–772
70. Pearse MJ, Drane D (2005) ISCOMATRIX® adjuvant for antigen delivery. Adv Drug Deliv Rev 57(3):465–474
71. Schnurr M et al (2009) ISCOMATRIX adjuvant induces efficient cross-presentation of tumor antigen by dendritic cells via rapid cytosolic antigen delivery and processing via tripeptidyl peptidase II. J Immunol 182(3): 1253–1259
72. Didierlaurent AM et al (2014) Enhancement of adaptive immunity by the human vaccine adjuvant AS01 depends on activated dendritic cells. J Immunol 193(4):1920–1930
73. Preis I, Langer RS (1979) A single-step immunization by sustained antigen release. J Immunol Methods 28(1–2):193–197

74. O'Hagan DT et al (1991) Biodegradable microparticles as controlled release antigen delivery systems. Immunology 73(2):239–242
75. Eldridge JH et al (1991) Biodegradable and biocompatible poly(DL-lactide-co-glycolide) microspheres as an adjuvant for staphylococcal enterotoxin B toxoid which enhances the level of toxin-neutralizing antibodies. Infect Immun 59(9):2978–2986
76. Jain S, O'Hagan DT, Singh M (2011) The long-term potential of biodegradable poly(lactide-co-glycolide) microparticles as the next-generation vaccine adjuvant. Expert Rev Vaccines 10(12):1731–1742
77. Wendorf J et al (2008) A comparison of anionic nanoparticles and microparticles as vaccine delivery systems. Hum Vaccin 4(1):44–49
78. Kazzaz J et al (2006) Encapsulation of the immune potentiators MPL and RC529 in PLG microparticles enhances their potency. J Control Release 110(3):566–573
79. Shah RR et al (2014) The impact of size on particulate vaccine adjuvants. Nanomedicine (Lond) 9(17):2671–2681
80. Fox CB et al (2011) Immunomodulatory and physical effects of oil composition in vaccine adjuvant emulsions. Vaccine 29(51):9563–9572
81. Shah RR et al (2015) The development of self-emulsifying oil-in-water emulsion adjuvant and an evaluation of the impact of droplet size on performance. J Pharm Sci 104(4):1352–1361
82. Calabro S et al (2011) Vaccine adjuvants alum and MF59 induce rapid recruitment of neutrophils and monocytes that participate in antigen transport to draining lymph nodes. Vaccine 29(9):1812–1823
83. Lal H et al (2015) Efficacy of an adjuvanted herpes zoster subunit vaccine in older adults. N Engl J Med 372(22):2087–2096
84. Efficacy and safety of RTS,S/AS01 malaria vaccine with or without a booster dose in infants and children in Africa: final results of a phase 3, individually randomised, controlled trial. Lancet 386(9988):31–45
85. Garcon N et al (2011) Development of an AS04-adjuvanted HPV vaccine with the adjuvant system approach. BioDrugs 25(4):217–226
86. Eng NF et al (2013) The potential of 1018 ISS adjuvant in hepatitis B vaccines. Hum Vaccin Immunother 9(8):1661–1672
87. Dynavax announces FDA acceptance for review of biologics license application and PDUFA action date for HEPLISAV-B(TM). 2016. http://investors.dynavax.com/releasedetail.cfm?ReleaseID=962813
88. Melero I et al (2014) Therapeutic vaccines for cancer: an overview of clinical trials. Nat Rev Clin Oncol 11(9):509–524
89. Update on phase III clinical trial of investigational MAGE-A3 antigen-specific cancer immunotherapeutic in non-small cell lung cancer. 2014 [cited 2016 3/18/2016]. https://us.gsk.com/en-us/media/press-releases/2014/update-on-phase-iii-clinical-trial-of-investigational-mage-a3-antigen-specific-cancer-immunotherapeutic-in-non-small-cell-lung-cancer/
90. Wu TY, Singh M et al (2014) Rational design of small molecules as vaccine adjuvants. Sci Transl Med 6(263):263ra160
91. Knipe DM et al (2014) Summary and recommendations from a National Institute of Allergy and Infectious Diseases (NIAID) workshop on "Next Generation Herpes Simplex Virus Vaccines". Vaccine 32(14):1561–1562
92. Skoberne M et al (2013) An adjuvanted herpes simplex virus 2 subunit vaccine elicits a T cell response in mice and is an effective therapeutic vaccine in Guinea pigs. J Virol 87(7): 3930–3942
93. Nohynek H et al (2012) AS03 adjuvanted AH1N1 vaccine associated with an abrupt increase in the Incidence of Childhood Narcolepsy in Finland. PLoS One 7(3):e33536
94. Winstone AM et al (2014) Clinical features of narcolepsy in children vaccinated with AS03 adjuvanted pandemic A/H1N1 2009 influenza vaccine in England. Dev Med Child Neurol 56(11):1117–1123
95. Ahmed SS et al (2015) Antibodies to influenza nucleoprotein cross-react with human hypocretin receptor 2. Sci Transl Med 7(294):294

Chapter 2

Development of the CpG Adjuvant 1018: A Case Study

John D. Campbell

Abstract

The development of aluminum salts (alum) as vaccine adjuvants was an empirical process with little understanding of the mechanism of action and, with decades of use, it has become clear that there is a need for alternatives where alum-based adjuvants are suboptimal. Oligonucleotides containing unmethylated CpG sequences represent one alternative as they are potent stimulators of the vertebrate innate immune system through activation of Toll-like receptor-9. This chapter outlines the methods used by Dynavax Technologies to progress a CpG-containing oligonucleotide sequence termed 1018 through preclinical and clinical testing as an adjuvant for immunization against hepatitis B virus (HBV). 1018 is a short (22-mer) oligonucleotide sequence containing CpG motifs active in both rodents and primates. Preclinical testing of hepatitis B surface antigen (HBsAg) + 1018 in comparison to HBsAg + alum demonstrated induction of substantially higher antibody titers and a favorable safety profile for 1018. Most importantly, clinical studies with HBsAg vaccination consistently demonstrate more rapid induction of protective antibody titers with 1018 compared to alum in all populations studied, including groups that are harder to immunize such as the elderly and immunocompromised individuals. These studies represent the basis for use of the CpG-motif-containing oligonucleotide 1018 as an improved adjuvant for HBsAg immunogenicity. HBsAg + 1018 (HEPLISAV-B™) is currently in late-stage clinical testing for prophylactic immunization against HBV.

Key words 1018, Adjuvant, CpG, HBsAg, HEPLISAV-B™, TLR-9, Vaccine

1 Introduction

Vaccines have proven to be one of the most successful medical advances in history in terms of increasing human health and longevity. Both inactivated or attenuated whole-pathogen vaccines have proven efficacious worldwide in preventing infection and disease caused by several pathogens despite reactogenicity being an issue with a subset of whole-pathogen vaccines (e.g., pertussis) [1]. In contrast, protein subunit vaccines, being more well defined, result in less toxicity, but often at the price of reduced immunogenicity. As a solution to this, aluminum salts (alum) have been used routinely to adjuvant vaccine immunogenicity for antibody responses to both inactivated and protein subunit vaccines since the 1920s with considerable success and an impressive safety record [2].

Christopher B. Fox (ed.), *Vaccine Adjuvants: Methods and Protocols*, Methods in Molecular Biology, vol. 1494,
DOI 10.1007/978-1-4939-6445-1_2, © Springer Science+Business Media New York 2017

While originally thought to create an antigen depot effect, it is now recognized that alum's mechanism of action is more complicated and involves induction of danger signals, cellular recruitment and enhanced antigen uptake, as well as promotion of Th2 responses, all of which may contribute to the adjuvant effect [3]. However, alum has limitations as it is not an effective adjuvant for eliciting Th1-type immunity or cytotoxic T cell responses and is not always sufficiently potent for vaccination of the elderly and immunocompromised individuals [4].

Bacteria, viruses, protozoa, and fungi contain unique molecular motifs known as pathogen-associated molecular patterns (PAMPS) which potently stimulate cells of the innate immune system and have demonstrated potential as next generation vaccine adjuvants [5]. The Toll-Like Receptors (TLRs), found on antigen presenting cells such as dendritic cells and B cells, are the most well characterized of the pattern recognition receptors (PRR) that bind PAMPs. This family of ten receptors includes both surface (TLR-1, 2, 4, 5, 6, and 10) and endosomally localized (TLR-3, 7, 8, and 9) molecules that recognize a diverse range of PAMPs including viral dsRNA (TLR-3), bacterial lipopolysaccharide (LPS; TLR-4) and flagellin (TLR-5), as well as unmethylated CpG motifs (TLR-9) within virus and bacterial DNA [6]. While several TLR agonists have shown promise in the clinic, to date only the LPS-derivative monophosphoryl lipid A (a TLR4-agonist), adsorbed to alum, has been licensed for human vaccine use (GSK's AS04). Like TLR-4 agonists, CpG-containing oligodeoxynucleotides (CpG-ODN) have been extensively tested in the clinic and also promote Th1 responses [7]. CpG-ODN signal through TLR-9 on plasmacytoid dendritic cells to induce potent IFN-α production and, indirectly through natural killer cells, IFN-γ secretion [8, 9]. In addition, CpG-ODN also directly stimulate maturation in TLR9-expressing B cells [10]. As adjuvants for vaccines, CpG-ODN thus activate professional antigen-presenting cells, thereby enhancing the induction of antibody responses to co-administered protein antigens.

The CpG-ODN sequence 1018 is currently in advanced-stage clinical development by Dynavax Technologies as an adjuvant for hepatitis B surface antigen (HBsAg) immunization against hepatitis B virus (HBV). HBV is spread through infected blood or bodily fluids, with blood transfusion, sexual contact, injection drug use with contaminated needles, and mother to child being common modes of transmission [11]. Universal adoption of hepatitis B vaccination using alum-based vaccines has dramatically reduced HBV infections worldwide but prevalence is still high with chronic carriers at risk of developing hepatic cirrhosis and hepatocellular carcinoma [12]. Problematically, the current licensed vaccines are poorly immunogenic in several subpopulations including older adults and immunocompromised individuals [13]. Thus, immunization against HBV is an application for which the potentially strong immunogenic adjuvant effect of CpG-ODN is very attractive. This chapter focuses on the preclinical development and clinical testing of the CpG-ODN 1018 in combination with HbsAg (HEPLISAV-B™) by Dynavax Technologies as a new and improved prophylactic vaccine against HBV.

2 Drug Product: 1018 and HbsAg

CpG-containing sequences have been divided into three general classes based on structure and biological function (Table 1): CpG-A class, CpG-B class, and CpG-C class, with CpG-B class molecules being the most frequently used in clinical vaccine studies. Structure and function are closely related for CpG ODNs. Indeed, the higher order structure of the molecule determines whether the CpG ODN localizes intracellularly to early or late endosomes, compartments associated with different signaling pathways. Multimeric CpG-A ODNs predominantly localize to early endosomes, where in plasmacytoid dendritic cells they result in strong induction of IFN-α. Monomeric CpG-B ODNs concentrate in the late endosomal compartment and can promote cellular maturation of both plasmacytoid dendritic cells and B cells. CpG-C ODNs localize to both compartments, inducing IFN-α production and cellular maturation [14]. Additional structural modifications that influence the biological effects of CpG-containing sequences include linking two or more short phosphorothioate-backbone CpG-ODNs by non-nucleoside chemical linkers to produce linear chimeric immunomodulatory compounds and/or formulation of CpG-containing nanoparticle compounds [15–17].

Table 1
Comparative features of CpG classes A, B, and C

Class	Structural characteristics	Immunological characteristics
CpG-A	Phosphodiester CpG motif(s) Phosphorothioate poly-G at 5′ and 3′ Forms aggregates	Strong pDC IFN-α induction Moderate pDC maturation Weak B cell activation
CpG-B	Phosphorothioate backbone T-rich with CpG motifs Monomeric	Strong B cell activation Strong pDC maturation Weak pDC IFN-α induction
CpG-C	Phosphorothioate backbone 5′-TCG, CpG motif in central palindrome Forms duplexes	Good pDC IFN-α induction Good pDC maturation Good B cell activation

IFN interferon, *pDC* plasmacytoid dendritic cell

1018 is a synthetic CpG-B class oligonucleotide having a phosphorothioate-backbone and the sequence 5′-TGACTGTGAA CGTT**CG**AGATGA-3′. The first CpG motif (underlined) is a sequence active on mouse TLR-9, whereas the second CpG motif (bold) is active on human and nonhuman primate TLR-9. Protocols have been established to confirm the quality and safety of the 1018 adjuvant and focus on characteristics regarded as appropriate for ensuring safety and immunogenicity of the HEPLISAV-B™ drug product. Oligonucleotide identity is tested by mass spectrometry, which includes confirmation of the correct nucleotide sequence. Purity and product-related impurities can be determined by complementary chromatographic test methods including RP-HPLC (reverse-phase-high performance liquid chromatography), IEX-HPLC (ion-exchange-HPLC), or LC-MS (liquid-chromatography-mass spectrometry). Testing for bioburden and endotoxin is performed to confirm the absence of microbial contaminants. The antigen used in the drug product, yeast-derived recombinant HbsAg, is also tested for characteristics such as purity, identity, and sterility in addition to assessment for antigenicity. For clinical use, 3 mg of 1018 mixed in a single vial with 20 mcg HbsAg in phosphate-buffered saline and is administered in a volume of 0.5 mL into the deltoid muscle.

3 Preclinical Development of 1018

In preclinical models, CpG-B 1018 has been shown to augment mouse humoral immune responses to a variety of antigens including influenza hemagglutinin and HIVgp120 [18, 19], and these responses are largely IgG2a dominated as a consequence of the Th1-promoting bias of CpG motifs. As an adjuvant for HbsAg vaccination, 1018 has been evaluated in mice, dogs, cynomolgus monkeys, and baboons [20]. In addition to augmenting anti-HbsAg antibody responses in mice and dogs, intramuscular injection of HbsAg+1018 substantially raised anti-HbsAg-specific antibody levels in nonhuman primates compared to immunization with HbsAg alone. A single immunization with 10 mcg HbsAg+500 mcg 1018-induced seroprotection (defined as antibody titers greater than 10 mIU/mL) in 80% of the animals compared to 20% in the group receiving only HbsAg (N=5/group). In a separate nonhuman primate study, all HbsAg+1018-immunized animals (3/3) achieved seroprotection following one immunization and further demonstrated 3- to 50-fold higher titers than the HbsAg-only immunized group following the third immunization. Importantly, HbsAg+1018 immunization induced approximately 45-fold higher titers in nonhuman primates compared to immunization with HbsAg+alum, i.e., the constituents of the currently licensed vaccine [21]. Taken together, these immunogenicity studies demonstrated strong adjuvant activity of 1018 for anti-HbsAg antibody responses in different species including nonhuman primates.

Preclinical studies also evaluated the safety profile of 1018 in different species, taking into consideration the known differences between species in terms of responsiveness to CpG-ODN. In addition to the well-known class effects of phosphorothioate-containing ODNs [22], the toxicity profile of CpG-containing ODNs such as 1018 is also influenced by the immunostimulatory effects of the sequences. These effects are much more pronounced in mice and rats due to the wider cellular distribution of TLR-9 expression in these animals when compared to primates [23]. For example, studies in which high-dose 1018 (5 mg/kg) was delivered to the lungs of mice have shown that the increased sensitivity of rodents (as measured by lung inflammation/pathology and body weight loss) was strictly dependent on tumor necrosis factor (TNF) production [24]. These effects were absent in TNF-deficient mice or in mice lacking TNF receptors. As humans and nonhuman primates do not have TLR-9 expression in the principal TNF-producing cells such as monocytes and macrophages, they lack the TNF-mediated toxicity evident in rodents. This is supported by clinical studies using CpG-ODN therapy for asthma, where inhalation of 1018 by mildly asthmatic subjects stimulated expression of interferon-inducible genes *CXCL10* and *ISG-54* but did not induce appreciable *TNF* expression (as measured in induced sputum) [24].

A series of good laboratory practice-compliant preclinical toxicity studies have been conducted with 1018 in the presence or absence of HbsAg to evaluate its safety profile. These single- and multiple-dose studies in rodents and nonhuman primates have collectively shown that intramuscular injection of 1018 in doses up to 12.5 mg/kg produced no clinically significant toxicities [25]. By way of comparison to doses used in clinical studies, 1018 is administered at 3 mg to adults, which is 0.04 mg/kg for a 70 kg individual. Preclinical toxicity studies have demonstrated only mild and transient immune-related histopathological changes at the injection site, lymph nodes and spleen that were consistent with phosphorothioate ODN class effects at high doses but also reflected the immunostimulatory effects of 1018. Separate reproductive and genetic toxicity studies revealed no significant reproductive, mutagenic, or clastogenic signals and there has been no induction of anti-double-stranded DNA antibodies in mice or baboons immunized with 1018 vaccine formulations [25]. Together, preclinical immunogenicity and safety studies with 1018 demonstrated potent adjuvant activity combined with low toxicity and good tolerability, providing a solid basis for clinical studies.

4 Clinical Development of 1018

4.1 Phase 1 Studies

The adjuvant activity of 1018 for anti-HBsAg antibody induction has now been tested in a series of phase 1–3 clinical studies conducted by Dynavax Technologies. The initial phase 1 study evaluated safety and immunogenicity of a two dose regimen in healthy adults aged 18–55 years and was the first human trial to use a CpG-ODN as the sole adjuvant for improving HBsAg immunogenicity [26]. As in all HBsAg-1018 trials, study exclusion criteria included history of HBV infection, prior HBV vaccination or positive serological tests for HBsAg, or antibodies against HBsAg or HBcAg (core antigen). Four 1018 dosage groups were included in the Phase 1 study: 300, 650, 1000, or 3000 mcg. For each group, eight subjects received 20 mcg HBsAg + 1018, two control subjects received 1018 only, and two control subjects received 20 mcg HBsAg without adjuvant. Injections at 0 and 8 weeks were administered intramuscularly into opposite deltoid muscles and were well-tolerated with injection site reactions being mostly mild and of brief duration, albeit more frequent with higher 1018 doses. Antibody responses to immunization were quantified both as geometric mean antibody concentration (GMC) against HBsAg (anti-HBs) as well as proportions of subjects achieving seroprotection against HBV: defined as having post-immunization anti-HBs antibody levels of ≥10 mIU/mL [27]. The majority of subjects receiving HBsAg + 1000 or 3000 mcg 1018 were seroprotected by 28 days after the first immunization and all subjects in the top three dosage groups were seroprotected at 7 days after the second dose. Peak GMC of 3045 mIU/mL was achieved in the 3000 mcg group at 28 days post second dose. Two doses of HBsAg alone did not induce seroprotection in the study. Based on these results, 3 mg 1018 was chosen as the adjuvant dose for subsequent clinical studies including an additional Phase I study that compared an accelerated 0- and 4-week dosing schedule to a 0- and 8-week schedule [28]. The accelerated 0–4-week regimen resulted in 94% seroprotection in subjects at 8 weeks, compared to 70% seroprotection in the 0–8-week group at this time point with similar rates of adverse events between the groups. By 12 weeks, all subjects had achieved seroprotection with GMCs of 379 versus 3217 mIU/mL in the 0–4- and 0–8-week groups, respectively. The relative difference in GMCs was greatly reduced by 32 weeks. Thus, the 0–4-week dosing schedule potentially offers more rapid protection, which would be especially important for those at high risk of imminent exposure such as health care workers, injection drug users and others [29].

4.2 Comparison Between HEPLISAV-B™ and Engerix-B®

Engerix-B® (GSK) consists of 20 mcg HBsAg absorbed to 0.5 mg aluminum hydroxide and is currently licensed for vaccination against HBV in the USA and most countries worldwide. The standard regimen for healthy adults consists of intramuscular injections at 0, 1, and 6 months. As high rates of seroprotection

(85–100 % of subjects) generally require completion of the full three-dose regimen [30], there is an unmet need for a more rapid and potent vaccine not only for those at high risk of imminent exposure but also for difficult to immunize populations that respond poorly to alum-based vaccines such as Engerix-B®. Such groups include the elderly [31, 32], and patients with diabetes mellitus or chronic kidney disease who are at increased risk of nosocomial HBV transmission during assisted monitoring of blood sugar or hemodialysis, respectively [33, 34].

HBsAg + 1018 (HEPLISAV-B™) was first compared to Engerix-B® in a phase 2 study conducted with healthy, seronegative young adults (18–29 years old) which tested the hypothesis that the proportion of subjects achieving seroprotection (anti-HBs of ≥10 mIU/mL) 4 weeks after the first and second doses of vaccine would be greater for HEPLISAV-B™ (0–8 weeks; *N* = 48) versus Engerix-B® (0, 8, 24 weeks; *N* = 51) vaccinated subjects [35]. At 4 weeks post-first dose, 79 % of HEPLISAV-B™ recipients had protective antibody responses, whereas only 12 % of Engerix-B® recipients had demonstrated seroprotection. By 1 week post second dose (week 9), 100 % of HEPLISAV-B™ recipients had anti-HBs of ≥10 mIU/mL (and peak GMC of 2074 mIU/mL) whereas only 18 % of Engerix-B® subjects had protective antibody responses at this time point, increasing to 64 % at 1 month post-second dose (week 12) and 100 % at 1 month post-third dose (week 28) (Fig. 1). Peak GMC of 5239 mIU/mL were induced in Engerix-B® recipients at 4 weeks post-third dose. HEPLISAV-B™ subjects received placebo or meningococcal vaccine for the third injection. Both two dose HEPLISAV-B™ and three dose Engerix-B® regimens induced lasting antibody responses as indicated by GMCs of 851 and 617 mIU/mL, respectively, measured 1 year post-second dose.

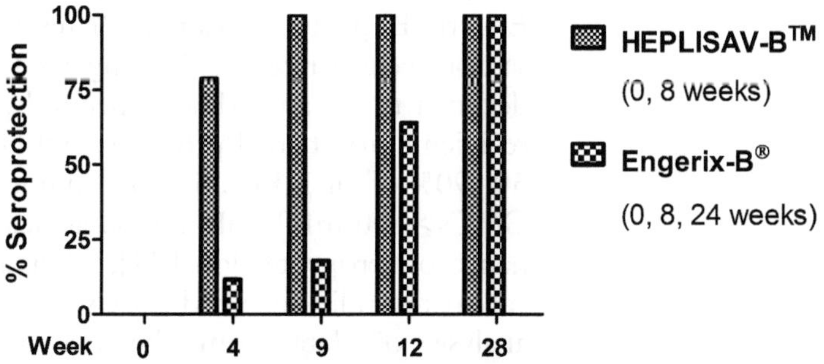

Fig. 1 Proportions of study participants with protective anti-HBsAg antibody responses at different time points following immunization. Healthy human subjects (18–29 years of age) were vaccinated with HEPLISAV-B™ (*N* = 48; 0, and 8 weeks, control injection at week 24) or Engerix-B® (*N* = 51; 0, 8, and 24 weeks) and serum anti-HBsAg antibody levels measured by ELISA. Percentages of vaccinated individuals with seroprotection (anti-HBsAg titers ≥ 10 mIU/mL) at specific time points are shown. Data from [35]

Subsequent phase 3 clinical studies have consistently shown more rapid and greater induction of protective immune responses in both healthy individuals and in more difficult to immunize groups. A double-blind, multicenter study of 2415 study participants (18–55 years of age) randomized 3:1 to HEPLISAV-B™ (0–4 weeks) or Engerix-B® (0, 4, 24 weeks) met its primary immunogenicity endpoint demonstrating superiority of seroprotection rate 8 weeks after the second dose of HEPLISAV-B™ (95%) versus 4 weeks after the third dose of Engerix-B® (81%) [36]. There was also a clear difference in magnitude of the anti-HBs antibody response between the two groups. In the Engerix-B® group, GMC only increased appreciably after the third dose, going from 7 to 348 mIU/mL whereas GMC in the HEPLISAV-B™ group rose from 82 mIU/mL at 4 weeks post-dose 2 to 137 mIU/mL at 8 weeks and 343 mIU/mL at 20 weeks post-dose 2. Age stratification of subjects into 18–39-year-old and 40–55-year-old cohorts revealed that the younger cohort had better seroprotection and GMCs than the older cohort for both Engerix-B® and HEPLISAV-B™ but that the 1018-containing vaccine induced more rapid responses in both age cohorts.

More rapid induction of protective antibody responses in older adults was demonstrated in two additional phase 3 studies conducted in Asia and North America, respectively [37, 38]. In the study of 40–70-year-old North American adults, HEPLISAV-B™ recipients (0–4 weeks; $N=1123$) achieved a seroprotective rate of 90% at 8 weeks post-second dose which was significantly higher than the 71% for Engerix-B® recipients (0, 4, 24 weeks, $N=359$) at 8 weeks post-third dose [38]. The primary endpoint for the study with Asian adults was seroprotective rate at 4 weeks after third active injection of either the 1018-containing vaccine or the current licensed product. At this time point (week 28) both the 40–55- and 56–70-year-old groups receiving HEPLISAV-B™ had 100% seroprotection, significantly greater than the corresponding Engerix-B® groups (78 and 56%, respectively) [37]. By week 50 the seroprotection rate for the Engerix-B®-recipient age cohorts had declined to 73 and 51%, respectively, whereas all HEPLISAV-B™ recipients maintained protective antibody responses. Also at week 50, 90% of all HEPLISAV-B™-immunized study participants had GMCs ≥ 100 mIU/mL, a level associated with long term maintenance of seroprotection [39], whereas only 44% of Engerix-B®-vaccinated individuals had GMCs ≥ 100 mIU/mL. In an exploratory analysis of data from the two phase 3 studies comparing HEPLISAV-B™ (0–4 weeks) to Engerix-B® (0, 4, 24 weeks), further stratification of subjects by age, body mass index and smoking status demonstrated significantly higher seroprotective rates in response to HEPLISAV-B™ not only in increasingly older cohorts, including 60–70-year-olds (Fig. 2), but also in smokers and the obese who have also been reported to be hyporesponsive to Engerix-B® [40].

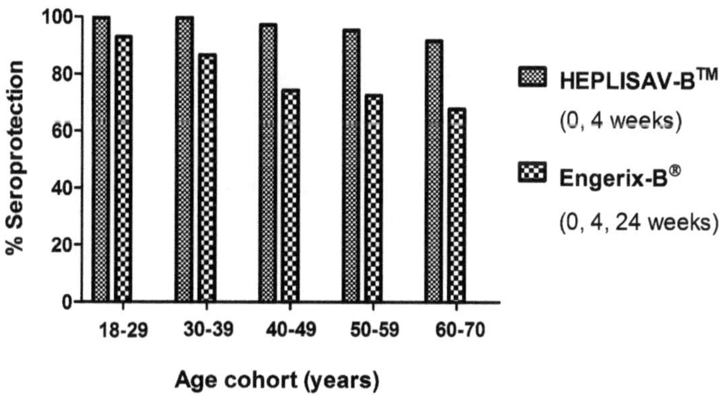

Fig 2 Peak seroprotection rates for different age cohorts of HEPLISAV-B™ or Engerix-B® immunized study participants. Healthy human subjects (18–70 years of age) were vaccinated twice (HEPLISAV-B™; 0, 4 weeks, placebo at week 24) or 3 times (Engerix-B®; 0, 4, and 24 weeks) and peak seroprotection rates measured at weeks 24 for HEPLISAV-B™ or week 28 for Engerix-B®. Data from [40]

Another population especially vulnerable to HBV infection is patients on dialysis because of chronic kidney disease (CKD). In addition to having impaired immune defenses and consequent poor responses to vaccines [41], CKD patients are at higher risk of developing chronic HBV infection and associated cirrhosis and hepatocellular carcinoma [34]. The current recommended Engerix-B® regimen for these hyporesponsive patients is four double doses (2×20 mcg HBsAg/dose) over 6 months (0, 4, 8, and 24 weeks) and was compared to a three dose regimen for HEPLISAV-B™ (0, 4, and 24 weeks) in a phase 3 study with CKD patients [42]. At the primary study endpoint (28 weeks), the HEPLISAV-B™ group ($N=247$) had 90% seroprotection (GMC of 587 mIU/mL) compared to 82% seroprotection (GMC of 157 mIU/mL) in the Engerix-B® group ($N=260$), which met the study's non-inferiority and superiority criteria for HEPLISAV-B™. HEPLISAV-B™ also induced significantly higher anti-HBs antibody responses, compared to Engerix-B®, in the subgroup of CKD with type 2 diabetes [43]. The percentage of all HEPLISAV-B™-immunized individuals in the study with anti-HBs ≥ 100 mIU/mL (74%) was significantly greater than that of the corresponding Engerix-B® group (63%) at 28 weeks, suggestive of more durable antibody responses in the HEPLISAV-B™-immunized group, and at 52 weeks (the last time point in the study) GMCs were 171 mIU/mL for the HEPLISAV-B™ group versus 51 mIU/mL for the Engerix-B® group. Across all phase 2–3 studies, HEPLISAV™ has been well tolerated with a safety profile similar to Engerix-B®.

5 Key Considerations for Novel Adjuvant Development

In developing a novel adjuvant, there are practical considerations that should be kept in mind for a roadmap to regulatory approval and to facilitate the process towards licensure for human use. Most importantly, the introduction of a novel adjuvant as part of a new vaccine for a given disease should have a clear rationale with a well-defined unmet medical need. This necessitates a thorough understanding of the adjuvant's mechanism of action and how this could influence humoral or cellular immune responses for improved prophylactic or therapeutic efficacy of a given vaccine. For many applications, the adjuvant would be used in combination with antigen to boost a specific immune response but, in some applications such as allergic diseases with natural exposure to environmental antigens, effects of an immunomodulatory adjuvant alone may be effective therapy.

Novel adjuvants, especially first in class products, will be expected to undergo extensive safety testing. In this context, a clear understanding of the adjuvant's molecular and cellular mechanisms of action and any potential or perceived safety implications will be crucial to address in comprehensive pharmacology and preclinical toxicity programs. In many cases, this will necessitate defining and establishing new protocols for evaluation of potency and other features specific to the novel adjuvant, in addition to meeting standard physiochemical characterization requirements and demonstration of product stability for regulatory approval. Other important factors to consider for novel adjuvant development include formulation of the product for optimal bio-distribution and efficacy as well as the intended delivery route, which could be parenteral or mucosal depending on the nature of the targeted immune response.

6 Conclusion

In the 20 years since the discovery of the immunostimulatory effects of unmethylated CpG sequences present in bacterial DNA [44], extensive preclinical and clinical work by multiple groups has gone into testing the potential of CpG-ODN as vaccine adjuvants. Collectively, these studies have shown that immunization with various protein antigens and CpG-ODN sequences strongly enhances specific antibody responses. Dynavax Technologies has advanced the clinical development of the CpG-B sequence 1018 in combination with HBsAg (HEPLISAV™) as an improved vaccine against HBV. Compared to alum, the adjuvant contained in Engerix-B®, 1018 significantly improves HBsAg immunogenicity in terms of rapidity of induction, magnitude and longevity of response.

As a representative of a new class of adjuvants, 1018 improves immunogenicity without increased safety signals, and will benefit not only healthy individuals, but also hypo-responsive populations that are underserved by the current licensed alum-based vaccines.

Acknowledgments

The author thanks Albert Candia and Robert Coffman for critical reading of the manuscript as well as Robert Janssen, Paula Traquina, Robert Milley, and Gary Ott for helpful discussions. HEPLISAV-B is a trademark of Dynavax Technologies Corporation.

References

1. Andre FE, Booy R, Bock HL, Clemens J, Datta SK, John TJ, Lee BW, Lolekha S, Peltola H, Ruff TA, Santosham M, Schmitt HJ (2008) Vaccination greatly reduces disease, disability, death and inequity worldwide. Bull World Health Organ 86(2):140–146
2. Lee S, Nguyen MT (2015) Recent advances of vaccine adjuvants for infectious diseases. Immune Netw 15(2):51–57. doi:10.4110/in.2015.15.2.51
3. Coffman RL, Sher A, Seder RA (2010) Vaccine adjuvants: putting innate immunity to work. Immunity 33(4):492–503. doi:10.1016/j.immuni.2010.10.002
4. Brady RC, Treanor JJ, Atmar RL, Keitel WA, Edelman R, Chen WH, Winokur P, Belshe R, Graham IL, Noah DL, Guo K, Hill H (2009) Safety and immunogenicity of a subvirion inactivated influenza A/H5N1 vaccine with or without aluminum hydroxide among healthy elderly adults. Vaccine 27(37):5091–5095. doi:10.1016/j.vaccine.2009.06.057
5. Mogensen TH (2009) Pathogen recognition and inflammatory signaling in innate immune defenses. Clin Microbiol Rev 22(2):240–273. doi:10.1128/CMR.00046-08.
6. Maisonneuve C, Bertholet S, Philpott DJ, De Gregorio E (2014) Unleashing the potential of NOD- and Toll-like agonists as vaccine adjuvants. Proc Natl Acad Sci U S A 111(34):12294–12299. doi:10.1073/pnas.1400478111
7. Toussi DN, Massari P (2014) Immune adjuvant effect of molecularly-defined toll-like receptor ligands. Vaccines 2(2):323–353. doi:10.3390/vaccines2020323
8. Krug A, Rothenfusser S, Hornung V, Jahrsdorfer B, Blackwell S, Ballas ZK, Endres S, Krieg AM, Hartmann G (2001) Identification of CpG oligonucleotide sequences with high induction of IFN-alpha/beta in plasmacytoid dendritic cells. Eur J Immunol 31(7):2154–2163, doi:10.1002/1521-4141(200107)31:7<2154::AID-IMMU2154>3.0.CO;2-U
9. Kranzer K, Bauer M, Lipford GB, Heeg K, Wagner H, Lang R (2000) CpG-oligodeoxynucleotides enhance T-cell receptor-triggered interferon-gamma production and up-regulation of CD69 via induction of antigen-presenting cell-derived interferon type I and interleukin-12. Immunology 99(2):170–178
10. Hartmann G, Krieg AM (2000) Mechanism and function of a newly identified CpG DNA motif in human primary B cells. J Immunol 164(2):944–953
11. Lee WM (1997) Hepatitis B virus infection. N Engl J Med 337(24):1733–1745. doi:10.1056/NEJM199712113372406
12. Chen DS (2009) Hepatitis B vaccination: the key towards elimination and eradication of hepatitis B. J Hepatol 50(4):805–816. doi:10.1016/j.jhep.2009.01.002
13. Shouval D (2003) Hepatitis B vaccines. J Hepatol 39(Suppl 1):S70–S76
14. Guiducci C, Ott G, Chan JH, Damon E, Calacsan C, Matray T, Lee KD, Coffman RL, Barrat FJ (2006) Properties regulating the nature of the plasmacytoid dendritic cell response to Toll-like receptor 9 activation. J Exp Med 203(8):1999–2008. doi:10.1084/jem.20060401
15. Marshall JD, Hessel EM, Gregorio J, Abbate C, Yee P, Chu M, Nest GV, Coffman RL, Fearon KL (2003) Novel chimeric immunomodulatory compounds containing short CpG oligodeoxyribonucleotides have differential activities in human cells. Nucleic Acids Res 31(17):5122–5133

16. Thomas SN, Vokali E, Lund AW, Hubbell JA, Swartz MA (2014) Targeting the tumor-draining lymph node with adjuvanted nanoparticles reshapes the anti-tumor immune response. Biomaterials 35(2):814–824. doi:10.1016/j.biomaterials.2013.10.003
17. Kachura MA, Hickle C, Kell SA, Sathe A, Calacsan C, Kiwan R, Hall B, Milley R, Ott G, Coffman RL, Kanzler H, Campbell JD (2016) A CpG-Ficoll nanoparticle adjuvant for anthrax protective antigen enhances immunogenicity and provides single-immunization protection against inhaled anthrax in monkeys. J Immunol 196(1):284–297. doi:10.4049/jimmunol.1501903
18. Roman M, Martin-Orozco E, Goodman JS, Nguyen MD, Sato Y, Ronaghy A, Kornbluth RS, Richman DD, Carson DA, Raz E (1997) Immunostimulatory DNA sequences function as T helper-1-promoting adjuvants. Nat Med 3(8):849–854
19. Horner AA, Datta SK, Takabayashi K, Belyakov IM, Hayashi T, Cinman N, Nguyen MD, Van Uden JH, Berzofsky JA, Richman DD, Raz E (2001) Immunostimulatory DNA-based vaccines elicit multifaceted immune responses against HIV at systemic and mucosal sites. J Immunol 167(3):1584–1591
20. Van Nest G, Tighe H, Raz E, Higgins D, Traquina P, Eiden JJ (1999) An immunostimulatory oligonucleotide (ISS ODN) enhances immune responses to HBV vaccine in a variety of animal species including primates. Paper presented at the 39th interscience conference on antimicrobial agents and chemotherapy (ICAAC), San Francisco, CA, 26–29 September 1999
21. Barry M, Cooper C (2007) Review of hepatitis B surface antigen-1018 ISS adjuvant-containing vaccine safety and efficacy. Expert Opin Biol Ther 7(11):1731–1737. doi:10.1517/14712598.7.11.1731
22. Iannitti T, Morales-Medina JC, Palmieri B (2014) Phosphorothioate oligonucleotides: effectiveness and toxicity. Curr Drug Targets 15(7):663–673
23. Ketloy C, Engering A, Srichairatanakul U, Limsalakpetch A, Yongvanitchit K, Pichyangkul S, Ruxrungtham K (2008) Expression and function of Toll-like receptors on dendritic cells and other antigen presenting cells from non-human primates. Vet Immunol Immunopathol 125(1–2):18–30. doi:10.1016/j.vetimm.2008.05.001
24. Campbell JD, Cho Y, Foster ML, Kanzler H, Kachura MA, Lum JA, Ratcliffe MJ, Sathe A, Leishman AJ, Bahl A, McHale M, Coffman RL, Hessel EM (2009) CpG-containing immunostimulatory DNA sequences elicit TNF-alpha-dependent toxicity in rodents but not in humans. J Clin Invest 119(9):2564–2576. doi:10.1172/JCI38294
25. Higgins D, Marshall JD, Traquina P, Van Nest G, Livingston BD (2007) Immunostimulatory DNA as a vaccine adjuvant. Expert Rev Vaccines 6(5):747–759. doi:10.1586/14760584.6.5.747
26. Halperin SA, Van Nest G, Smith B, Abtahi S, Whiley H, Eiden JJ (2003) A phase I study of the safety and immunogenicity of recombinant hepatitis B surface antigen co-administered with an immunostimulatory phosphorothioate oligonucleotide adjuvant. Vaccine 21(19–20):2461–2467
27. Mast EE, Weinbaum CM, Fiore AE, Alter MJ, Bell BP, Finelli L, Rodewald LE, Douglas JM Jr, Janssen RS, Ward JW, Advisory Committee on Immunization Practices Centers for Disease C, Prevention (2006) A comprehensive immunization strategy to eliminate transmission of hepatitis B virus infection in the United States: recommendations of the Advisory Committee on Immunization Practices (ACIP) Part II: immunization of adults. MMWR Recomm Rep 55(RR-16):1–33, quiz CE31-34
28. Halperin SA, McNeil S, Langley JM, Smith B, MacKinnon-Cameron D, McCall-Sani R, Heyward WL, Martin JT (2012) Safety and immunogenicity of different two-dose regimens of an investigational hepatitis B vaccine (hepatitis B surface antigen co-administered with an immunostimulatory phosphorothioate oligodeoxyribonucleotide) in healthy young adults. Vaccine 30(36):5445–5448. doi:10.1016/j.vaccine.2012.05.074
29. Komatsu H (2014) Hepatitis B virus: where do we stand and what is the next step for eradication? World J Gastroenterol 20(27):8998–9016. doi:10.3748/wjg.v20.i27.8998
30. Keating GM, Noble S (2003) Recombinant hepatitis B vaccine (Engerix-B): a review of its immunogenicity and protective efficacy against hepatitis B. Drugs 63(10):1021–1051
31. Wolters B, Junge U, Dziuba S, Roggendorf M (2003) Immunogenicity of combined hepatitis A and B vaccine in elderly persons. Vaccine 21(25–26):3623–3628
32. Chen WH, Kozlovsky BF, Effros RB, Grubeck-Loebenstein B, Edelman R, Sztein MB (2009) Vaccination in the elderly: an immunological perspective. Trends Immunol 30(7):351–359. doi:10.1016/j.it.2009.05.002
33. Reilly ML, Schillie SF, Smith E, Poissant T, Vonderwahl CW, Gerard K, Baumgartner J, Mercedes L, Sweet K, Muleta D, Zaccaro DJ, Klevens RM, Murphy TV (2012) Increased risk of acute hepatitis B among adults with

diagnosed diabetes mellitus. J Diabetes Sci Technol 6(4):858–866

34. Centers for Disease Control and Prevention (2001) Recommendations for preventing transmission of infections among chronic hemodialysis patients. MMWR Recomm Rep 50(RR-5):1–43
35. Halperin SA, Dobson S, McNeil S, Langley JM, Smith B, McCall-Sani R, Levitt D, Nest GV, Gennevois D, Eiden JJ (2006) Comparison of the safety and immunogenicity of hepatitis B virus surface antigen co-administered with an immunostimulatory phosphorothioate oligonucleotide and a licensed hepatitis B vaccine in healthy young adults. Vaccine 24(1):20–26. doi:10.1016/j.vaccine.2005.08.095
36. Halperin SA, Ward B, Cooper C, Predy G, Diaz-Mitoma F, Dionne M, Embree J, McGeer A, Zickler P, Moltz KH, Martz R, Meyer I, McNeil S, Langley JM, Martins E, Heyward WL, Martin JT (2012) Comparison of safety and immunogenicity of two doses of investigational hepatitis B virus surface antigen co-administered with an immunostimulatory phosphorothioate oligodeoxyribonucleotide and three doses of a licensed hepatitis B vaccine in healthy adults 18–55 years of age. Vaccine 30(15):2556–2563. doi:10.1016/j.vaccine.2012.01.087
37. Sablan BP, Kim DJ, Barzaga NG, Chow WC, Cho M, Ahn SH, Hwang SG, Lee JH, Namini H, Heyward WL (2012) Demonstration of safety and enhanced seroprotection against hepatitis B with investigational HBsAg-1018 ISS vaccine compared to a licensed hepatitis B vaccine. Vaccine 30(16):2689–2696. doi:10.1016/j.vaccine.2012.02.001
38. Heyward WL, Kyle M, Blumenau J, Davis M, Reisinger K, Kabongo ML, Bennett S, Janssen RS, Namini H, Martin JT (2013) Immunogenicity and safety of an investigational hepatitis B vaccine with a Toll-like receptor 9 agonist adjuvant (HBsAg-1018) compared to a licensed hepatitis B vaccine in healthy adults 40–70 years of age. Vaccine 31(46):5300–5305. doi:10.1016/j.vaccine.2013.05.068
39. Jilg W, Schmidt M, Deinhardt F (1988) Persistence of specific antibodies after hepatitis B vaccination. J Hepatol 6(2):201–207
40. Janssen JM, Jackson S, Heyward WL, Janssen RS (2015) Immunogenicity of an investigational hepatitis B vaccine with a toll-like receptor 9 agonist adjuvant (HBsAg-1018) compared with a licensed hepatitis B vaccine in subpopulations of healthy adults 18–70 years of age. Vaccine 33(31):3614–3618. doi:10.1016/j.vaccine.2015.05.070
41. Johnson DW, Fleming SJ (1992) The use of vaccines in renal failure. Clin Pharmacokinet 22(6):434–446. doi:10.2165/00003088-199222060 00003
42. Janssen RS, Mangoo-Karim R, Pergola PE, Girndt M, Namini H, Rahman S, Bennett SR, Heyward WL, Martin JT (2013) Immunogenicity and safety of an investigational hepatitis B vaccine with a toll-like receptor 9 agonist adjuvant (HBsAg-1018) compared with a licensed hepatitis B vaccine in patients with chronic kidney disease. Vaccine 31(46):5306–5313. doi:10.1016/j.vaccine.2013.05.067
43. Janssen JM, Heyward WL, Martin JT, Janssen RS (2015) Immunogenicity and safety of an investigational hepatitis B vaccine with a Toll-like receptor 9 agonist adjuvant (HBsAg-1018) compared with a licensed hepatitis B vaccine in patients with chronic kidney disease and type 2 diabetes mellitus. Vaccine 33(7):833–837. doi:10.1016/j.vaccine.2014.12.060
44. Krieg AM, Yi AK, Matson S, Waldschmidt TJ, Bishop GA, Teasdale R, Koretzky GA, Klinman DM (1995) CpG motifs in bacterial DNA trigger direct B-cell activation. Nature 374(6522): 546–549. doi:10.1038/374546a0

Chapter 3

Syntheses of Human TLR8-Specific Small-Molecule Agonists

Mallesh Beesu, Hari Prasad Kokatla, and Sunil A. David

Abstract

Human toll-like receptor (hTLR)-8 is expressed in myeloid dendritic cells, monocytes, and monocyte-derived dendritic cells. Engagement by TLR8 agonists evokes a distinct cytokine profile which favors the development of type 1 helper T cells. Focused exploration of structure-activity relationships in the imidazoquinolines has led to the identification of several novel human TLR8-specific agonists. The synthetic procedures for best-in-class analogues encompassing four chemotypes are described.

Key words TLR8, TLR8 agonists, Vaccine adjuvants, Innate immunity

1 Introduction

The majority of currently available vaccines contain a single adjuvant—"alum" (a mixture of aluminum phosphate and aluminum hydroxide), which was introduced by Alexander Glenny in 1926 [1]. Although aluminum salts have been in widespread use and have a good safety record, they are weak adjuvants for antibody induction and induce a T helper-2 (Th2)-skewed, rather than a T helper-1 (Th1) response [2, 3], an attribute that has been implicated in the rapidly waning humoral responses to alum-adjuvanted pertussis subunit vaccines [4–6], and the recent re-emergence of pertussis in the USA [7, 8] and elsewhere in the world [9, 10].

Antigens in modern subunit vaccines are highly purified and poorly immunogenic proteins, inducing feeble, short-lived immune responses. Indeed, as early as 1962, Dresser observed that the administration of purified soluble proteins not only failed to stimulate an immune response, but also induced tolerance in animals, unless a bacterial extract was admixed with the protein immunogen [11]. This led him to redefine adjuvanticity as "a property of a substance which can act as a physiological switch, directing at least some immunologically competent cells to respond by making

Christopher B. Fox (ed.), *Vaccine Adjuvants: Methods and Protocols*, Methods in Molecular Biology, vol. 1494,
DOI 10.1007/978-1-4939-6445-1_3, © Springer Science+Business Media New York 2017

antibody rather than by becoming immunologically paralyzed by the antigen [12]." Dresser's observations confirmed Johnson's earlier observations that lipopolysaccharide (LPS) from Gram-negative bacteria exerted potent adjuvant properties [13], which is now acknowledged to be due to the engagement of innate immune responses mediated by the recognition of LPS by toll-like receptor 4 (TLR4) [14, 15], and the consequent amplification of antigen-specific adaptive immune responses.

Innate immune signals evoked by vaccine adjuvants include those originating from toll-like receptors (TLRs) [16–18], as well as RIG-I-like receptors [19] and NOD-like receptors (NLRs) [20, 21]. There are ten functional TLRs encoded in the human genome, which are trans-membrane proteins with an extracellular domain having leucine-rich repeats (LRR) and a cytosolic domain called the toll/IL-1 receptor (TIR) domain [17]. The ligands for these receptors are highly conserved molecules such as lipopolysaccharides (LPS) (recognized by TLR4), lipopeptides (TLR2 in combination with TLR1 or TLR6), flagellin (TLR5), single stranded RNA (TLR7 and TLR8), double-stranded RNA (TLR3), CpG motif-containing DNA (recognized by TLR9), and profilin present on uropathogenic bacteria (TLR11) [17]. TLR1, -2, -4, -5, and -6 recognize extracellular stimuli, while TLR3, -7, -8, and -9 function within the endolysosomal compartment.

The need for the development of safe and effective vaccine adjuvants has provided an impetus for the systematic exploration of a variety of innate immune stimuli, including small-molecule agonists of TLR2 [22–24], TLR7 [25–33], TLR8 [33–38], nucleotide oligomerization domain 1 (NOD1) [39], as well as C-C chemokine receptor type 1 (CCR1) [40]. Structure-activity relationship studies have proven useful in providing tools with which to examine how these different classes of innate immune signaling molecules affect and modulate pathways linking the innate and adaptive immune systems.

TLR8 is expressed predominantly in myeloid dendritic cells, monocytes, and monocyte-derived dendritic cells [41, 42]. Engagement by TLR8 agonists evokes a dominant proinflammatory cytokine profile, including tumor necrosis factor-α (TNF-α), interleukin (IL)-12, and IL-18, and appears uniquely potent in enhancing the production of Th1-polarizing cytokines TNF-α and IL-12 in antigen-presenting cells [41, 43–45]. Our interest in small-molecule agonists of TLR8 has led to the exploration of the 4-amino-furo[2,3-*c*]quinolines [36], 3-alkyl-quinoline-2-amines [37], 5-(5-aminoalkyl)-3-pentylquinolin-2-amines [46], and 1-alkyl-2-aminobenzimidazoles [38], all of which are pure TLR8 agonists with no detectable activity at TLR7 (*see* Table 1 and Fig. 1). The synthetic procedures for best-in-class analogues encompassing these four chemotypes are described.

Table 1
EC_{50} values of compounds in human TLR 8-specific reporter gene assays

Structure number	Structure	TLR8 agonistic activity (μM)
5	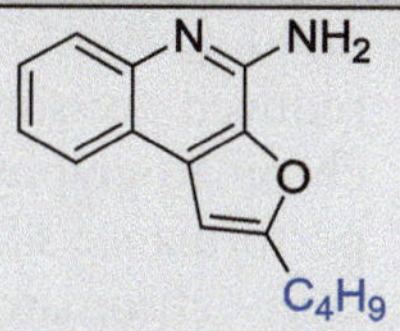	1.60
9	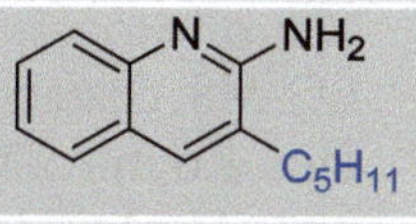	0.20
13	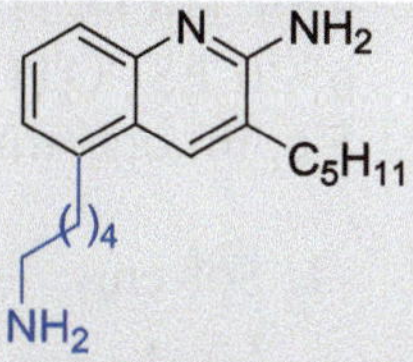	0.009
17	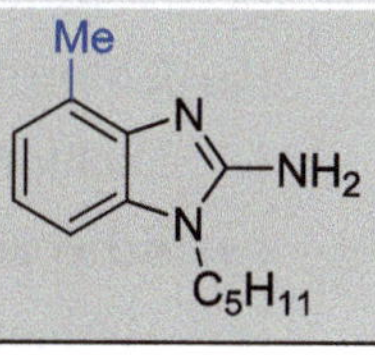	1.13

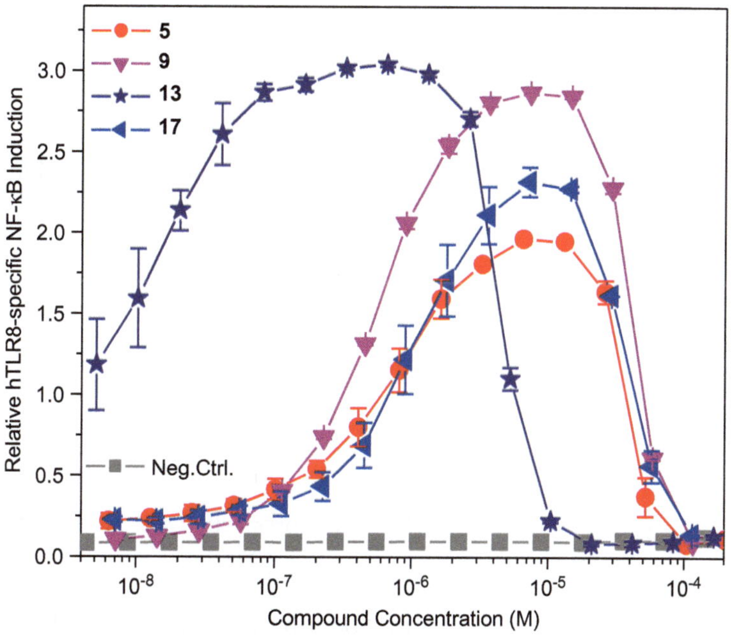

Fig. 1 Agonistic activities of analogues **5**, **9**, **13**, and **17** in human TLR8 reporter gene assays. Means ± SD on quadruplicates are shown

2 Materials

All of the solvents and reagents used were obtained commercially and used as such unless noted otherwise. Moisture- or air-sensitive reactions were conducted under nitrogen atmosphere in oven-dried (120 °C) glass apparatus. Solvents were removed under reduced pressure using standard rotary evaporators. Flash column chromatography was carried out using RediSep Rf "Gold" high-performance silica columns on CombiFlash Rf instruments. Thin-layer chromatography was carried out on silica gel CCM (Chromatographie sur couche mince) pre-coated aluminum sheets. LC-MS characterization was performed using a Zorbax Eclipse Plus 4.6 mm × 150 mm, 5 μm analytical reverse-phase C_{18} column with H_2O-CH_3CN and H_2O-MeOH gradients and an Agilent 6520 ESI-QTOF Accurate Mass spectrometer (mass accuracy of 5 ppm) operating in the positive ion acquisition mode.

2.1 Synthesis of 2-Butylfuro[2,3-c]quinolin-4-amine (Compound 5)

1. Solvents:
   (a) Acetonitrile.
   (b) Chloroform ($CHCl_3$).
   (c) Dichloromethane (CH_2Cl_2).
   (d) Ethyl acetate (EtOAc).
   (e) Methanol (MeOH).
2. Reagents:
   (a) 3-Hydroxyquinoline.
   (b) Sodium hydroxide (NaOH).
   (c) Iodine.
   (d) 20% Aqueous potassium iodide.
   (e) Glacial acetic acid.
   (f) Triethylamine.
   (g) 1-Hexyne.
   (h) *Tetrakis*(triphenylphosphine)palladium(0) ($Pd(PPh_3)_4$).
   (i) Copper(I) iodide (CuI)
   (j) Sodium sulfate (Na_2SO_4).
   (k) *m*-Chloroperbenzoic acid (*m*-CPBA).
   (l) Benzoyl isocyanate.
   (m) Sodium methoxide (NaOMe).

2.2 Synthesis of 3-Pentylquinolin-2-amine (Compound 9)

1. Solvents:
   (a) Chloroform ($CHCl_3$).
   (b) Dichloromethane (CH_2Cl_2).
   (c) Ethyl acetate (EtOAc).
   (d) Methanol (MeOH).
   (e) 1,4-Dioxane.
2. Reagents:
   (a) 3-Bromoquinoline.
   (b) *m*-Chloroperbenzoic acid (*m*-CPBA).
   (c) Sodium sulfate (Na_2SO_4).
   (d) n-Pentylboronic acid.
   (e) Tetrakis(triphenylphosphine)palladium(0) ($Pd(PPh_3)_4$).
   (f) Potassium carbonate (K_2CO_3).

2.3 Synthesis of 5-(5-Aminopentyl)-3-pentylquinolin-2-amine (Compound 13)

1. Solvents:
   (a) Dimethyl sulfoxide (DMSO).
   (b) Ethyl acetate (EtOAc).
   (c) Hexanes.
   (d) Tetrahydrofuran (THF).
2. Reagents:
   (a) 2-Amino-6-bromobenzaldehyde.
   (b) Heptanenitrile.
   (c) Potassium tert-butoxide (*t*-BuOK).
   (d) Sodium sulfate (Na_2SO_4).
   (e) 4-Cyanobutylzinc bromide solution (0.5 M in THF).
   (f) Tetrakis(triphenylphosphine)palladium(0) ($Pd(PPh_3)_4$).
   (g) Lithium aluminum hydride ($LiAlH_4$, 1.0 M solution in THF).
   (h) Sodium hydroxide (NaOH).

2.4 Synthesis of 3-Methyl-2-nitro-*N*-pentylaniline (Compound 15)

1. Solvents:
   (a) Dimethyl sulfoxide (DMSO).
   (b) Ethyl acetate (EtOAc).
   (c) Hexanes.
   (d) Methanol (MeOH).
   (e) Water.
2. Reagents:
   (a) 1-Fluoro-3-methyl-2-nitrobenzene.
   (b) Amyl amine.

(c) Diisopropylethylamine (DIPEA).
(d) Sodium sulfate (Na_2SO_4).
(e) 5% Platinum on carbon (Pt/C).
(f) Hydrogen (H_2).
(g) Cyanogen bromide (CNBr).
(h) Sodium hydroxide (NaOH).

3 Methods

3.1 Synthesis of 2-Butylfuro[2,3-c]quinolin-4-amine (Compound 5)

Compound **5** can be synthesized from commercially available 3-hydroxyquinoline in four steps via a tandem, one-pot Sonogashira coupling and intramolecular 5-*endo-dig* cyclization strategy as depicted in Fig. 2 [36]. The furo[2,3-*c*]quinolone **5** is a pure TLR8 agonist, and structure-activity relationship studies served to identify that the C2-butyl group is optimal. The EC_{50} value of **5** is 1.6 μM in human TLR8 reporter gene assays, and this compound displays prominent proinflammatory cytokine induction (including interleukin-12 and interleukin-18) in human PBMCs (but is bereft of interferon-α inducing properties), confirming its high selectivity for human TLR8.

3.1.1 Synthesis of 4-Iodoquinolin-3-ol (Compound 2)

1. Dissolve 1.0 g (6.89 mmol) of 3-hydroxyquinoline in 20 mL of 2 N NaOH in an oven-dried round-bottomed flask with a stirring bar.
2. To this mixture, add dropwise a solution of iodine (8.27 mmol) in 20% aqueous potassium iodide (20 mL), and stir for 3 h at room temperature.
3. Slowly add sufficient quantity of glacial acetic acid to neutralize the NaOH and acidify the mixture. A precipitate forms.
4. Filter the precipitate. Wash the precipitate with water, and then dry the precipitate thoroughly in vacuum. Approximately 1.50 g (80% yield) of **2** (crude) is expected, which can be used for the next step without purification.
5. Characterization of **2**: ^1H NMR (500 MHz, DMSO) δ 11.19 (s, 1H), 8.50 (s, 1H), 7.98–7.85 (m, 2H), 7.65–7.60 (m, 1H), 7.60–7.55 (m, 1H). ^{13}C NMR (126 MHz, DMSO) δ 152.2, 142.6, 141.3, 130.9, 129.9, 129.2, 128.5, 126.6, 94.5. MS (ESI) calculated for C_9H_6INO (*m/z*), 270.95; observed mass: 271.96 $[M+H]^+$

3.1.2 Synthesis of 2-Butylfuro[2,3-c]quinolone (Compound 3)

1. Dissolve 203 mg (0.75 mmol) of compound **2** in acetonitrile/triethylamine (2:1)
2. Sequentially add 129 μL (1.125 mmol) of 1-hexyne, 42 mg (0.036 mmol) of $Pd(PPh_3)_4$ (*see* **Note 1**) and 6.8 mg (0.036 mmol) of CuI.

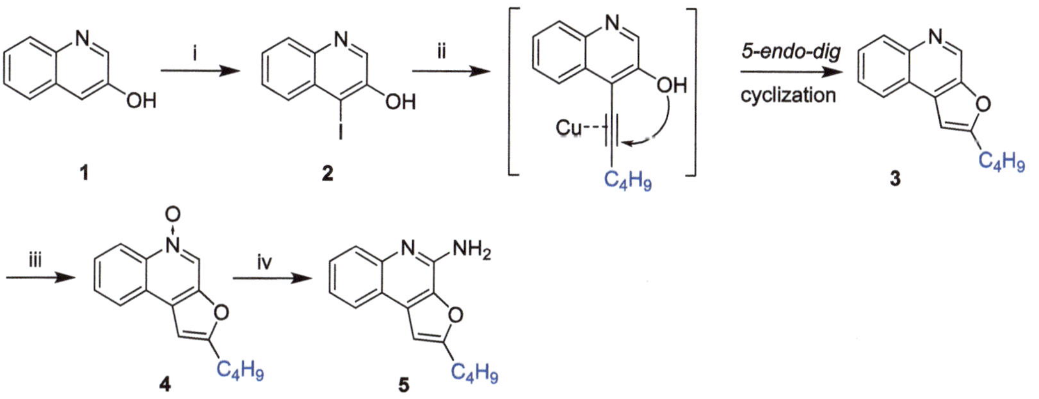

Reagents: (i) I_2, KI, NaOH; (ii) $Pd(PPh_3)_4$, CuI,1-hexyne, $Et_3N:CH_3CN$ (1:2); (iii) *m*-CPBA, $CHCl_3$; (iv) (a) benzoyl isocyanate, CH_2Cl_2, (b) $NaOCH_3$, MeOH.

Fig. 2 Synthesis of **5** (2-butylfuro[2,3-*c*]quinolin-4-amine)

3. Stir the resulting reaction mixture at 70 °C under a nitrogen atmosphere for 12 h.
4. Dilute the reaction mixture with water and extract with ethyl acetate (3 × 10 mL) in a separating funnel.
5. Pool the organic layer, and dry the solution by adding solid Na_2SO_4; evaporate the solvent using a rotary evaporator and purify the crude material using flash chromatography using a gradient of CH_2Cl_2 and MeOH (0–15 %).
6. Compound **3** is obtained as a yellow solid (140 mg, 83 % yield).

Characterization of **3**: ^1H NMR (500 MHz, $CDCl_3$) δ 9.08 (d, *J* = 0.5 Hz, 1H), 8.19 (dd, *J* = 8.4, 0.5 Hz, 1H), 8.09 – 8.05 (m, 1H), 7.66 (ddd, *J* = 8.4, 6.9, 1.5 Hz, 1H), 7.60 (ddd, *J* = 8.1, 7.0, 1.2 Hz, 1H), 6.90 (d, *J* = 0.8 Hz, 1H), 2.92 (t, 2H), 1.82 (ddd, *J* = 15.2, 8.5, 6.7 Hz, 2H), 1.51 – 1.42 (m, 2H), 0.99 (t, *J* = 7.4 Hz, 3H). ^{13}C NMR (126 MHz, $CDCl_3$) δ 163.2, 148.8, 144.3, 136.4, 131.4, 130.1, 127.3, 126.5, 123.7, 123.2, 101.0, 29.9, 28.5, 22.4, 13.9. MS (ESI) calculated for $C_{15}H_{15}NO$ (*m/z*), 225.11; observed mass: 226.13 $[M+H]^+$

3.1.3 Synthesis of 2-Butylfuro[2,3-c]quinoline 5-oxide (Compound 4)

1. Dissolve 119.3 mg (0.53 mmol) compound **3** in $CHCl_3$, and add 182.8 mg (1.06 mmol) of *m*-CPBA. Stir the reaction mixture at room temperature for 4 h.
2. After completion of the reaction, extract the reaction mixture with water (10 mL) and CH_2Cl_2 (3 × 10 mL).
3. Dry the pooled organic fractions over Na_2SO_4, remove solvent in a rotary evaporator, and purify the crude material by flash chromatography using a gradient of CH_2Cl_2 and MeOH (0–15 %). Compound **4** is obtained as a white solid (89 mg, 70 % yield).

4. Characterization of **4**: ^{1}H NMR (500 MHz, $CDCl_3$) δ 8.86 (d, J=0.5 Hz, 1H), 8.85–8.83 (m, 1H), 8.08–8.04 (m, 1H), 7.75–7.68 (m, 2H), 6.86 (d, J=0.9 Hz, 1H), 2.90–2.86 (m, 2H), 1.82–1.76 (m, 2H), 1.46 (dq, J=14.7, 7.4 Hz, 2H), 0.98 (t, J=7.4 Hz, 3H). ^{13}C NMR (126 MHz, CDC13) δ 164.0, 147.1, 138.7, 128.9, 128.5, 124.5, 124.2, 124.2, 122.8, 121.0, 101.3, 29.8, 28.5, 22.4, 13.9. MS (ESI) calculated for $C_{15}H_{15}NO_2$ (m/z), 241.11; observed mass: 242.12 $[M+H]^+$.

3.1.4 Synthesis of 2-Butylfuro[2,3-c]quinolin-4-amine (Compound 5)

1. To a solution of compound **4** (48 mg, 0.2 mmol) in CH_2Cl_2, slowly add benzoyl isocyanate (88 mg, 0.6 mmol) and stir the reaction mixture at 55 °C for 2 h.
2. Evaporate the solvent in a rotary evaporator and re-dissolve the residue in 4 mL of MeOH in a round-bottomed flask. Add 54 mg (1.0 mmol) of NaOMe, and reflux at 80 °C for 4 h.
3. Remove the solvent and purify the crude material by flash chromatography using 10% MeOH/CH_2Cl_2 as the eluent. Compound **5** is obtained as a white solid (39 mg, 81% yield).
4. Characterization of compound **5**: ^{1}H NMR (500 MHz, $CDCl_3$) δ 7.87 (ddd, J=8.0, 1.4, 0.4 Hz, 1H), 7.80– 7.76 (m, 1H), 7.52 (ddd, J=8.4, 7.0, 1.5 Hz, 1H), 7.34 (ddd, J=8.1, 7.0, 1.2 Hz, 1H), 6.80 (t, J=0.8 Hz, 1H), 5.11 (s, 2H), 2.90–2.83 (m, 2H), 1.79 (ddd, J=13.3, 8.5, 6.7 Hz, 2H), 1.51–1.40 (m, 2H), 0.98 (t, J=7.4 Hz, 3H). ^{13}C NMR (126 MHz, $CDCl_3$) δ 161.9, 144.8, 144.1, 138.6, 131.3, 127.6, 126.5, 123.4, 122.8, 120.4, 101.7, 30.0, 28.4, 22.4, 13.9. HRMS (ESI) calculated for $C_{15}H_{16}N_2O$ (m/z), 240.1263; observed mass: 241.1349 $[M+H]^+$.

3.2 Synthesis of 3-Pentylquinolin-2-amine (Compound 9)

A disconnection strategy on compound **5** lead to the evaluation of 3-substituted 2-aminoquinolines, of which compound **9** was found to be a potent human TLR8-specific agonist (EC_{50}: 200 nM in human TLR8-specific reporter gene assays) [37]. Compound **9** can be efficiently synthesized in three steps from commercially available 3-bromoquinoline as shown in Fig. 3.

3.2.1 Synthesis of 3-Bromoquinoline 1-oxide (Compound 7)

1. Dissolve 400 mg of 3-bromoquinoline (1.92 mmol) in $CHCl_3$, add 994 mg of m-CPBA (5.76 mmol), and stir for 4 h at room temperature.
2. Extract the reaction mixture with water (10 mL) and CH_2Cl_2 (3×10 mL); combine the organic fractions and dry over Na_2SO_4.
3. Remove solvent and purify the crude material by flash chromatography using a gradient of CH_2Cl_2 and MeOH (0–15%) to obtain compound **7** as white solid (360 mg, 84% yield).

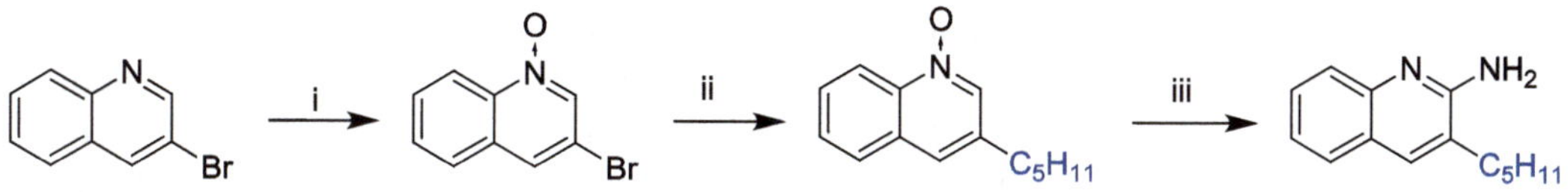

6 7 8 9

Reagents: (i) *m*-CPBA, CHCl3; (ii) $Pd(PPh_3)_4$, C_5H_{11}-$B(OH)_2$, K_2CO_3, 1,4-dioxane; (iii) (a) benzoyl isocyanate, CH_2Cl_2; (b) NaOMe, MeOH.

Fig. 3 Synthesis of **9** (3-pentylquinolin-2-amine)

4. Characterization of compound 7: ^{1}H NMR (500 MHz, $CDCl_3$) δ 8.66 (d, *J*=8.8 Hz, 1H), 8.62 (d, *J*=1.6 Hz, 1H), 7.89 (s, 1H), 7.81–7.73 (m, 2H), 7.66 (ddd, *J*=8.1, 7.0, 1.1 Hz, 1H). ^{13}C NMR (126 MHz, $CDCl_3$) δ 140.7, 137.3, 130.7, 130.4, 130.0, 127.8, 127.5, 120.0, 114.5. MS (ESI) *m/z* $[M+H]^+$ calculated for C_9H_6BrNO: 223.9706; observed mass: 223.9662.

3.2.2 Synthesis of 3-Pentylquinoline 1-oxide (Compound 8)

1. Dissolve 100 mg of compound 7 (0.446 mmol) in 1,4-dioxane in a round-bottomed flask.
2. Sequentially add n-pentylboronic acid (103 mg, 0.892 mmol), $Pd(PPh_3)_4$ (26 mg, 0.0223 mmol) (*see* **Note 1**), and K_2CO_3 (184 mg, 1.33 mmol).
3. Stir the mixture at 90 °C under an atmosphere of dry nitrogen for 12 h.
4. Dilute the reaction mixture with water and extract with ethyl acetate (3×10 mL); dry the combined organic layer fractions over Na_2SO_4 and remove solvent using a rotary evaporator.
5. Purify the crude material by flash chromatography using 10% MeOH/CH_2Cl_2 as an eluent to obtain compound **8** as a white solid (80 mg, 84% yield).
6. Characterization of compound **8**: ^{1}H NMR (500 MHz, $CDCl_3$) δ 8.69 (d, *J*=8.7 Hz, 1H), 8.45 (d, *J*=1.2 Hz, 1H), 7.82–7.77 (m, 1H), 7.69 (ddd, *J*=8.5, 6.9, 1.3 Hz, 1H), 7.64–7.58 (m, 1H), 7.53 (s, 1H), 2.70 (t, 2H), 1.75–1.66 (m, 2H), 1.38–1.30 (m, 4H), 0.89 (t, *J*=7.0 Hz, 3H). ^{13}C NMR (126 MHz, $CDCl_3$) δ 140.0, 137.0, 136.4, 130.4, 129.6, 128.9, 127.8, 125.2, 119.8, 33.3, 31.9, 30.4, 22.6, 14.1. MS (ESI) *m/z* [M+H]+calculated for $C_{14}H_{17}NO$: 216.1383; observed mass: 216.1380.

3.2.3 Synthesis of 3-Pentylquinolin-2-amine (Compound 9)

1. To a stirred solution of compound **8** (53 mg, 0.248 mmol) in CH_2Cl_2, add benzoylisocyanate (109 mg, 0.741 mmol), and stir the mixture at 55 °C for 1 h.
2. Evaporate the solvent, and re-dissolve the residue in 5 mL of MeOH (5 mL); add 67 mg of NaOMe (1.24 mmol), and reflux at 80 °C for 2 h.

3. Evaporate the solvent and purify the crude material by flash chromatography using 10% $MeOH/CH_2Cl_2$ as an eluent to obtain compound **9** as a white solid (44 mg, 83% yield). Characterization of compound **9**: ^{1}H NMR (500 MHz, $CDCl_3$) δ 7.68 (s, 1H), 7.65 (d, *J*=8.4 Hz, 1H), 7.60 (d, *J*=8.0 Hz, 1H), 7.51 (ddd, *J*=8.4, 7.0, 1.4 Hz, 1H), 7.26–7.22 (m, 1H), 4.83 (s, 2H), 2.58 (t, 2H), 1.78–1.68 (m, 2H), 1.46–1.34 (m, 4H), 0.93 (t, *J*=7.0 Hz, 3H). ^{13}C NMR (126 MHz, CDCl3) δ 156.3, 146.6, 135.5, 128.9, 127.1, 125.7, 124.7, 123.8, 122.7, 31.8, 31.3, 27.7, 22.7, 14.2. MS (ESI) *m/z* $[M+H]^+$ calculated for $C_{14}H_{18}N_2$: 215.1543; observed mass: 215.1407.

3.3 Synthesis of 5-(5-Aminopentyl)-3-pentylquinolin-2-amine (Compound 13)

Crystal structures of the ectodomain of human TLR8 (hTLR8) cocrystallized with two regioisomers of N^1-aminomethylbenzyl-substituted imidazoquinolines showed subtle differences in their interactions in the binding site of hTLR8, which led to a focused and hypothesis-driven exploration of introducing alkylamino groups at all possible positions on the quinoline core. These studies led to the identification of a novel TLR8-specific agonist (compound **13**), with an EC_{50} of 9 nM [46]. This compound can be conveniently synthesized from commercially available 2-amino-6-bromobenzaldehyde (compound **10**) in three steps as shown in Fig. 4.

3.3.1 Synthesis of 5-Bromo-3-pentylquinolin-2-amine (Compound 11)

1. Dissolve 200 mg (1 mmol) of 2-amino-6-bromobenzaldehyde (compound **10**) in 3 mL of DMSO in a round-bottomed flask; add sequentially heptanenitrile (275 μL, 2 mmol) and *t*-BuOK (224 mg, 2 mmol), and stir the reaction mixture for 3 h at 60 °C under nitrogen atmosphere.
2. Dilute the reaction mixture with water and extract with EtOAc (3×50 mL); dry the combined organic layer fractions over Na_2SO_4 and evaporate the solvent in a rotary evaporator.
3. Purify the crude material by flash chromatography using a gradient of hexanes and EtOAc (0–50%) to obtain compound **11** as an off-white solid (220 mg, 75% yield).
4. Characterization of compound **11**: ^{1}H NMR (500 MHz, DMSO-d_6) δ 7.82 (s, 1H), 7.49–7.40 (m, 2H), 7.34 (dd, *J*=7.6, 8.3 Hz, 1H), 6.58 (s, 2H), 2.62 (t, *J*=7.8 Hz, 2H), 1.66–1.57 (m, 2H), 1.44–1.29 (m, 4H), 0.89 (t, *J*=7.0 Hz, 3H). ^{13}C NMR (126 MHz, DMSO-d_6) δ 157.75, 147.59, 132.61, 128.85, 126.08, 124.89, 124.73, 121.98, 120.40, 30.96, 30.29, 27.42, 22.06, 14.01. MS (ESI-TOF) for $C_{14}H_{17}BrN_2$ $[M+H]^+$ calculated 293.0648; observed mass: 293.0684.

3.3.2 Synthesis of 5-(2-Amino-3-pentyl quinolin-5-yl)pentanenitrile (Compound 12)

1. To a solution of compound **11** (58.8 mg, 0.2 mmol) in 2 mL of tetrahydrofuran (THF), slowly add 0.8 mL (0.4 mmol) of 4-cyanobutylzinc bromide solution (0.5 M in THF) with a syringe fitted with a stainless steel needle. Observe safety

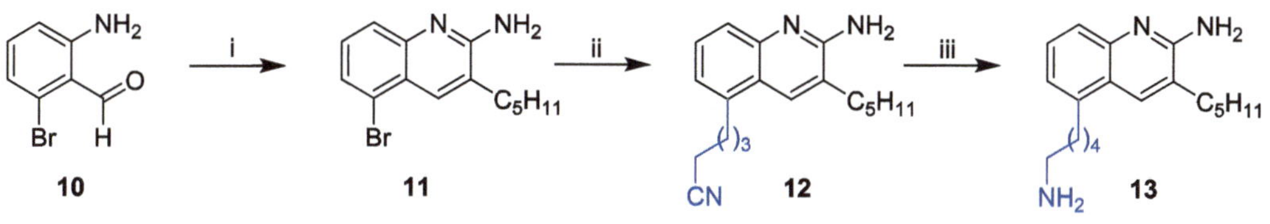

Reagents: (i) heptanenitrile, *t*-BuOK, DMSO; (ii) 4-cyanobutylzinc bromide, $Pd(PPh_3)_4$, THF; (iii) $LiAlH_4$, THF, 4 h.

Fig. 4 Synthesis of **13** (5-(5-aminopentyl)-3-pentylquinolin-2-amine)

precautions, and note health hazard codes associated with the reagent (GHS07, GHS08).

2. Next, add 11.6 mg (0.01 mmol) of $Pd(PPh_3)_4$ to the reaction mixture and stir at 65 °C under nitrogen atmosphere for 12 h (*see* **Note 1**).
3. Dilute the reaction mixture gradually with water and extract with EtOAc (3 × 10 mL).
4. Dry the combined organic fractions over Na_2SO_4 and remove solvent in a rotary evaporator.
5. Purify the crude material by flash chromatography (60% EtOAc/hexanes) to obtain compound **12** as an off-white solid (45 mg, 76% yield).
6. Characterization of compound **12**: ^{1}H NMR (500 MHz, $CDCl_3$) δ 7.84 (s, 1H), 7.54 (d, *J* = 8.4 Hz, 1H), 7.43 (dd, *J* = 7.1, 8.4 Hz, 1H), 7.07 (dd, *J* = 1.1, 7.1 Hz, 1H), 4.80 (s, 2H), 3.02 (t, *J* = 7.5 Hz, 2H), 2.62 (t, *J* = 7.6 Hz, 2H), 2.37 (t, *J* = 7.1 Hz, 2H), 1.93–1.83 (m, 2H), 1.80–1.69 (m, 4H), 1.47–1.36 (m, 4H), 0.93 (t, *J* = 7.1 Hz, 3H). ^{13}C NMR (126 MHz, $CDCl_3$) δ 155.86, 147.12, 136.99, 131.59, 128.56, 124.66, 123.49, 123.01, 122.83, 119.68, 31.82, 31.77, 31.69, 29.93, 27.97, 25.25, 22.67, 17.27, 14.22. MS (ESI-TOF) for $C_{19}H_{25}N_3$ $[M+H]^+$ calculated 296.2121; observed mass: 296.2068.

3.3.3 Synthesis of 5-(5-Aminopentyl)-3-pentylquinolin-2-amine (Compound 13)

1. Take 3 mL of THF in a round-bottomed flask, and cool it to 0 °C in a ice-bath.
2. To the flask containing THF, gently add 0.5 mL of a 1.0 M solution of $LiAlH_4$ in THF; maintain 0 °C temperature.
3. Prepare a solution of compound **12** (29.5 mg, 0.1 mmol) in 5 mL of THF, and add it dropwise to the flask containing the solution of $LiAlH_4$ in THF. Observe all precautions, as this reaction is exothermic.
4. Stir the reaction mixture for 2 h at 25 °C, and then for an additional 2 h at 75 °C.

5. Quench the reaction mixture carefully quenched with ice-cold water (1 mL) at 0 °C, and then add 1 mL of 10% NaOH; stir for 10 min at room temperature.
6. Filter the mixture through celite and wash the celite with at least 15 mL of CH_2Cl_2 to elute all bound organic material.
7. Dry the filtrate over Na_2SO_4 and remove solvent.
8. Purify the crude material by flash chromatography (using a gradient of CH_2Cl_2 and MeOH (0–15%)); the presence of a primary aliphatic amine necessitates the use of a neutral-alumina column. Compound **13** is obtained as a white solid (21 mg, 70%).
9. Characterization of compound **13**: ^{1}H NMR (500 MHz, MeOD) δ 7.94 (s, 1H), 7.42 – 7.32 (m, 2H), 7.06 (dd, J=2.9, 5.4 Hz, 1H), 2.98 (t, J=7.6 Hz, 2H), 2.67 (t, J=7.6 Hz, 2H), 2.62 (t, J=7.0 Hz, 2H), 1.78 – 1.65 (m, 4H), 1.57 – 1.47 (m, 2H), 1.49 – 1.39 (m, 6H), 0.95 (t, J=7.0 Hz, 3H). ^{13}C NMR (126 MHz, MeOD) δ 157.96, 147.46, 139.91, 133.37, 129.57, 125.12, 123.73, 123.58, 123.39, 42.53, 33.77, 33.35, 32.69, 32.39, 32.04, 29.03, 27.94, 23.68, 14.47. MS (ESI-TOF) for $C_{19}H_{29}N_3$ $[M+H]^+$ calculated 300.2434, observed mass: 300.2374.

3.4 Synthesis of 4-Methyl-1-pentyl-1H-benzo[d]imidazol-2-amine (Compound 17*)*

Detailed structure–activity relationship exploration in the 3-substituted 2-aminoquinolines class (typified by compound **9**) also resulted in the ring-contracted 1-alkyl-1*H*-benzimidazol-2-amines. The best-in-class compound of this novel chemotype, 4-methyl-1-pentyl-1*H*-benzo[d]imidazol-2-amine (compound **17**), was found to retain a pure TLR8 agonistic activity profile with an EC_{50} of 1.13 μM [38], and is obtained in three steps from commercially available starting material as shown in Fig. 5.

3.4.1 Synthesis of 3-Methyl-2-nitro-N-pentylaniline (Compound 15)

1. Dissolve 155 mg (1 mmol) of 1-fluoro-3-methyl-2-nitrobenzene in 2 mL DMSO.
2. Add 116 μL (1 mmol) amyl amine and 174 μL (1 mmol) diisopropylethylamine (DIPEA), and stir for 6 h at 60 °C.
3. After the completion of the reaction (monitored by TLC), dilute the reaction mixture with water and extract with EtOAc (3×20 mL).
4. Dry the combined organic layer fractions over Na_2SO_4 and remove solvent.
5. Purify the crude material by flash chromatography (10% EtOAc/hexanes) to obtain compound **15** as a red oil (200 mg, 90% yield).
6. Characterization of compound **15**: R_f=0.70 (10% EtOAc/hexanes). ^{1}H NMR (500 MHz, $CDCl_3$) δ 7.25 – 7.14 (m,

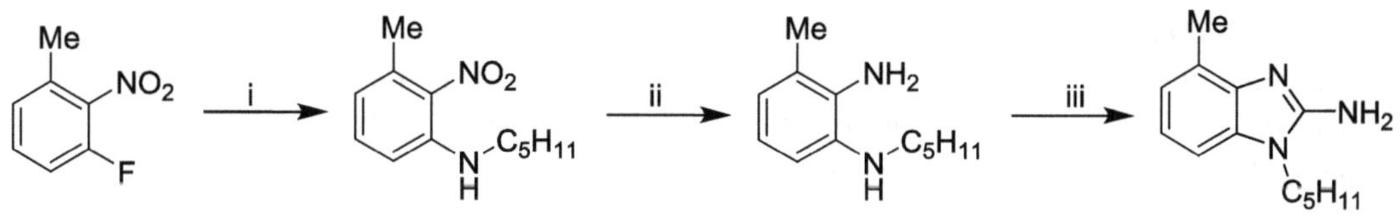

14 **15** **16** **17**

Reagents: (i) $C_5H_{11}NH_2$, DIPEA, DMSO; (ii) H_2, Pt/C, EtOAc; (iii) CNBr, MeOH:H_2O (1:1).

Fig. 5 Synthesis of **17** (4-methyl-1-pentyl-1H-benzo[*d*]imidazol-2-amine)

1H), 6.65 (d, *J*=8.5 Hz, 1H), 6.60 (bs, 1H), 6.50 (d, *J*=7.4 Hz, 1H), 3.19 (td, *J*=7.1, 5.1 Hz, 2H), 2.47 (s, 3H), 1.73–1.60 (m, 2H), 1.46–1.31 (m, 4H), 0.92 (t, *J*=7.1 Hz, 3H). ^{13}C NMR (126 MHz, $CDCl_3$) δ 144.34, 135.92, 135.59, 133.41, 119.09, 111.31, 43.55, 29.36, 28.86, 22.55, 21.71, 14.13. MS (ESI-TOF) for $C_{12}H_{18}N_2O_2$ $[M+H]^+$ calculated 223.1441; observed mass: 223.1400.

3.4.2 Synthesis of 4-Methyl-1-pentyl-1H-benzo[d]imidazol-2-amine (Compound 17)

1. To a solution of compound **15** (44.4 mg, 0.2 mmol) in anhydrous EtOAc (10 mL), add a catalytic amount of 5% Pt on carbon (16 mg, 2 mol%).
2. The reaction mixture is subjected to hydrogenation at 30 psi H_2 pressure for 3 h in a Parr apparatus (*see* **Note 2**).
3. Filtered the reaction mixture, and remove solvent to obtain crude **16** (*see* **Note 3**).
4. To a solution of compound **16** in a 1:1 mixture of MeOH (1 mL) and water (1 mL), add CNBr (64 mg, 0.6 mmol), and stir for 3 h at 60 °C.
5. Cool the reaction mixture to room temperature, and remove solvent in a rotary evaporator.
6. Add sufficient quantity of 1.0 M aq. NaOH to obtain a pH of ~8.0, and then extract with EtOAc (3×10 mL).
7. Dry the combined organic layer fractions over Na_2SO_4, and remove solvent.
8. Purify the crude material by flash chromatography (10% MeOH/CH_2Cl_2) to obtain compound **17** as a white solid (33 mg, 76% yield).
9. Characterization of compound **17**: R_f=0.50 (10% MeOH/CH_2Cl_2). ^{1}H NMR (500 MHz, DMSO) δ 6.93 (dd, *J*=7.3, 1.2 Hz, 1H), 6.82–6.61 (m, 2H), 6.34 (s, 2H), 3.92 (t, *J*=7.2 Hz, 2H), 2.34 (s, 3H), 1.70–1.46 (m, 2H), 1.40–1.10 (m, 4H), 0.83 (t, *J*=7.1 Hz, 3H). ^{13}C NMR (126 MHz, DMSO) δ 154.21, 141.56, 133.59, 123.77, 120.83, 117.83, 105.20, 41.44, 28.30, 28.21, 21.95, 16.41, 13.95. MS (ESI-TOF) for $C_{13}H_{19}N_3$ $[M+H]^+$ calculated 218.1652; observed mass: 218.1657.

3.5 Human TLR8-Specific Reporter Gene Assays (NF-kB Induction), and TLR-2/-3/-4/-5/-7/-9- and NOD-1/NOD-2 Counter-Screens

1. The induction of NF-kB is quantified using human TLR-2/3/-4/-5/-7/-8/-9 and NOD-1/NOD-2-specific, rapid-throughput, liquid handler-assisted reporter gene assays as previously described [26, 39, 40].
2. HEK293 cells stably co-transfected with the appropriate hTLR (or NOD) and secreted alkaline phosphatase (sAP) are maintained in HEK-Blue™ Selection medium.
3. Stable expression of secreted alkaline phosphatase (sAP) under control of NF-kB/AP-1 promoters is inducible by appropriate TLR/NOD agonists, and extracellular sAP in the supernatant is proportional to NF-kB induction.
4. Reporter cells are incubated at a density of ~10^5 cells/mL in a volume of 80 μL/well, in 384-well, flat-bottomed, cell culture-treated microtiter plates in the presence of graded concentrations of stimuli.
5. sAP is assayed spectrophotometrically using an alkaline phosphatase-specific chromogen (present in HEK-detection medium as supplied by InvivoGen) at 620 nm (*see* Fig. 1).

4 Notes

1. All reaction using palladium catalysts should ensure that solvents are first purged with nitrogen, and the reactions should be carried out in a nitrogen atmosphere (using a N_2-filled balloon, for instance).
2. Observe all safety precautions when using a Parr apparatus, according to the manufacturer's directions.
3. Note that platinum-on-carbon is potentially flammable and must be disposed of safely.

Acknowledgments

This work was supported by NIH/NIAID contracts HSN272200900033C and HHSN272201400056C.

References

1. Glenny AT, Pope CG, Waddington H, Wallace V (1926) The antigenic value of toxoid precipitated by potassium-alum. J Pathol Bacteriol 29:38–45
2. Gupta RK, Siber GR (1995) Adjuvants for human vaccines—current status, problems and future prospects. Vaccine 13:1263–1276
3. Gupta RK (1998) Aluminum compounds as vaccine adjuvants. Adv Drug Deliv Rev 32:155–172
4. Sheridan SL, Frith K, Snelling TL, Grimwood K, McIntyre PB, Lambert SB (2014) Waning vaccine immunity in teenagers primed with whole cell and acellular pertussis vaccine: recent epidemiology. Expert Rev Vaccines 13:1081–1106

5. Lavine JS, Bjornstad ON, de Blasio BF, Storsaeter J (2012) Short-lived immunity against pertussis, age-specific routes of transmission, and the utility of a teenage booster vaccine. Vaccine 30:544–551
6. Suryadevara M, Domachowske JB (2015) Prevention of pertussis through adult vaccination. Hum Vaccin Immunother 11:1744–1747
7. Clark TA (2014) Changing pertussis epidemiology: everything old is new again. J Infect Dis 209:978–981
8. Cherry JD (2012) Epidemic pertussis in 2012—the resurgence of a vaccine-preventable disease. New Engl J Med 367:785–787
9. Zepp F, Heininger U, Mertsola J, Bernatowska E, Guiso N, Roord J, Tozzi AE, Van Damme P (2011) Rationale for pertussis booster vaccination throughout life in Europe. Lancet Infect Dis 11:557–570
10. Hara M, Fukuoka M, Tashiro K, Ozaki I, Ohfuji S, Okada K, Nakano T, Fukushima W, Hirota Y (2015) Pertussis outbreak in university students and evaluation of acellular pertussis vaccine effectiveness in Japan. BMC Infect Dis 15:45
11. Dresser DW (1962) Specific inhibition of antibody production. II. Paralysis induced in adult mice by small quantities of protein antigen. Immunology 5:378–388
12. Dresser DW (1968) An assay for adjuvanticity. Clin Exp Immunol 3:877–888
13. Johnson AJ, Gaines S, Landy M (1956) Studies on the O antigen of Salmonella typhosa. V. Enhancement of the antibody response to protein antigens by the purified lipopolysaccharide. J Exp Med 103:225–233
14. Beutler B (2000) Tlr4: central component of the sole mammalian LPS sensor. Curr Opin Immunol 12:20–26
15. Beutler B, Poltorak A (2001) The sole gateway to endotoxin response: how *LPS* was identified as *TLR4*, and its role in innate immunity. Drug Metab Dispos 29:474–478
16. Hoffmann J, Akira S (2013) Innate immunity. Curr Opin Immunol 25:1–3
17. Kumagai Y, Akira S (2010) Identification and functions of pattern-recognition receptors. J Allergy Clin Immunol 125:985–992
18. Kawai T, Akira S (2010) The role of pattern-recognition receptors in innate immunity: update on Toll-like receptors. Nat Immunol 11:373–384
19. Loo YM, Gale M Jr (2011) Immune signaling by RIG-I-like receptors. Immunity 34:680–692
20. Kersse K, Bertrand MJ, Lamkanfi M, Vandenabeele P (2011) NOD-like receptors and the innate immune system: coping with danger, damage and death. Cytokine Growth Factor Rev 22:257–276
21. Clarke TB, Weiser JN (2011) Intracellular sensors of extracellular bacteria. Immunol Rev 243:9–25
22. Salunke DB, Shukla NM, Yoo E, Crall BM, Balakrishna R, Malladi SS, David SA (2012) Structure-activity relationships in human Toll-like receptor 2-specific monoacyl lipopeptides. J Med Chem 55:3353–3363
23. Salunke DB, Connelly SW, Shukla NM, Hermanson AR, Fox LM, David SA (2013) Design and development of stable, water-soluble, human Toll-like receptor 2 specific monoacyl lipopeptides as candidate vaccine adjuvants. J Med Chem 56:5885–5900
24. Wu W, Li R, Malladi SS, Warshakoon HJ, Kimbrell MR, Amolins MW, Ukani R, Datta A, David SA (2010) Structure-activity relationships in toll-like receptor-2 agonistic diacylthioglycerol lipopeptides. J Med Chem 53:3198–3213
25. Shukla NM, Kimbrell MR, Malladi SS, David SA (2009) Regioisomerism-dependent TLR7 agonism and antagonism in an imidazoquinoline. Bioorg Med Chem Lett 19:2211–2214
26. Shukla NM, Malladi SS, Mutz CA, Balakrishna R, David SA (2010) Structure-activity relationships in human toll-like receptor 7-active imidazoquinoline analogues. J Med Chem 53:4450–4465
27. Shukla NM, Mutz CA, Ukani R, Warshakoon HJ, Moore DS, David SA (2010) Syntheses of fluorescent imidazoquinoline conjugates as probes of Toll-like receptor 7. Bioorg Med Chem Lett 20:6384–6386
28. Shukla NM, Lewis TC, Day TP, Mutz CA, Ukani R, Hamilton CD, Balakrishna R, David SA (2011) Toward self-adjuvanting subunit vaccines: model peptide and protein antigens incorporating covalently bound toll-like receptor-7 agonistic imidazoquinolines. Bioorg Med Chem Lett 21:3232–3236
29. Shukla NM, Malladi SS, Day V, David SA (2011) Preliminary evaluation of a 3H imidazoquinoline library as dual TLR7/TLR8 antagonists. Bioorg Med Chem 19:3801–3811
30. Shukla NM, Mutz CA, Malladi SS, Warshakoon HJ, Balakrishna R, David SA (2012) Toll-like receptor (TLR)-7 and -8 modulatory activities of dimeric imidazoquinolines. J Med Chem 55:1106–1116
31. Shukla NM, Salunke DB, Balakrishna R, Mutz CA, Malladi SS, David SA (2012) Potent adjuvanticity of a pure TLR7-agonistic imidazoquinoline dendrimer. PLoS One 7, e43612

32. Yoo E, Crall BM, Balakrishna R, Malladi SS, Fox LM, Hermanson AR, David SA (2013) Structure-activity relationships in Toll-like receptor 7 agonistic 1*H*-imidazo[4,5-*c*]pyridines. Org Biomol Chem 11:6526–6545
33. Yoo E, Salunke DB, Sil D, Guo X, Salyer AC, Hermanson AR, Kumar M, Malladi SS, Balakrishna R, Thompson WH, Tanji H, Ohto U, Shimizu T, David SA (2014) Determinants of activity at human Toll-like receptors 7 and 8: quantitative structure-activity relationship (QSAR) of diverse heterocyclic scaffolds. J Med Chem 57:7955–7970
34. Salunke DB, Yoo E, Shukla NM, Balakrishna R, Malladi SS, Serafin KJ, Day VW, Wang X, David SA (2012) Structure-activity relationships in human Toll-like receptor 8-active 2,3-diamino-furo[2,3-*c*]pyridines. J Med Chem 55:8137–8151
35. Kokatla HP, Yoo E, Salunke DB, Sil D, Ng CF, Balakrishna R, Malladi SS, Fox LM, David SA (2013) Toll-like receptor-8 agonistic activities in C2, C4, and C8 modified thiazolo[4,5-*c*] quinolines. Org Biomol Chem 11:1179–1198
36. Kokatla HP, Sil D, Malladi SS, Balakrishna R, Hermanson AR, Fox LM, Wang X, Dixit A, David SA (2013) Exquisite selectivity for human toll-like receptor 8 in substituted furo[2,3-*c*] quinolines. J Med Chem 56:6871–6885
37. Kokatla HP, Sil D, Tanji H, Ohto U, Malladi SS, Fox LM, Shimizu T, David SA (2014) Structure-based design of novel human Toll-like receptor 8 agonists. ChemMedChem 9:719–723
38. Beesu M, Malladi SS, Fox LM, Jones CD, Dixit A, David SA (2014) Human Toll-like receptor 8-selective agonistic activities in 1-alkyl-1*H*-benzimidazol-2-amines. J Med Chem 57:7325–7341
39. Agnihotri G, Ukani R, Malladi SS, Warshakoon HJ, Balakrishna R, Wang X, David SA (2011) Structure-activity relationships in nucleotide oligomerization domain 1 (Nod1) agonistic gamma-glutamyldiaminopimelic acid derivatives. J Med Chem 54:1490–1510
40. Ukani R, Lewis TC, Day TP, Wu W, Malladi SS, Warshakoon HJ, David SA (2012) Potent adjuvantic activity of a CCR1-agonistic bis-quinoline. Bioorg Med Chem Lett 22:293–295
41. Bekeredjian-Ding I, Roth SI, Gilles S, Giese T, Ablasser A, Hornung V, Endres S, Hartmann G (2006) T cell-independent, TLR-induced IL-12p70 production in primary human monocytes. J Immunol 176:7438–7446
42. Warshakoon HJ, Hood JD, Kimbrell MR, Malladi S, Wu WY, Shukla NM, Agnihotri G, Sil D, David SA (2009) Potential adjuvantic properties of innate immune stimuli. Hum Vaccin 5:381–394
43. Bohnenkamp HR, Papazisis KT, Burchell JM, Taylor-Papadimitriou J (2007) Synergism of Toll-like receptor-induced interleukin-12p70 secretion by monocyte-derived dendritic cells is mediated through p38 MAPK and lowers the threshold of T-helper cell type 1 responses. Cell Immunol 247:72–84
44. Philbin VJ, Levy O (2007) Immunostimulatory activity of Toll-like receptor 8 agonists towards human leucocytes: basic mechanisms and translational opportunities. Biochem Soc Trans 35:1485–1491
45. Saruta M, Michelsen KS, Thomas LS, Yu QT, Landers CJ, Targan SR (2009) TLR8-mediated activation of human monocytes inhibits TL1A expression. Eur J Immunol 39:2195–2202
46. Beesu M, Caruso G, Salyer AC, Khetani KK, Sil D, Weerasinghe M, Tanji H, Ohto U, Shimizu T, David SA (2015) Structure-based design of human TLR8-specific agonists with augmented potency and adjuvanticity. J Med Chem 58:7833–7849

Chapter 4

Semisynthesis of Analogues of the Saponin Immunoadjuvant QS-21

Alberto Fernández-Tejada, William E. Walkowicz, Derek S. Tan, and David Y. Gin

Abstract

Saponins are triterpene glycoside natural products that exhibit many different biological properties, including activation and modulation of the immune system, and have therefore attracted significant interest as immunological adjuvants for use in vaccines. QS-21 is the most widely used and promising saponin adjuvant but suffers from several liabilities, such as scarcity, dose-limiting toxicity, and hydrolytic instability. Chemical synthesis has emerged as a powerful approach to obtain homogeneous, pure samples of QS-21 and to improve its properties and therapeutic profile by providing access to optimized, synthetic saponin variants. Herein, we describe a general method for the semisynthesis of these molecules from QS-21, with detailed synthetic protocols for two saponin variants developed in our recent work.

Key words Vaccine, Immunoadjuvant, QS-21, Saponin, Natural product, Semisynthesis, Carbohydrate, Glycosylation

1 Introduction

Saponins are a class of plant-derived, natural products consisting of a triterpenoid or steroidal core glycosylated with a variety of sugar units and having important biological and pharmacological properties. Saponin extracts from the bark of the South American tree *Quillaja saponaria* (QS) have long been known for their immunoadjuvant activities. A purified QS-21 fraction from this extract [1] has been widely used as an adjuvant to potentiate the immune response to classical whole-organism and modern subunit vaccines. Despite thesunique potency and promise of QS-21 in numerous vaccine clinical trials, its inherent limitations in terms of scarcity and heterogeneity, dose-limiting toxicity, and chemical instability [2] have hindered its further clinical advancement, with the notable exceptions of the recent malaria (Mosquirix) and shingles

David Y. Gin was deceased at the time of publication.

Christopher B. Fox (ed.), *Vaccine Adjuvants: Methods and Protocols*, Methods in Molecular Biology, vol. 1494, DOI 10.1007/978-1-4939-6445-1_4, © Springer Science+Business Media New York 2017

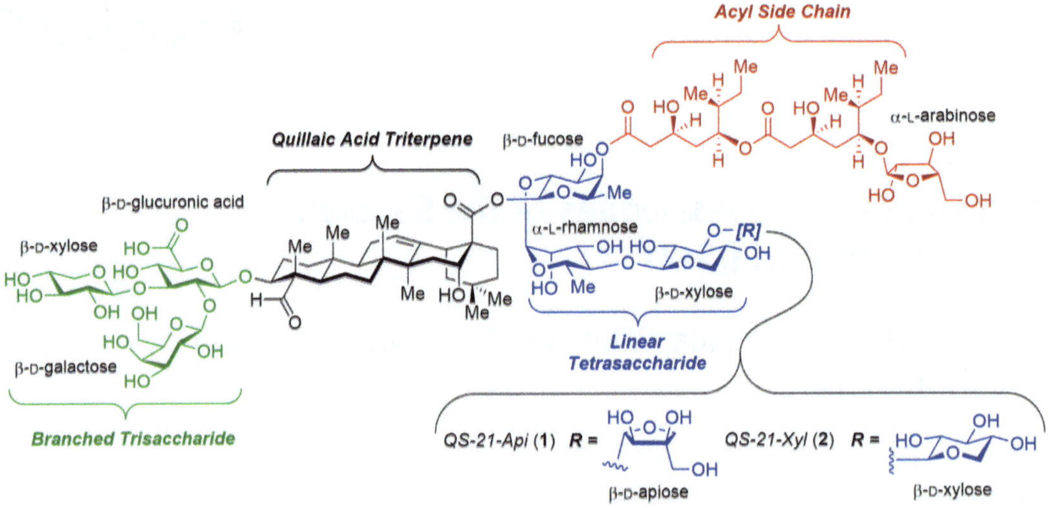

Fig. 1 Chemical structure of the QS-21 saponin adjuvant and its four structural domains

vaccines developed by GSK [3, 4]. Structural modification of the natural product at the molecular level via *de novo* chemical synthesis has become a powerful approach to address these liabilities.

QS-21 (Fig. 1) comprises four structural domains, with a central quillaic acid triterpene core flanked by a branched trisaccharide, a bridging linear tetrasaccharide, and a glycosylated acyl side chain. The natural product is not a single compound but a ≈2:1 mixture of apiose and xylose isomers (QS-21-Api, **1** and QS-21-Xyl, **2**) at the terminal sugar in the linear tetrasaccharide domain. The total syntheses of each of these QS-21 isomers provided a robust method to produce this potent adjuvant in high purity and homogeneous composition [5–7]. These efforts involved the synthesis of all four structural domains of QS-21 in protected form, followed by late-stage coupling, global deprotection, and HPLC purification to provide synthetic QS-21-Api [5, 6] and QS-21-Xyl [7] in a highly modular fashion. To streamline the rather lengthy, multistep preparation of these molecules, a novel semisynthetic route was then developed [8]. In this route, the branched trisaccharide–triterpene conjugate (prosapogenin), which is common to both QS-21 isomers, was obtained via basic hydrolysis and chromatographic purification of commercially available Quil-A, a semipurified, saponin-rich extract from *Q. saponaria*. Installation of the bridging linear tetrasaccharide and acyl chain domains then provided access to a variety of QS-21 analogues.

The technology gained from the chemical synthesis of QS-21 and the establishment of the new semisynthetic route has enabled the application of this saponin chemistry to design and synthesize novel, synthetically accessible QS-21 variants that exhibit increased stability and potency, and attenuated in vivo toxicity [9–14].

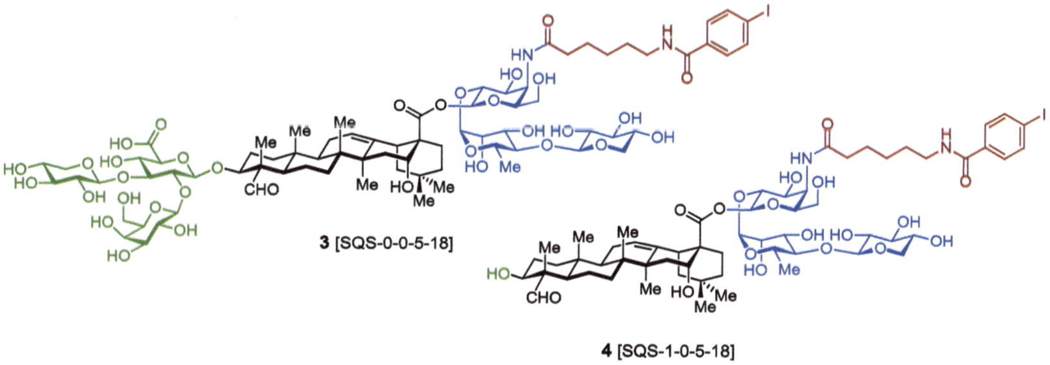

Fig. 2 Chemical structures of semisynthetic saponin adjuvants based on QS-21

Our studies have revealed that significant structural modifications of the bridging fucose residue within the linear tetrasaccharide and of the acyl chain of QS-21 cause little or no impairment of adjuvant activity [9, 10, 12]. Additionally, systematic structure–function studies of the carbohydrate regions have indicated that the terminal sugar within the linear tetrasaccharide as well as the entire branched trisaccharide domain are not required for adjuvant activity [10, 11]. This led us to identify highly simplified acyl chain variants and a truncated linear trisaccharide congener that were equipotent to QS-21 in a preclinical vaccination model. More recently, structure–activity investigations around the central glycosidic ester linkage revealed that relatively conservative modifications result in significant differences in adjuvant activity that correlate with local and global conformational changes observed in molecular dynamics studies [14].

In this chapter, we present a general approach to the semisynthesis of saponin variants based on the QS-21 parent architecture. Syntheses of two saponin adjuvants, **3** (SQS-0-0-5-18) and **4** (SQS-1-0-5-18) (Fig. 2), which include and lack the branched trisaccharide domain, respectively, are provided as examples. We describe protocols for the controlled hydrolysis and purification of *Quillaja* extracts to isolate sufficient quantities of the prosapogenin and triterpene substructures of QS-21 and their selective protection. We also detail synthetic routes to the requisite structural domains (prosapogenin and triterpene substructures, as well as simplified acyl chain and truncated linear oligosaccharide domains) and their late-stage, convergent assembly to protected saponin scaffolds, followed by global deprotection.

2 Materials

1. All chemicals are obtained from commercial vendors (Aldrich Chemical, Acros Organics, or Fisher Scientific) and used without further purification unless otherwise noted.

2. Lyophilized QS saponin Quil A, obtained from Brenntag Biosector (Frederikssund, Denmark) via distribution by Accurate Chemical and Scientific Corporation (Westbury, NY).
3. Dichloromethane (DCM), tetrahydrofuran (THF), acetonitrile (MeCN), toluene, and benzene, purified by passage through two packed columns of neutral alumina under an argon (Ar) atmosphere using a solvent drying system.
4. Methanol (MeOH), distilled from magnesium turnings under nitrogen (N_2) atmosphere at 760 Torr.
5. *N*,*N*-Dimethylformamide (DMF), dried over freshly activated 4 Å molecular sieves (MS) or as purchased from Acros Organics (*N*,*N*-dimethylformamide 99.8 %, Extra Dry over Molecular Sieve, AcroSeal™).
6. Triethylamine (Et_3N), pyridine, and boron trifluoride diethyl etherate ($BF_3 \cdot OEt_2$), distilled from calcium hydride (CaH_2) under N_2 atmosphere at 760 Torr.
7. Trifluoromethanesulfonic anhydride (Tf_2O), distilled from phosphorus pentoxide (P_2O_5) under N_2 atmosphere at 760 Torr.
8. Acetic acid (AcOH).
9. Acetone.
10. Acetyl chloride (AcCl).
11. Activated charcoal.
12. Allyl alcohol.
13. Allyl bromide.
14. Aluminum foil.
15. Benzoyl chloride (BzCl).
16. Benzyl bromide (BnBr).
17. Benzyl chloroformate (CbzCl).
18. Brine (saturated solution of sodium chloride (NaCl) in distilled water).
19. *tert*-Butanol (*t*BuOH).
20. 6-[(*tert*-Butoxycarbonyl)amino]hexanoic acid (6-(Boc-amino) hexanoic acid).
21. Celite.
22. Chloroform ($CHCl_3$).
23. 1,8-Diazabicyclo[5.4.0]undec-7-ene (DBU).
24. Diethyl ether (Et_2O).
25. Diethylamine (Et_2NH).
26. 2,2-Dimethoxypropane (DMP).
27. 4-Dimethylaminopyridine (DMAP).

28. Diphenyldiselenide (PhSeSePh).
29. Ethanol (EtOH).
30. Ethyl acetate (EtOAc).
31. Ethyl chloroformate (EtOCOCl).
32. D-Glucal.
33. Hydrochloric acid, concentrated (HCl, 37%, 12.1 N).
34. HCl (1 N aqueous).
35. Hexanes.
36. Hypophosphorous acid (H_3PO_2), 50% solution in water.
37. Imidazole.
38. 4-Iodobenzoic acid *N*-hydroxysuccinimide ester.
39. 2,6-Lutidine.
40. Magnesium sulfate ($MgSO_4$).
41. Methanesulfonyl chloride (MsCl).
42. Methanol (MeOH).
43. Methanol-d_4 (deuterated methanol).
44. *N*-Methylmorpholine *N*-oxide (NMO).
45. Osmium tetroxide (OsO_4).
46. Palladium (II) acetate ($Pd(OAc)_2$).
47. Palladium on carbon (Pd/C), 10% dry basis, wet Degussa type E101 NE/W.
48. Phenylselenol (PhSeH).
49. Phenyl sulfoxide (Ph_2SO).
50. Potassium bicarbonate ($KHCO_3$).
51. Potassium hydroxide (KOH).
52. Pyrrolidine.
53. L-Rhamnose monohydrate.
54. Sodium azide (NaN_3).
55. Sodium bicarbonate ($NaHCO_3$).
56. $NaHCO_3$, saturated solution in distilled water.
57. Sodium hydride (NaH), 60% dispersion in mineral oil.
58. Sodium hydroxide (NaOH).
59. Sodium sulfate (Na_2SO_4).
60. Sodium sulfite (Na_2SO_3).
61. Tetrabutylammonium chloride (Bu_4NCl).
62. Tetrabutylammonium fluoride (TBAF), solution in THF (1 M).
63. Tetrakis(triphenylphosphine)palladium(0) ($Pd(PPh_3)_4$).
64. *p*-Toluenesulfonic acid monohydrate (pTsOH).

65. Trichloroacetonitrile (Cl_3CCN).
66. Triethylsilyltrifluoromethanesfulonate (TESOTf).
67. Trifluoroacetic acid (TFA).
68. Triisopropylsilyl chloride (TIPSCl).
69. Triphenylphosphine (PPh_3).
70. Water, distilled.
71. D-Xylose.

3 Methods

3.1 General Experimental Methods

1. Reactions are performed in a flame-dried, modified Schlenk flask (Kjeldahl shape), equipped with a Teflon-coated, magnetic stir bar, and fitted with a glass stopper under positive pressure of Ar, unless otherwise noted.
2. Air- and moisture-sensitive liquids are transferred via glass syringe or stainless-steel cannula, which are oven-dried and cooled under Ar prior to use.
3. Gas-tight syringes are dried and stored in a desiccator and purged with Ar prior to use.
4. Carbohydrate and sulfoxide reagents are dried via azeotropic removal of water with toluene (~2 mL/0.10 mmol scale) under high vacuum. This process is repeated three times and the residue is further dried under vacuum.
5. Molecular sieves (MS) are activated at 350 °C, then crushed and flame-dried under vacuum immediately prior to use.
6. 2,4,6-Tri-*tert*-butylpyridine (TBP) used for dehydrative glycosylation reactions is stored and weighed out in a glovebox, then added from a vial under Ar.
7. Cooling baths are generated as follows: 0 °C, wet ice/water; −10 °C, wet ice/acetone; −42 °C, dry ice/EtOH:water (1:1) or dry ice/MeCN; −60 °C, dry ice/$CHCl_3$; −78 °C, dry ice/acetone.
8. Organic solutions are concentrated by rotary evaporation below 35 °C.
9. Analytical thin-layer chromatography (TLC) is performed using glass plates precoated to a depth of 0.25 mm with 230–400 mesh silica gel (E. Merck) impregnated with a fluorescent indicator (254 nm). Compounds are visualized using UV light (254 nm) or by dipping the plates in a ceric ammonium molybdate (CAM) solution followed by heating.
10. Flash column chromatography is performed using 230–400 mesh silica gel (E. Merck) under positive pressure of nitrogen.

11. Automated silica gel column chromatography is performed on an Isco Combiflash Rf with Isco columns (Teledyne Isco, Lincoln, Nebraska). Gradient elutions are performed with a linear gradient of the indicated solvents.
12. Reverse-phase high performance liquid chromatography (RP-HPLC) purification and analyses are carried out on a Waters 2545 binary gradient HPLC system equipped with a Waters 2996 photodiode array detector (Waters Corporation, Milford, Massachusetts). Absorbances are monitored at wavelengths of 210–600 nm. RP-HPLC purifications are performed on an XBridge Prep BEH300 C18 column (5 μm, 10×250 mm) using a linear gradient of acetonitrile/water at a flow rate of 5 mL/min.

3.2 Isolation and Selective Protection of Branched Trisaccharide–Triterpene Prosapogenin

3.2.1 Isolation of Branched Trisaccharide–Triterpene Prosapogenins **5** and **6** (Fig. 3) from Quil A

1. In a 250-mL round-bottomed flask equipped with a reflux condenser, Quil A (1.15 g) and potassium hydroxide (0.97 g, 17 mmol) are suspended in EtOH/water (1:1) (50 mL), then the mixture is heated to 80 °C for 7 h.
2. The reaction is cooled to 0 °C, neutralized with 1.0 N HCl, and concentrated to approximately one-half volume (*see* **Note 1**).
3. The mixture is frozen and lyophilized, and the resulting dry solid is purified by silica gel chromatography ($CHCl_3$/MeOH/water/AcOH, 15:9:2:1). The major product corresponding to the main spot observed by TLC is isolated by concentrating the desired fractions.
4. The resulting solid is dried by azeotropic removal of solvents with toluene (2×20 mL) and lyophilized in MeCN/water (1:1) (3×15 mL) (*see* **Note 2**) to provide a mixture of prosapogenins

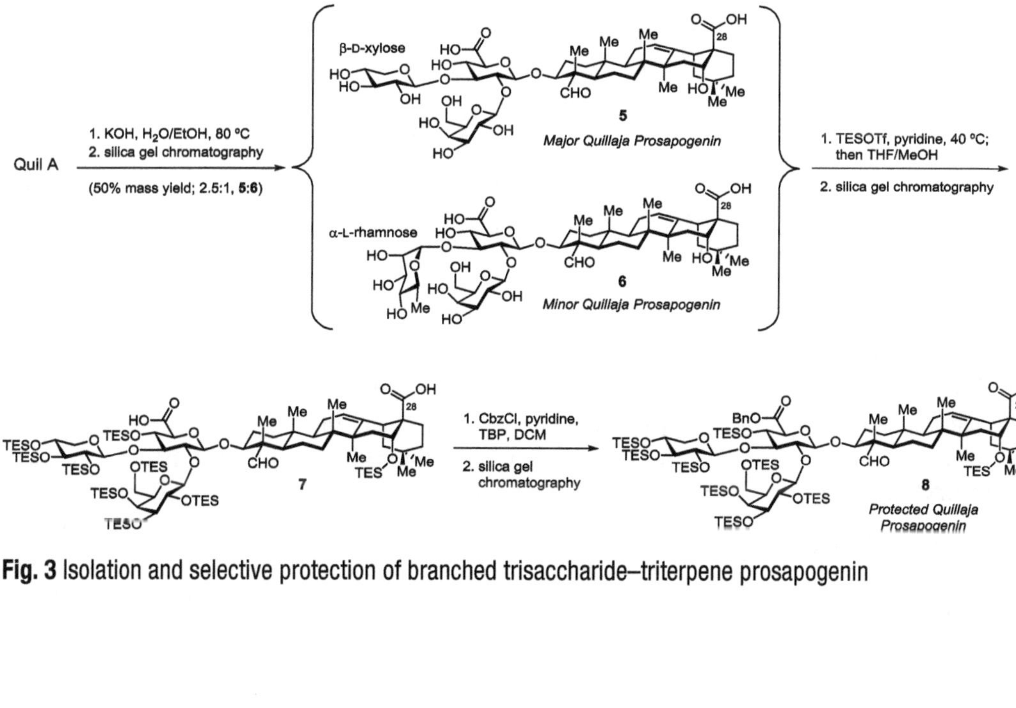

Fig. 3 Isolation and selective protection of branched trisaccharide–triterpene prosapogenin

(**5**:**6**, 2.5:1) as a light tan foam (~0.55 g, 50% mass yield). These xylose and rhamnose-containing prosapogenins **5** and **6** (Fig. 3), respectively, correspond to the two most abundant trisaccharide–triterpene fragments found in QS saponins, and are advanced to the next protection step without further purification.

3.2.2 Synthesis of Triethylsilyl (TES)-Protected Prosapogenin 7 (Fig. 3) by Selective Protection of Prosapogenin Hydroxyl Groups

1. In a 25-mL modified Schlenk flask, the solid mixture of prosapogenins **5** and **6** (~0.55 g) is azeotroped from pyridine (5 mL), then additional pyridine (8 mL) is added, followed by TESOTf (2.0 mL, 8.8 mmol).
2. The reaction mixture is stirred for 2.75 days, then TESOTf (0.3 mL, 1.3 mmol) is added, followed by two further additions (0.1 mL each, 0.44 mmol each) 24 h and 48 h later, respectively (*see* **Note 3**).
3. After a total of 5 days, the mixture is concentrated and passed through a short plug of silica gel eluted with hexanes/EtOAc (4:1 to 2:1). The eluate is concentrated, the resulting yellow oil is dissolved in MeOH/THF (1:1) (20 mL), and the solution is stirred for 3.5 days to remove the silyl esters by solvolysis.
4. The reaction mixture is concentrated and the resulting mixture of xylose- and rhamnose-containing $(TES)_9$-protected prosapogenin diacids is separated by silica gel chromatography (hexanes/EtOAc, 4:1 to 2:1) to afford purified xylose-containing protected prosapogenin 7 (~0.25 g, ~22% yield) as a white solid.

3.2.3 Synthesis of Protected Quillaja Prosapogenin 8 (Fig. 3) by Selective Esterification of Glucuronic Acid Carboxylic Acid in Protected Prosapogenin 7

1. In a 10-mL modified Schlenk flask, the prosapogenin diacid 7 (81 mg, 41 μmol, 1.0 equiv.) is dissolved in DCM (0.7 mL) and pyridine (30 μL, 0.37 mmol, 9.0 equiv.) and TBP (102 mg, 0.41 mmol, 10 equiv.) are added, followed by benzyl chloroformate (15 μL, 0.11 mmol, 2.6 equiv.).
2. The reaction is stirred for 6 h, additional benzyl chloroformate (3.0 μL, 21 μmol, 0.51 equiv.) is added (*see* **Note 4**) and the reaction is stirred for another 20 h.

The mixture is concentrated and purified by silica gel chromatography (hexanes/EtOAc, 20:1 to 7:1) to afford selectively glucuronate-protected prosapogenin (**8** in Fig. 3) (58 mg, 68%) as a white solid.

3.3 Isolation and Selective Protection of Quillaic Acid Triterpene, Lacking the Branched Trisaccharide Domain

3.3.1 Isolation of Quillaic Acid Triterpene 9 (Fig. 4) from Quil A

1. In a 250-mL round-bottomed flask equipped with a reflux condenser, Quil A (5 g) is suspended in distilled water (25 mL) and concentrated HCl (17 mL) is added.
2. The mixture is slowly heated to reflux for 7 h (*see* **Note 5**), then removed from heat, and filtered through filter paper. The dark brown solid is washed with hot (~65 °C) distilled water (2 × 50 mL), collected and dried under high vacuum overnight.
3. The dry solid is placed into a Soxhlet thimble and subjected to continuous extraction with diethyl ether (200 mL) for 24 h.

4. The ether solution is concentrated, the residue is dissolved in MeOH (20 mL), and activated charcoal (~5 g) is added. The mixture is filtered through celite, the solids are washed with MeOH (50 mL), and the solvent is removed by rotary evaporation.
5. The resulting residue is purified by silica gel chromatography ($CHCl_3$/MeOH, 30:1 to 20:1 to 10:1) to afford the quillaic acid triterpene **9** (~0.5 g, ~10% mass yield) (*see* **Note 6**).

*3.3.2 Synthesis of Quillaic Acid Allyl Ester **10** (Fig. 4) by Allylation of C28 Carboxylic Acid of Quillaic Acid **9***

1. In a 50-mL round-bottomed flask, the quillaic acid triterpene **9** (100 mg, 0.20 mmol, 1.0 equiv.) is dissolved in DMF (5 mL) and the solution is cooled to 0 °C.
2. Potassium bicarbonate (205 mg, 2.05 mmol, 10 equiv.) and allyl bromide (23 μL, 0.27 mmol, 1.3 equiv.) are added and the mixture is stirred and allowed to warm to room temperature (rt) overnight.
3. The reaction is diluted with water (25 mL) and extracted with hexanes/EtOAc (1:1) (3 × 15 mL). The organic extracts are combined, washed with brine (15 mL), dried over anhydrous Na_2SO_4, filtered, and concentrated.
4. Purification by silica gel chromatography (hexanes/EtOAc, 8:1 to 2:1) affords quillaic acid allyl ester **10** (77 mg, 71%) as a white solid.

*3.3.3 Synthesis of Protected Quillaic Acid Triterpene **11** (Fig. 4) by Silylation of C3 and C16 Hydroxyl Groups of Quillaic Acid Allyl Ester **10***

1. In a 25-mL modified Schlenk flask, quillaic allyl ester **10** (77 mg, 0.15 mmol, 1.0 equiv.) is dissolved in DCM (5 mL) and the solution is cooled to 0 °C. 2,6-Lutidine (0.17 mL, 1.46 mmol, 10 equiv.) is added, followed by TESOTf (0.17 mL, 0.73 mmol, 5.0 equiv.) via gas-tight syringe, and the mixture is stirred while the ice bath is allowed to melt.
2. The reaction progress is monitored by TLC using $CHCl_3$/MeOH (10:1) as eluent. If the reaction is not complete after 3 h, more TESOTf (33 μL, 0.15 mmol, 1.0 equiv.) is added and the mixture is stirred until the reaction is complete.

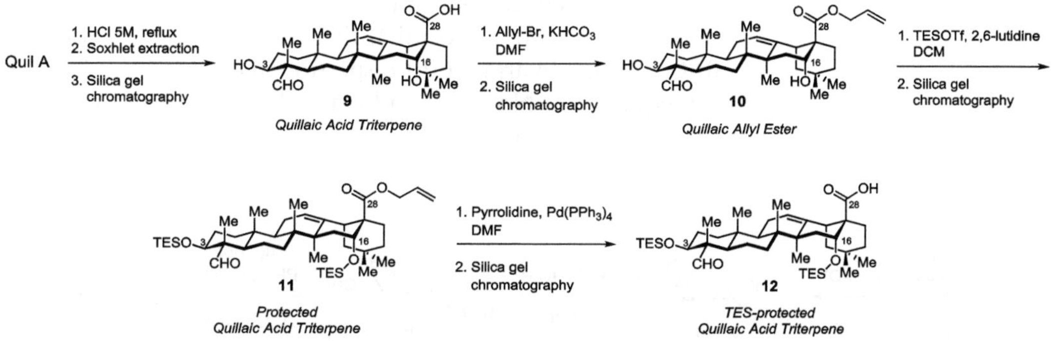

Fig. 4 Isolation and selective protection of quillaic acid triterpene lacking branched trisaccharide domain

3. The reaction mixture is diluted with water (10 mL) and the aqueous phase is extracted with EtOAc (10 mL × 3). The combined organic phases are dried (anhydrous Na_2SO_4), filtered, and concentrated.
4. Purification by silica gel chromatography (hexanes/acetone, 1:0 to 10:1) yields the TES-protected quillaic allyl ester **11** (93 mg, 84 %) as a white solid.

*3.3.4 Synthesis of TES-Protected Quillaic Acid Triterpene **12** (Fig. 4) by Deallylation of Protected Quillaic Acid **11***

1. In a 10-mL round-bottomed flask, fully protected quillaic acid **11** (93 mg, 0.12 mmol, 1.0 equiv.) is dissolved in DCM (2 mL) and pyrrolidine (51 μL, 0.61 mmol, 5.0 equiv.) is added, followed by $Pd(PPh_3)_4$ (7.0 mg, 0.006 mmol, 0.05 equiv.).
2. The reaction mixture is stirred for 15 min, then directly subjected to purification by silica gel chromatography (hexanes/EtOAc, 2:1), to afford TES-protected quillaic acid **12** (88 mg, >99 %) as a white solid.

3.4 Synthesis of Truncated Linear Oligosaccharide Domain

*3.4.1 Synthesis of Selectively Protected Monosaccharide Precursor 2,3,4-tri-O-Benzyl-D-xylose **15** (Fig. 5) from D-Xylose*

1. *Step A: Synthesis of 1-O-allyl-D-xylose* 13 *by selective allylation of D-xylose.* In a 500-mL round-bottomed flask, a solution of allyl alcohol (50 mL, 0.74 mol, 9.0 equiv.) and AcCl (12.7 mL, 0.17 mol, 2.1 equiv.) is cooled to −10 °C, then solid D-xylose (12.3 g, 0.08 mol, 1.0 equiv.) is added.
2. Once all xylose has been added, the cooling bath is removed and the reaction mixture is stirred for 19 h at rt.
3. Solid $NaHCO_3$ (25 g) is added, the mixture is filtered through a pad of celite, and the volatile materials are removed by rotary evaporation.
4. The residue is passed through a plug of silica gel eluted with DCM/MeOH (9:1) and the eluate is concentrated to afford the anomeric allyl xylose **13** (11.5 g), which is used in the next step without further purification.
5. *Step B: Synthesis of 1-O-allyl-2,3,4-tri-O-benzyl-D-xylose* 14 *by benzylation of 1-O-allyl-D-xylose* 13. In a 500-mL round-bottomed flask, allyl xylose **13** (11.5 g, 60.5 mmol, 1.0 equiv.) is dissolved in DMF (200 mL), then the solution is cooled to 0 °C. Sodium hydride (60 % dispersion in oil, 15.7 g, 0.39 mol, 6.5 equiv.) (*see* **Note 7**) is added and the reaction mixture is stirred for 10 min.

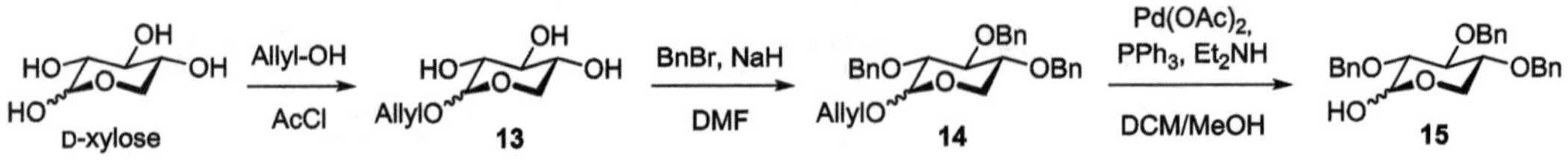

Fig. 5 Selective protection of D-xylose

6. Benzyl bromide (47 mL, 0.39 mol, 6.5 equiv.) is added dropwise at 0 °C, and the resulting suspension is stirred at rt for 16 h.
7. The reaction mixture is cooled to 0 °C and quenched by slow addition of MeOH (150 mL) followed by water (600 mL). The mixture is extracted with hexanes/EtOAc (1:1) (3 × 250 mL) and the combined organic layers are washed with water (100 mL), brine (100 mL), dried with anhydrous $MgSO_4$, filtered, and concentrated.
8. Purification by silica gel chromatography (hexanes/EtOAc, 9:1) affords the fully protected xylose **14** (23 g, 83%).
9. *Step C: Synthesis of selectively protected 2,3,4-tri-O-benzyl-D-xylose* 15 *by deallylation of 1-O-allyl-2,3,4-tri-O-benzyl-D-xylose* 14. In a 100-mL round-bottomed flask covered in aluminum foil, PPh_3 (3.4 g, 13 mmol, 1.2 equiv.) and $Pd(OAc)_2$ (0.45 g, 2.2 mmol, 0.2 equiv.) are dissolved in DCM/MeOH (1:1) (20 mL), then Et_2NH (15.8 mL, 0.15 mol, 14.0 equiv.) is added.
10. A solution of the fully protected xylose **14** (5.0 g, 10.9 mmol, 1.0 equiv.) in DCM (100 mL) is added by cannula transfer, and the reaction mixture is stirred at 30 °C for 18 h.
11. The solution is passed through a plug of silica gel eluted with hexanes/EtOAc (1:1) and the eluate is concentrated.
12. Purification by silica gel chromatography (hexanes/EtOAc, 8:2 to 7:3) affords 2,3,4,-tri-*O*-benzyl xylose **15** (4.1 g, 90%) as a mixture of anomers (α:β, 2:1).

*3.4.2 Synthesis of Selectively Protected Monosaccharide Precursor 1-O-Allyl-2,3-O-isopropylidene-L-rhamnose **16** (Fig. 6) from L-Rhamnose*

1. In a 250-mL round-bottomed flask, a solution of allyl alcohol (34 mL, 0.50 mol, 9.0 equiv.) and AcCl (8.1 mL, 0.12 mol, 2.1 equiv.) is cooled at −10 °C, then L-rhamnose monohydrate (10 g, 0.055 mol, 1.0 equiv.) is added.
2. The mixture is stirred for 20 h at rt, neutralized with Et_3N, and concentrated.
3. The residue is dissolved in toluene and the solution is concentrated to remove allyl alcohol; this process is repeated two more times.
4. The residual syrup is dissolved in dry acetone (75 mL), and DMP (27 mL, 0.22 mol, 4.0 equiv.) and pTsOH monohydrate (95 mg, 0.5 mmol, 0.01 equiv.) are added.

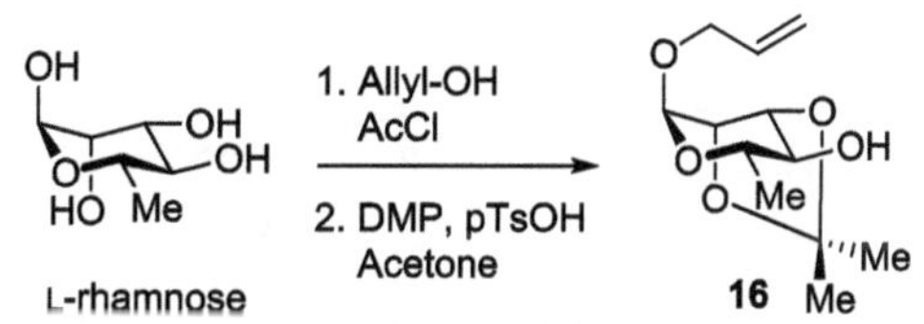

Fig. 6 Selective protection of L-rhamnose

5. The reaction mixture is stirred for 16 h at rt and Et_3N is then added.
6. The reaction mixture is concentrated and purified by silica gel chromatography (hexanes/EtOAc, 8:2) to afford 1-*O*-allyl-2,3-*O*-isopropylidene-α-L-rhamnose (**16**) (8.9 g, 66%) as a colorless oil.

*Synthesis of Selectively Protected Monosaccharide Precursor 4-Azido-4-deoxy-3,6-di-O-benzyl-1-O-triisopropylsilyl-D-galactose **21** (Fig. 7) from D-Glucal*

1. *Step A: Synthesis of 3,6-di-O-benzoyl-4-O-mesyl-D-glucal* 17 *by selective protection of* D*-glucal.* In a 500-mL round-bottomed flask, D-glucal (10.0 g, 67.1 mmol, 1.0 equiv.) is dissolved in pyridine (165 mL) and the solution is cooled to 0 °C, then BzCl (17 mL, 0.15 mol, 2.2 equiv.) is added dropwise.
2. The reaction mixture is stirred at 0 °C for 1.5 h, then MsCl (10.3 mL, 0.13 mol, 2.0 equiv.) is added. The reaction mixture is stirred for 0.5 h while allowing the ice bath warm to rt, then quenched by slow addition of MeOH (20 mL) at 0 °C (*see* **Note 8**).
3. The mixture is concentrated and the residue is partitioned between EtOAc (200 mL) and water (200 mL). The organic layer is washed with water (100 mL), brine (100 mL), dried with anhydrous $MgSO_4$, filtered, and concentrated.
4. Purification by silica gel chromatography (hexanes/EtOAc, 8:2) affords 3,6-di-*O*-benzoyl-4-*O*-mesyl-D-glucal (**17**) (19.4 g, 67%) as a syrup.
5. *Step B: Synthesis of 4-azido-4-deoxy-3,6-di-O-benzoyl-D-galactal* 18 *by azide substitution of mesylate* 17. In a 250 mL round-bottomed flask, the mesyl-glucal **17** (5.1 g, 11.8 mmol, 1.0 equiv.) is dissolved in toluene (55 mL), then sodium azide (*see* **Note 9**) (2.8 g, 43.3 mmol, 3.7 equiv.) is added, followed by Bu_4NCl (7.1 g, 25.6 mmol, 2.2 equiv.), and the flask is equipped with a reflux condenser.

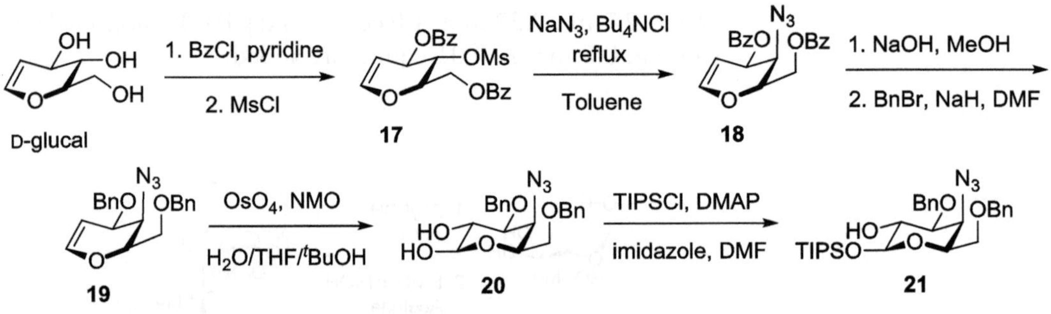

Fig. 7 Synthesis of protected 4-azido-4-deoxygalactose (**21**) from D-glucal

6. The reaction mixture is heated to reflux (110 °C) for 20 h. The resulting brown suspension is washed with water (2 × 100 mL), dried with anhydrous $MgSO_4$, filtered, and concentrated to give an orange oil.
7. Purification by silica gel chromatography (hexanes/EtOAc, 19:1 to 8:2) provides 4-azido-4-deoxy-3,6-di-*O*-benzoyl-D-galactal (**18**) (2.9 g, 66%) as a light yellow oil.
8. *Step C: Synthesis of 4-azido-4-deoxy-3,6-di-O-benzyl-*D*-galactal* 19 *by saponification and benzylation of dibenzoate* 18. In 250-mL round-bottomed flask, the benzoyl-protected azidogalactal **18** (2.9 g, 8.1 mmol, 1.0 equiv.) is dissolved in MeOH (40 mL) and the solution is cooled to 0 °C.
9. Sodium hydroxide (0.12 g, 2.9 mmol, 0.36 equiv.) is added and the reaction mixture is stirred for 14 h at rt.
10. The reaction mixture is concentrated to afford a sticky tan solid, then evaporated again from toluene (7 mL) to remove trace solvent.
11. DMF (40 mL) is added to the residue and the resulting brown suspension is cooled to 0 °C. Sodium hydride (60% dispersion in mineral oil, 0.98 g, 24.4 mmol, 3.0 equiv.) (*see* **Note 7**) is added, followed by benzyl bromide (4.8 mL, 40.3 mmol, 5.0 equiv.), and the mixture is stirred at 0 °C for 3 h.
12. The resulting orange suspension is stirred for another 16 h at rt, and the reaction is quenched with MeOH (20 mL), diluted with DCM (100 mL), and washed with water (100 mL).
13. The aqueous layer is extracted with DCM (80 mL), and the combined organic layers are washed with water (100 mL), dried with anhydrous $MgSO_4$, filtered, and concentrated.
14. Purification by silica gel chromatography (hexanes/EtOAc, 9:1 to 4:1) affords 4-azido-4-deoxy-3,6-di-*O*-benzyl-D--galactal (**19**) (2.2 g, 78%) as a yellow oil.
15. *Step D: Synthesis of 4-azido-4-deoxy-3,6-di-O-benzyl-*D*-galactose* 20 *by dihydroxylation of galactal* 19. The benzyl-protected azidogalactal **19** (5.8 g, 16.5 mmol, 1.0 equiv.) is dissolved in a mixture of water/THF/*t*BuOH (1:3:7) (400 mL), then OsO_4 (2.5 wt% in *t*BuOH) (5.1 mL, 0.4 mmol, 0.025 equiv.) is added. NMO (50% in water) (10.2 mL, 44.5 mmol, 3.0 equiv.) is added in three portions (1.0 equiv. each) over 8 h.
16. The reaction mixture is stirred at rt overnight, then quenched with saturated aqueous Na_2SO_3 solution (30 mL) and EtOAc (200 mL).
17. After 5 min, the phases are separated and the aqueous layer is extracted with EtOAc (2 × 75 mL) and DCM (2 × 50 mL). The combined organic phases are dried over anhydrous sodium sulfate, filtered, and concentrated.

18. Purification by silica gel chromatography (hexanes/EtOAc, 4:1 to 1:1) affords 4-azido-4-deoxy-3,6-di-*O*-benzyl-D-galactose (**20**) (5.5 g, 88 %) as a colorless oil.
19. *Step E: Synthesis of 4-azido-4-deoxy-3,6-di-O-benzyl-1-O-triisopropylsilyl-*D*-galactose* 21 *by selective silylation of diol* 20. In a 10-mL modified Schlenk flask, the galactose diol **20** (0.96 g, 2.5 mmol, 1.0 equiv.) is dissolved in DMF (2.5 mL), then imidazole (0.41 g, 6.0 mmol, 2.4 equiv.) and DMAP (29 mg, 0.24 mmol, 0.1 equiv.) are added.
20. TIPSCl (0.63 mL, 3.0 mmol, 1.2 equiv.) is added and the reaction mixture is stirred for 19 h at rt.
21. The yellow solution is concentrated and purified by silica gel chromatography (hexanes/EtOAc, 19:1 to 9:1) to afford 4-azido-4-deoxy-3,6-di-*O*-benzyl-1-*O*-triisopropylsilyl-D-galactose (**21**) (0.8 g, 59 %) as a colorless oil.

*3.4.3 Synthesis of Protected Xylose–Rhamnose Disaccharide Hemiacetal **23** (Fig. 8) ([2,3,4-Tri-O-benzyl-β-D-xylopyranosyl-(1→ 4)]-2,3-di-O-isopropylidene-L-rhamnopyranose) from protected D-xylose **15** and protected L-rhamnose **16***

1. *Step A: Dehydrative glycosylation of protected rhamnose* 16 *with protected xylose* 15 *(22 in Fig. 8)*: In a 25-mL modified Schlenk flask, azeotropically dried 2,3,4-tri-*O*-benzyl xylose (**15**) (52 mg, 0.12 mmol, 1.7 equiv.), Ph_2SO (69 mg, 0.34 mmol, 4.9 equiv.), and TBP (85 mg, 0.34 mmol, 4.9 equiv.) are dissolved in DCM (2 mL), injected via glass syringe.
2. The solution is cooled to −78 °C, Tf_2O (29 μL, 0.17 mmol, 2.4 equiv.) is added via gas-tight syringe, and the reaction mixture is stirred for 2 h at −78 °C.
3. A precooled solution of protected rhamnose **16** (17 mg, 70 μmol, 1.0 equiv.) in toluene (1 mL) is then cannula transferred from a flame dried, 10-mL modified Schlenk flask, then additional toluene (1 mL) is added to rinse the source flask and transferred to the reaction flask.
4. The reaction mixture is stirred at −60 °C for 12 h, at −42 °C for 30 min, and finally at 0 °C for 2 min.
5. The reaction is quenched by addition of Et_3N (0.1 mL) at −42 °C, diluted with DCM (90 mL) and transferred to a separatory funnel. The organic layer is washed with saturated aqueous $NaHCO_3$ solution (30 mL) and the aqueous layer is

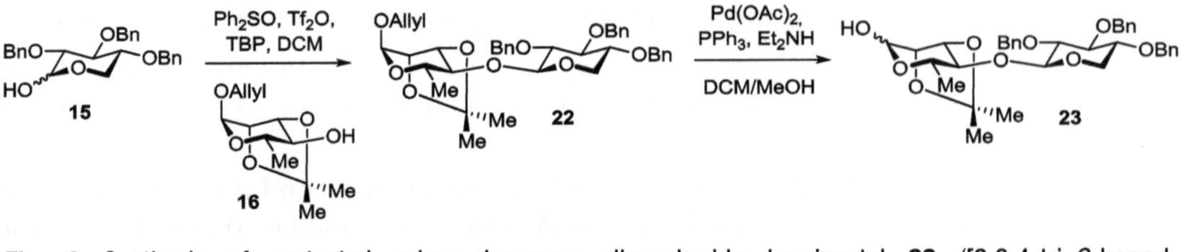

Fig. 8 Synthesis of protected xylose–rhamnose disaccharide hemiacetal **23** ([2,3,4-tri-*O*-benzyl-β-D-xylopyranosyl-(1 → 4)]-2,3-*O*-isopropylidene-L-rhamnopyranose)

extracted with DCM (2×80 mL). The organic phases are combined, dried over anhydrous Na_2SO_4, filtered, and concentrated to afford the crude product as a tan oil (160 mg).

6. Purification by silica gel chromatography (hexanes/EtOAc, 50:1 to 25:1) affords *O*-allyl [2,3,4-tri-O-benzyl-β-D-xylopyranosyl-(1→4)]-2,3-*O*-isopropylidene-L-rhamnopyranoside (**22**) as a clear oil (32.1 mg, 71% yield).
7. *Step B: Anomeric deallylation of protected xylose–rhamnose disaccharide* (**23** in Fig. 8): In a 5-mL pear-shaped Schlenk flask equipped with a triangular stir bar, PPh_3 (13 mg, 51 μmol, 1.2 equiv.) and $Pd(OAc)_2$ (2.4 mg, 11 μmol, 0.25 equiv.) are placed. A solution of DCM/MeOH (1:1) (0.2 mL) is added via syringe followed by Et_2NH (62 μL, 0.6 mmol, 14.0 equiv.), which results in a change from a clear yellow-orange to a bright yellow solution.
8. Allyl-protected disaccharide **22** (29 mg, 43 μmol, 1.0 equiv.) dissolved in DCM (0.4 mL) is cannula transferred to the reaction Schlenk flask and the source flask is rinsed with additional DCM (0.2 mL) that is transferred to the reaction flask.
9. The solution is degassed by performing three freeze-thaw-pump cycles (*see* **Note 10**) and then stirred at 30 °C for 18 h, at which point the turbid solution turns clear, dark yellow.
10. The reaction mixture is passed through a plug of silica gel eluted with hexanes/EtOAc (2:1, 50 mL) and the eluate is concentrated to afford the crude product as a bright yellow oil (29 mg).
11. Purification by silica gel chromatography (hexanes/EtOAc, 2:1) affords disaccharide hemiacetal (**23** in Fig. 8) as an inseparable mixture of anomers (α:β, 9:1) as a clear oil (25.9 mg, >99%).

*3.4.4 Synthesis of Protected Xylose–Rhamnose–Azidogalactose Trisaccharide Imidate (**26** in Fig. 9) (O-Trichloroacetimidoyl {[2,3,4-tri-O-Benzyl-β-D-xylopyranosyl-(1→4)]-2,3-O-isopropylidene-L-rhamnopyranosyl-(1→2)}-4-azido-4-deoxy-3,6-O-benzyl-β-D-galactopyranoside)*

1. *Step A: Synthesis of protected xylose–rhamnose–azidogalactose trisaccharide* 24 *by dehydrative glycosylation of protected 4-azido-4-deoxygalactose* 21 *with protected xylose–rhamnose disaccharide* 23 (**24** in Fig. 9): In a 25-mL modified Schlenk flask, Ph_2SO (171 mg, 0.85 mmol, 3.2 equiv.) is dissolved in DCM (3.2 mL). To this clear, colorless solution, Tf_2O (76 μL, 0.45 mmol, 1.7 equiv.) is injected via gas-tight syringe at −78 °C. After 10 s, the solution turns pink, then purple, and quickly dissipates back to a clear, colorless solution.
2. A precooled solution of azeotropically dried disaccharide hemiacetal **23** (185 mg, 0.30 mmol, 1.1 equiv.) in DCM (1 mL) is added to the reaction mixture at −42 °C via cannula from a flame-dried, 5-mL pear-shaped Schlenk flask; then additional DCM (1 mL) is added to rinse the source flask and transferred to the reaction flask.

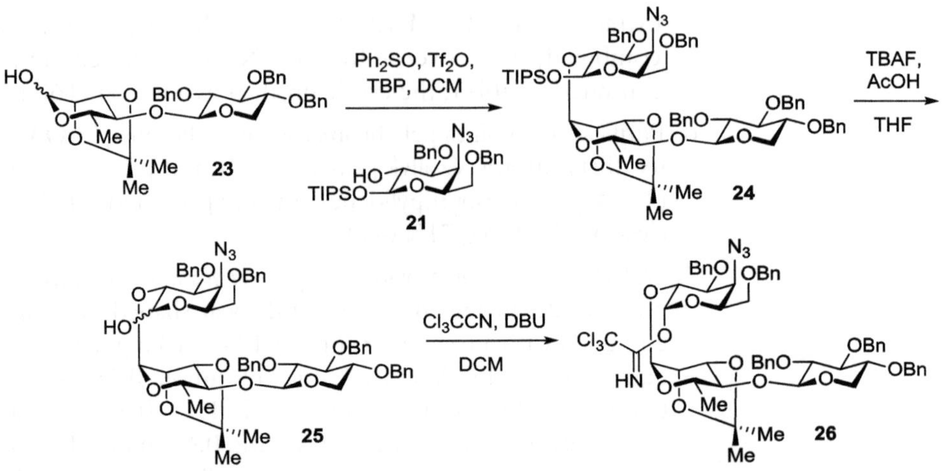

Fig. 9 Synthesis of protected xylose–rhamnose–azidogalactose trisaccharide imidate **26** (*O*-trichloroacetimidoyl {[2,3,4-tri-*O*-benzyl-β-D-xylopyranosyl-(1 → 4)]-2,3-*O*-isopropylidene-L-rhamnopyranosyl-(1 → 2)}-4-azido-4-deoxy-3,6-di-*O*-benzyl-β-D-galactopyranoside)

3. The reaction mixture is stirred at –42 °C for 15 min, then TBP (190 mg, 0.77 mmol, 3.0 equiv.) is added, and the mixture is further stirred at –42 °C for 1 h.
4. A precooled solution of protected 4-azido-4-deoxygalactose **21** (141 mg, 0.26 mmol, 1.0 equiv.) in DCM (1 mL) is added to the reaction mixture via cannula from a flame-dried, 5-mL pear-shaped Schlenk flask, at which point white fumes develop. Additional DCM (1 mL) is added to rinse the source flask and transferred to the reaction flask.
5. The reaction mixture is stirred at –42 °C for 16.5 h and at 0 °C for 1 h, then concentrated.
6. Purification by silica gel chromatography (hexanes/EtOAc, 99:1 to 50:1 to 6:1) gives a mixture of monosaccharide starting material (**21**) and trisaccharide product (**24**) as a yellow oil (460 mg). Additional purification of this mixture by silica gel chromatography (hexanes/EtOAc, 10:1 to 6:1) provides the protected trisaccharide **24** (231 mg, 79%) as a clear oil.
7. *Step B: Synthesis of trisaccharide hemiacetal* 25 *by anomeric desilylation of protected xylose–rhamnose–azidogalactose trisaccharide* 24. In a 250-mL modified Schlenk flask, the protected trisaccharide **24** (575 mg, 0.51 mmol, 1.0 equiv.) is dissolved in THF (50 mL) and the solution is cooled to 0 °C.
8. A precooled (0 °C) solution of commercially available TBAF (1 M in THF) (0.76 mL, 0.76 mmol, 1.5 equiv.) and AcOH (35 μL, 0.61 mmol, 1.2 equiv.) in THF (50 mL) is added dropwise via cannula to the reaction flask over 50 min at 0 °C.

9. The reaction mixture is stirred for an additional 5 min at 0 °C, then quenched by addition of saturated aqueous $NaHCO_3$ solution (20 mL).
10. The contents are transferred to a separatory funnel, EtOAc (125 mL) and brine (50 mL) are added, and the organic phase is separated. The aqueous layer is extracted with EtOAc (2 × 200 mL) and the combined organic phases are dried over anhydrous magnesium sulfate, filtered, and concentrated.
11. The resulting oil is passed through a plug of silica gel eluted with EtOAc, and the eluate is concentrated to afford the trisaccharide hemiacetal **25** (402 mg, 82 %) as a white foam, which is taken directly to the next step without further purification.
12. *Step C: Synthesis of protected xylose–rhamnose–azidogalactose trisaccharide trichloroacetimidate* 26 *by activation of protected xylose–rhamnose–azidogalactose trisaccharide* 25. In a 100-mL round-bottomed flask, the hemiacetal **25** (200 mg, 0.21 mmol, 1.0 equiv.) is dissolved in DCM (32 mL) and the solution is cooled to 0 °C.
13. Cl_3CCN (0.32 mL, 3.2 mmol, 1.6 equiv.) is added followed by DBU (0.1 mL, 0.67 mmol, 3.3 equiv.) and the reaction is allowed to warm to rt.
14. After stirring for 13.5 h, the mixture is concentrated to afford an oil.
15. Purification by silica gel chromatography (hexanes/EtOAc, 6:1 with 0.5 vol% Et_3N) (*see* **Note 11**) affords the linear trisaccharide imidate **26** (230 mg, >99 %) as a yellow foam.

3.5 Modular, Convergent Assembly of Saponin Domain Fragments

3.5.1 Synthesis of Protected Aminogalactose Saponin *28* (Fig. 10) by Glycosylation of Prosapogenin *8* with Linear Trisaccharide *26* and Azide Reduction

1. *Step A: Synthesis of protected azidogalactose saponin* 27 *by glycosylation of branched trisaccharide–triterpene prosapogenin* 8 *with protected xylose–rhamnose–azidogalactose linear trisaccharide* 26. In a 50-mL modified Schlenk flask, the selectively protected prosapogenin **8** (653 mg, 0.32 mmol, 1.5 equiv.) and the trisaccharide imidate **26** (230 mg, 0.21 mmol, 1.0 equiv.) are azeotropically dried from toluene (3 × 3 mL) under high vacuum, then dissolved in DCM (10 mL).
2. Powdered 4 Å MS (1 g) is added and the suspension is stirred for 2 h at rt. The opaque, white mixture is then cooled to −78 °C and freshly distilled $BF_3{\cdot}OEt_2$ (15 μL, 0.23 mmol, 1.1 equiv.) is injected via gas-tight syringe.
3. The reaction mixture is stirred at −78 °C for 6 h, passed through a plug of silica gel, and the filtrate is concentrated.
4. Purification by silica gel chromatography (hexanes/EtOAc, 9:1 to 4:1) affords the prosapogenin – linear trisaccharide conjugate **27** (322 mg, 73 %) as a glassy solid.

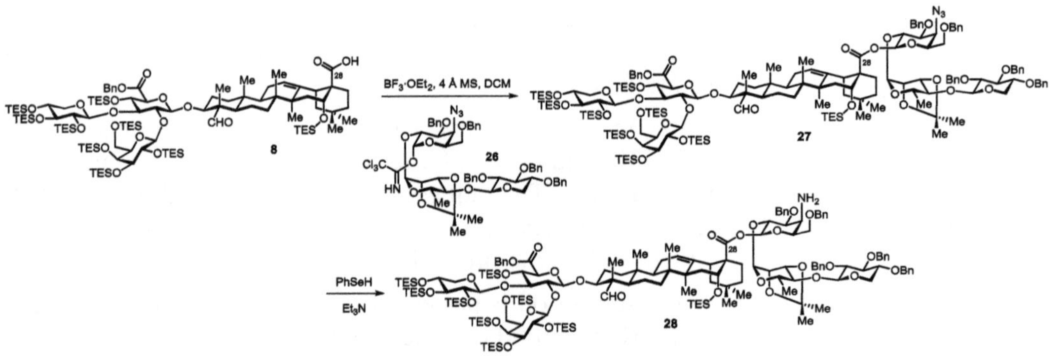

Fig. 10 Glycosylation of prosapogenin **8** with linear trisaccharide **26** and azide reduction (**28**)

5. *Step B: Synthesis of protected aminogalactose saponin* 28 *by reduction of protected azidogalactose saponin* 27. In a 50-mL modified Schlenk flask, PhSeSePh (313 mg, 1.0 mmol, 1.0 equiv.) (*see* **Note 12**) is dissolved in THF (8 mL) and H_3PO_2 (50% in water) (1.2 mL, 11.0 mmol, 11 equiv.) is then added via syringe.
6. The yellow solution is heated at 40 °C for 1 h until it turns colorless.
7. The reaction mixture is removed from the heat, diluted with benzene (8 mL) and distilled water (8 mL), and stirred vigorously for 5 min under Ar. The lower aqueous phase of the resulting biphasic suspension is removed by syringe (or glass pipette) under positive pressure of Ar, and anhydrous sodium sulfate is added to the Schlenk flask to dry the remaining organic layer while stirring.
8. This freshly prepared solution of PhSeH (~1.9 mmol) is then added under Ar via cannula transfer to a 250-mL reaction Schlenk flask containing a solution of the azeotropically dried saponin azide **27** (322 mg, 0.11 mmol, 1.0 equiv.) in Et_3N (50 mL). Upon addition, a white precipitate is formed and the solution turns bright yellow.
9. The reaction mixture is stirred for 3 h at 40 °C, then concentrated to give a yellow-white solid.
10. Purification by silica gel chromatography (hexanes/EtOAc, 4:1 to EtOAc with 0.5 vol% Et_3N) affords the saponin amine **28** (256 mg, 87%) as a glassy solid (*see* **Note 13**).

3.5.2 Synthesis of Protected Aminogalactose Saponin **30** (Fig. 11), Lacking the Branched Trisaccharide Domain, by Glycosylation of Protected Quillaic Acid **12** with Linear Trisaccharide **26** and Azide Reduction

1. *Step A: Synthesis of protected azidogalactose saponin* 29 *by glycosylation of protected quillaic acid* 12 *with protected xylose–rhamnose–azidogalactose linear trisaccharide* 26. In a 25-mL modified Schlenk flask, the selectively protected quillaic acid triterpene **12** (38 mg, 49 μmol, 1.05 equiv.) and the trisaccharide imidate **26** (52 mg, 47 μmol, 1.0 equiv.) are azeotroped from toluene (3 × 1 mL) under high vacuum, then dissolved in DCM (7 mL) and powdered 4 Å MS (80 mg) is added to the solution.
2. The mixture is stirred for 30 min at rt, then cooled to −42 °C. Freshly distilled $BF_3{\cdot}OEt_2$ (1.2 μL, 9.0 μmol, 0.2 equiv.) is injected via gas-tight syringe and the reaction mixture is stirred for another 30 min at −42 °C.
3. The reaction is quenched by addition of Et_3N (0.2 mL) and the mixture is concentrated by rotary evaporation.
4. Purification by silica gel chromatography (benzene with 0.5 vol% Et_3N to benzene/EtOAc, 97:3) affords the triterpene-linear trisaccharide conjugate **29** (56 mg, 72%) as a white solid.
5. *Step B: Synthesis of protected aminogalactose saponin* 30 *by reduction of protected azidogalactose saponin* 29. In a 50-mL modified Schlenk flask, PhSeSePh (187 mg, 0.6 mmol, 1.0 equiv.) is dissolved in THF (6 mL) and H_3PO_2 (50% in water) (0.72 mL, 6.6 mmol, 11 equiv.) is added via syringe.
6. The yellow solution is heated at 40 °C for 1 h until it turns colorless.
7. The reaction mixture is removed from the heat, diluted with benzene (6 mL) and distilled water (6 mL), and stirred vigorously for 5 min under Ar. The lower aqueous phase of the resulting biphasic suspension is removed by glass pipette and the remaining organic layer is dried over anhydrous sodium sulfate while stirring.
8. This freshly prepared solution of PhSeH (~1.1 mmol, 30 equiv.) is then cannula transferred under Ar to a 100-mL reaction

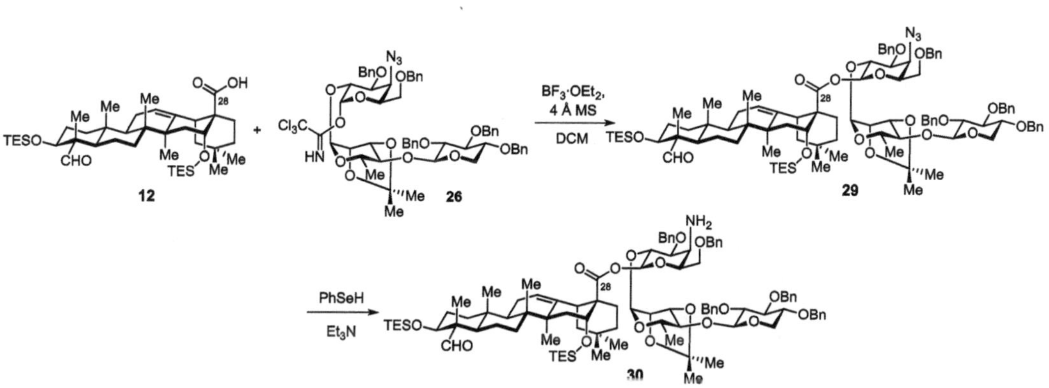

Fig. 11 Glycosylation of protected quillaic acid **12** with linear trisaccharide **26** and azide reduction (**30**)

Schlenk flask containing a solution of the azeotropically dried saponin azide **29** (62 mg, 37 μmol, 1.0 equiv.) in Et_3N (28 mL). Upon addition, a white precipitate is formed and the solution becomes bright yellow.

9. The reaction mixture is stirred for 8 h at 38 °C, then concentrated to afford a yellow-white solid.
10. Purification by silica gel chromatography (benzene/EtOAc, 90:10 to 85:15) affords the truncated saponin amine **30** (49 mg, 80%) as a glassy solid.

*3.5.3 Synthesis of Protected Aminoacyl Saponin **31** (Fig. 12) by Acylation of Protected Aminogalactose Saponin **28***

1. In a 5-mL pear-shaped Schlenk flask, commercially available 6-(Boc-amino)hexanoic acid ($HO_2C(CH_2)_5NHBoc$) (19.9 mg, 86 μmol, 10 equiv.) is dissolved in THF (0.9 mL), then Et_3N (0.11 mL, 0.77 mmol, 90 equiv.) is added. To this clear, colorless solution at 0 °C, EtOCOCl (7.3 μL, 77 μmol, 9.0 equiv.) is injected via gas-tight syringe.
2. The turbid white mixture is stirred for 3 h at 0 °C. The prosapogenin–linear trisaccharide saponin amine **28** (26 mg, 8.6 μmol, 1.0 equiv.) is then added, and the reaction is stirred for 1.5 h at rt.
3. Water (0.1 mL) is added to quench the reaction, at which point the solution turns from turbid white to clear yellow. After addition of more water (0.1 mL), the resulting immiscible mixture is concentrated.

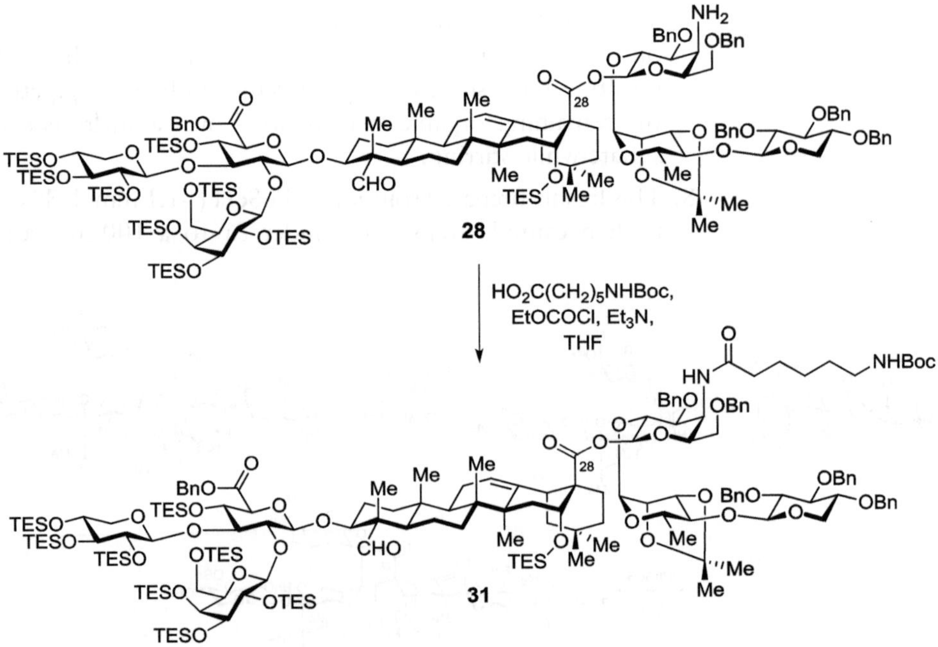

Fig. 12 Installation of acyl chain domain on aminogalactose residue by acylation of protected branched trisaccharide–triterpene–linear trisaccharide (**31**)

4. Purification by silica gel chromatography (toluene/EtOAc, 20:1 to 11:1) affords the aminoacyl, branched trisaccharide-containing saponin **31** (22 mg, 81 %) as a white glassy solid.

3.5.4 Synthesis of Protected Aminoacyl Saponin 32 (Fig. 13), Lacking the Branched Trisaccharide Domain, by Acylation of Protected Aminogalactose Saponin 30

1. In a 10-mL pear-shaped Schlenk flask, 6-(Boc-amino)hexanoic acid (45.0 mg, 0.20 mmol, 11.5 equiv.) is dissolved in THF (2.5 mL), then Et_3N (213 μL, 1.53 mmol, 90 equiv.) is added. To this clear, colorless solution at 0 °C, EtOCOCl (16 μL, 0.17 mmol, 10 equiv.) is injected via gas-tight syringe.
2. The resulting turbid white mixture is stirred for 2.5 h at 0 °C, and then cannula transferred at 0 °C into a 10-mL, Schlenk flask containing a neat film of azeotropically dried (3 × 1 mL toluene) saponin amine **30** (28 mg, 17.0 μmol, 1.0 equiv.).
3. The turbid white reaction mixture is stirred for 1.5 h at 0 °C, then quenched with water (0.2 mL) to give a clear, colorless solution.
4. The mixture is diluted with saturated aqueous $NaHCO_3$ solution (30 mL) and the aqueous phase is extracted with DCM (3 × 25 mL). The combined organic layers are dried over anhydrous sodium sulfate, filtered, and concentrated (*see* **Note 14**).
5. Purification by silica gel chromatography (hexanes/EtOAc, 2:1 with 0.5 vol% Et_3N) (*see* **Note 15**) affords the truncated, fully protected aminoacyl saponin **32** (28 mg, 88 %) as a white glassy solid.

3.6 Global Deprotection of Protected Aminoacylated Saponins

3.6.1 Synthesis of Aminoacyl Saponin 33, SQS-0-0-5-11 (Fig. 14) by Hydrogenolysis and Acid Hydrolysis of Protected Aminoacyl Saponin 31

1. In a 100-mL round-bottomed flask, fully protected, branched trisaccharide-containing saponin **31** (240 mg, 75 μmol, 1.0 equiv.) is dissolved in THF/EtOH (1:1) (20 mL), then 10% (dry basis) Pd/C, wet, Degussa type E101 NE/W (140 mg, 66 μmol, 0.9 equiv.) is added (*see* **Note 16**).
2. The reaction mixture is stirred under H_2 atmosphere (50 psi) for 24 h at rt using a high-pressure bomb reactor, and the suspension is filtered through a 0.45 μm nylon syringe filter.
3. The palladium is washed thoroughly with MeOH (3 × 100 mL) and the clear filtrate is concentrated. Successful debenzylation is assessed by disappearance of aromatic resonances by ^1H-NMR in methanol-d_4.

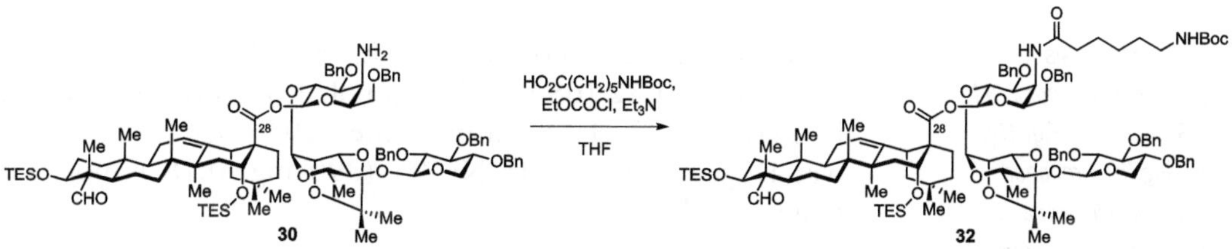

Fig. 13 Installation of acyl chain domain on amino galactose residue by acylation of protected triterpene–linear trisaccharide lacking branched trisaccharide domain (**32**)

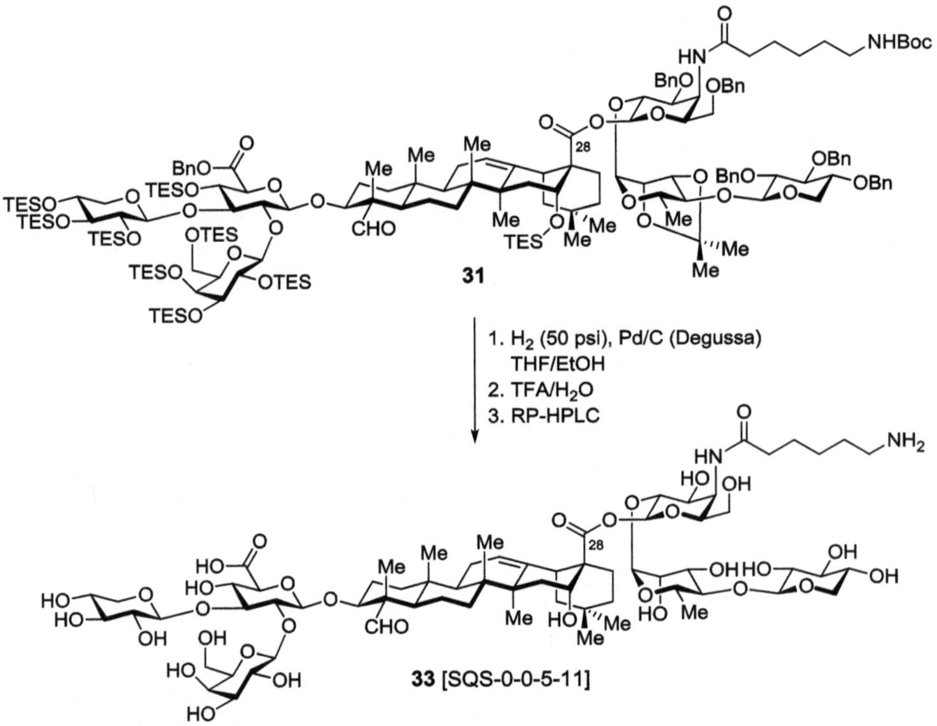

Fig. 14 Global deprotection of branched trisaccharide-containing aminoacylated saponin precursor

4. In a 50-mL round-bottomed flask, the resulting crude mixture of partially desilylated products is dissolved in a precooled (0 °C) solution of TFA/water (4:1) (10 mL).
5. The reaction mixture is stirred for 3 h at 0 °C and then concentrated under high vacuum at 0 °C to give a white solid residue (140 mg).
6. This crude product is dissolved in a solution of water/MeCN (4:1) and purified by RP-HPLC using a linear gradient of 20→35 % MeCN in water (0.05 vol% TFA) over 10 min. The fraction containing the major, single peak is collected and lyophilized to dryness to afford the fully deprotected, free amine-containing saponin **33** (SQS-0-0-5-11) (88 mg, 78 %) as a fluffy white solid.

*3.6.2 Synthesis of Aminoacyl Saponin **34**, SQS-1-0-5-11 (Fig. 15), Lacking the Branched Trisaccharide Domain, by Hydrogenolysis and Acid Hydrolysis of Protected Aminoacyl Saponin **32***

1. In a 50-mL round-bottomed flask, the fully protected truncated saponin **32** (68 mg, 36.6 μmol, 1.0 equiv.) is dissolved in THF/EtOH (1:1) (20 mL), then 10% (dry basis) Pd/C, wet Degussa type E101 NE/W (390 mg, 0.18 mmol, 5.0 equiv.) is added.
2. The reaction mixture is stirred under an atmosphere of H_2 (50 psi) for 24 h at rt using a high-pressure bomb reactor (*see* **Note 17**).

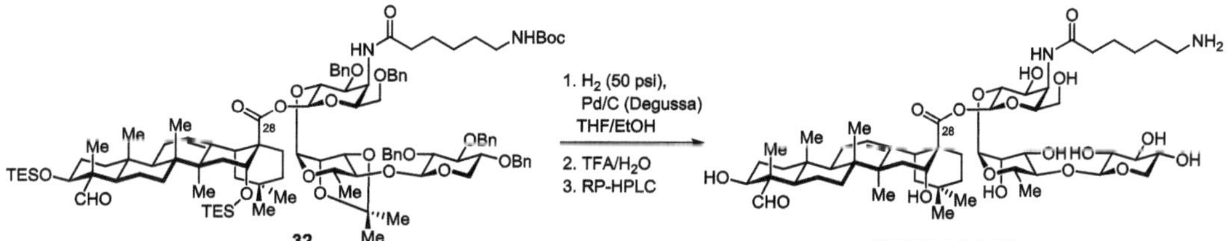

Fig. 15 Global deprotection of truncated aminoacylated saponin precursor lacking branched trisaccharide domain (**34**)

3. The suspension is filtered through a 0.45 μm nylon syringe filter, washed with MeOH (3 × 30 mL) and concentrated. Successful debenzylation is assessed by the disappearance of aromatic resonances by ^{1}H-NMR in methanol-d_4.
4. In a 25-mL round-bottomed flask, the resulting crude mixture is dissolved in a precooled (0 °C) solution of TFA/water (3:1) (8 mL).
5. The reaction mixture is stirred for 2 h at 0 °C and then concentrated under high vacuum at 0 °C to give a white solid residue.
6. This crude product is dissolved in water/MeCN (4:1) (20 mL) and purified by RP-HPLC using a linear gradient of 30 → 70% MeCN in water (0.05 vol% TFA) over 15 min. The fully deprotected, truncated saponin **34** (SQS-1-0-5-11) elutes as a main, single peak and is obtained as a fluffy white solid (28 mg, 74%) after lyophilization.

3.7 Late-Stage Acylation of Acyl Chain Domain Amine to form Fully Elaborated Saponins 3 (SQS-0-0-5-18) and 4 (SQS-1-0-5-18)

*3.7.1 Synthesis of Fully Elaborated Saponin **3**, SQS-0-0-5-18 (Fig. 16) by Selective 4-Iodobenzoylation of Free Amine in Aminoacyl Saponin **33***

1. In a 10-mL round-bottomed flask equipped with a rubber septum fitted with an Ar inlet needle, amine-terminating saponin **33** (9.0 mg, 6.0 μmol, 1.0 equiv.) is dissolved in DMF (2.0 mL) and Et_3N (50 μL, 0.36 mmol, 60 equiv.) is injected via gas-tight syringe.
2. The mixture is stirred for 50 min at rt and commercially available *N*-succinimidyl 4-iodobenzoate (20 mg, 60 μmol, 10 equiv.), dissolved in DMF (0.6 mL) under Ar, is then added dropwise via syringe from a 5-mL pear-shaped flask equipped with a rubber septum.
3. The reaction mixture is stirred for 1 h at rt, diluted with water/MeCN (4:1) (10 mL), and directly purified by RP-HPLC using a linear gradient of 20 → 70% MeCN in water over 30 min.
4. The fraction corresponding to the peak containing the desired product, as assessed by mass spectrometry, is collected and lyophilized to dryness to afford the fully elaborated saponin **3** (SQS-0-0-5-18) (5.4 mg, 52%) as a white powder.

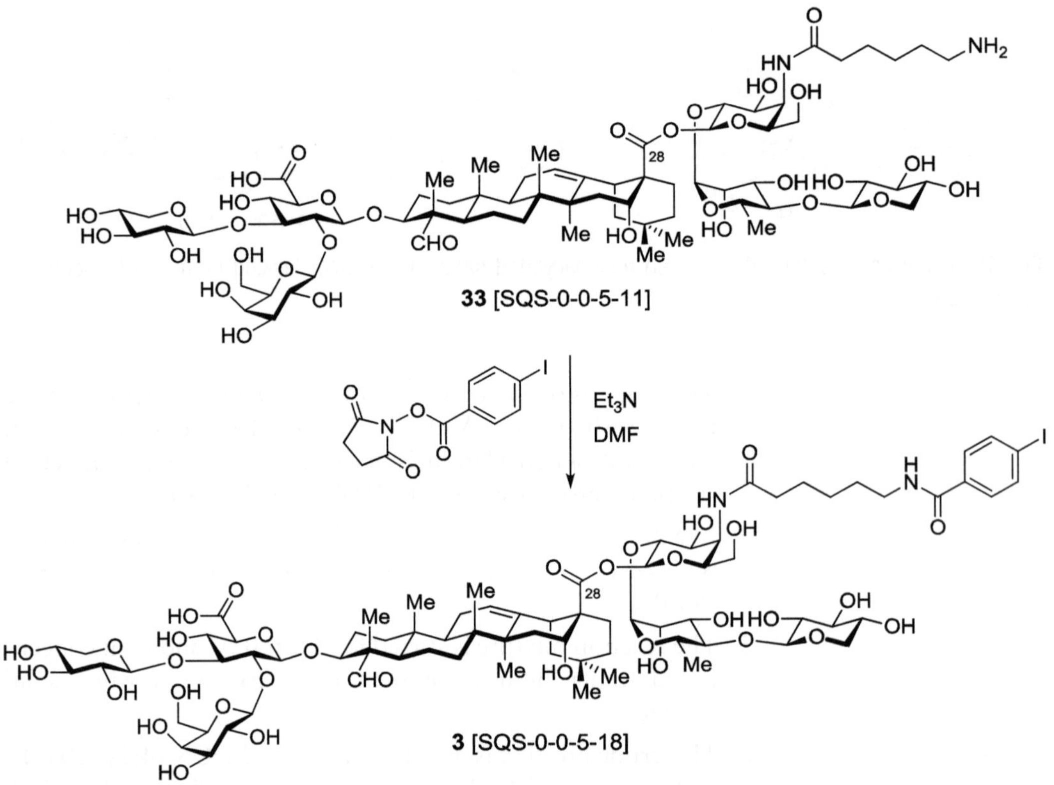

Fig. 16 4-Iodobenzoylation of free amine in branched trisaccharide–triterpene–linear trisaccharide–acyl chain saponin precursor (**3**, SQS-0-0-5-18)

*3.7.2 Synthesis of Fully Elaborated Saponin **4**, SQS-1-0-5-18 (Fig 17), Lacking the Branched Trisaccharide Domain, by Selective 4-Iodobenzoylation of Free Amine in Aminoacyl Saponin **34***

1. In a 5-mL pear-shaped flask equipped with a rubber septum fitted with an Ar inlet needle, amine-terminating truncated saponin **34** (2.1 mg, 2.0 μmol, 1.0 equiv.) is dissolved in DMF (0.4 mL). Et_3N (11 μL, 0.08 mmol, 40 equiv.) is injected followed by dropwise addition of a solution of *N*-succinimidyl 4-iodobenzoate (4.0 mg, 10 μmol, 5.8 equiv.) in DMF (0.2 mL) under Ar via gas-tight syringe.
2. The reaction mixture is stirred for 2 h at rt, then diluted with 30% MeCN/water (2.3 mL), and directly purified by RP-HPLC using a linear gradient of 30→70% MeCN in water (0.05 vol% TFA) over 15 min.
3. The fully elaborated, truncated saponin **4** (SQS-1-0-5-18) (1.7 mg, 67%) is obtained as a white powder after lyophilization.

4 Notes

1. Care must be taken to avoid excessive foaming and bumping. Water bath should be kept at 35 °C and pressure decreased slowly.

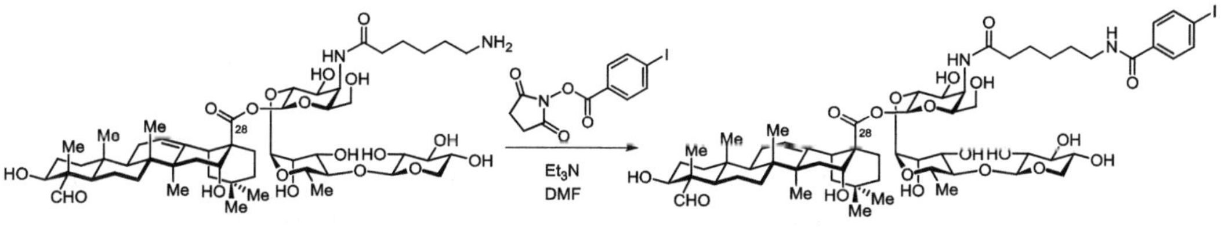

Fig. 17 4-Iodobenzoylation of free amine in triterpene–linear trisaccharide–acyl chain saponin precursor (**4**, SQS-1-0-5-18)

2. At this point, compare crude ^{1}H-NMR in methanol-d_4 with reference spectrum [15]. Since there is significant variability present in the *Quillaja* bark extracts, some extracts do not contain any of the desired prosapogenin. The best supplier (Brenntag) is mentioned in the Materials section.
3. The last extra addition of TESOTf is situation-dependent and only required if the reaction is still incomplete after the first 4 days.
4. The extra addition of CbzCl after the first 6 h depends on the progress of the reaction in each particular case. When purifying by silica gel chromatography, elution with benzene/EtOAc (100:0 to 24:1) can also be considered.
5. Heating should be done slowly to avoid a foam-over when approaching reflux.
6. Quillaic acid triterpene product is ~80% pure. High purity is achieved after allylation reaction.
7. *Caution*: sodium hydride reacts violently with water.
8. *Caution*: exothermic reaction.
9. *Caution*: sodium azide is a toxic, hazardous substance that should not be acidified to avoid poisonous, explosive hydrazoic acid (HN_3). The reaction should be carried out behind a blast shield due to risk of explosion of sodium azide when heated near its decomposition temperature (300 °C).
10. This degassing technique involves freezing the solvent under liquid nitrogen, evacuating the headspace for 4–5 min, and letting the solvent thaw under static vacuum, thereby allowing any gas bubbles trapped in the solvent to escape into the headspace of the flask. After the last cycle, the flask is refilled with Ar.
11. In absence of Et$_3$N, prolonged chromatography on silica gel when purifying glycosyl trichloroacetimidates leads to progressive hydrolysis of the product.
12. *Caution*: selenium compounds are highly toxic and have an unpleasant odor. Phenylselenol itself is extremely noxius. The in situ preparation of phenylselenol solution by reduction of diphenyldiselenide circumvents the need to handle phenylselenol

directly, but manipulation of the selenide-containing solution that will be added to the reaction flask is necessary. Care should be taken when handling selenium reagents and all manipulations should be performed in a fumehood wearing protective gloves and safety glasses, including weighing of the diphenyldiselenide starting material. A bleach solution should be prepared in advance to treat all used glassware and possibly early column fractions as well, to oxidize any remaining trace selenides. Bleach solution should also be placed in the solvent trap of the rotary evaporator, which should be thoroughly cleaned after use and ideally contained within the fumehood.

13. Another alternative experimental procedure to perform this azide reduction step to give the corresponding saponin amine is the treatment of the starting material in Et_3N with hydrogen sulfide (gas) as follows. An excess of hydrogen sulfide from a steel cylinder is bubbled via cannula (long steel needle) through an ice-cooled solution of the saponin azide (~45 mg, ~0.015 mmol, 1.0 equiv.) in pyridine/Et_3N (3.5:1) (4.5 mL) for 2 min. Vent needle and cannula are removed from septum, which is sealed with Teflon tape and parafilm, and the reaction mixture is stirred overnight at rt. The dark green solution is then purged of excess hydrogen sulfide with a stream of nitrogen, and the resulting light-orange solution is concentrated by rotary evaporation. Purification of the residue by silica gel chromatography (hexanes/EtOAc, 1.0 vol% Et_3N) yields the desired saponin amine product (~40 mg, 80–90 % yield).
14. After quenching the reaction with water, the mixture can also be directly concentrated by rotary evaporation without the need for performing the described aqueous work-up.
15. Elution with 9:1 to 5:1 benzene/EtOAc (0.5 vol% Et_3N) can also be used for the silica gel chromatography purification.
16. *Caution*: hydrogenolysis reactions pose a significant fire hazard. Caution should be taken when handling flammable palladium on carbon as well as hydrogen gas, which increases the risk of explosion.
17. In similar saponin triterpene variants lacking the branched trisaccharide domain, hydrogenolysis under hydrogen atmosphere at balloon pressure for 12 h is sufficient to provide the corresponding debenzylated products.

Acknowledgements

Dedicated to the memory of our mentor and colleague, Professor David Y. Gin (1967–2011). We thank Dr. George Sukenick, Rong Wang, Dr. Hui Liu, Hui Fang, and Dr. Sylvi Rusli (MSKCC) for expert mass spectral analyses. A. F.-T. thanks the Spanish Ministry of Education (ME–Fulbright postdoctoral fellowship) and the European Commission (Marie Curie Individual Fellowship) for postdoctoral funding. Financial support from the NIH (R01 AI085622 to D. Y. G., R01 GM058833 to D. S. T. and D. Y. G., and P30 CA008748 to C. B. Thompson), William and Alice Goodwin and the Commonwealth Foundation for Cancer Research, and the MSKCC Center for Experimental Therapeutics is gratefully acknowledged.

References

1. Kensil CR, Patel U, Lennick M, Marciani D (1991) Separation and characterization of saponins with adjuvant activity from *Quillaja saponaria* Molina cortex. J Immunol 146:431–437
2. Ragupathi G, Gardner JR, Livingston PO, Gin DY (2011) Natural and synthetic saponin adjuvant QS-21 for vaccines against cancer. Expert Rev Vaccines 10:463–470
3. RTS,S Clinical Trials Partnership (2015) Efficacy and safety of RTS, S/AS01 malaria vaccine with or without a booster dose in infants and children in Africa: final results of a phase 3, individually randomised, controlled trial. Lancet 386:31–45
4. Lal H, Cunningham AL, Godeaux O, Chlibek R, Diez-Domingo J, Hwang SJ, Levin MJ, McElhaney JE, Poder A, Puig-Barberà J, Vesikari T, Watanabe D, Weckx L, Zahaf T, Heineman TC, ZOE-50 Study Group (2015) Efficacy of an adjuvanted herpes zoster subunit vaccine in older adults. N Engl J Med 372:2087–2096
5. Wang P, Kim YJ, Navarro-Villalobos M, Rohde BD, Gin DY (2005) Synthesis of the potent immunostimulatory adjuvant QS-21A. J Am Chem Soc 127:3256–3257
6. Kim YJ, Wang P, Navarro-Villalobos M, Rohde BD, Derryberry J, Gin DY (2006) Synthetic studies of complex immunostimulants from *Quillaja saponaria*: synthesis of the potent clinical immunoadjuvant QS-21A_{api}. J Am Chem Soc 128:11906–11915
7. Deng K, Adams MM, Damani P, Livingston PO, Ragupathi G, Gin DY (2008) Synthesis of QS-21-xylose: establishment of the immunopotentiating activity of synthetic QS-21 adjuvant with a melanoma vaccine. Angew Chem Int Ed 47:6395–6398
8. Deng K, Adams MM, Gin DY (2008) Synthesis and structure verification of the vaccine adjuvant QS-7-Api. Synthetic access to homogeneous Quillaja saponaria immunostimulants. J Am Chem Soc 130:5860–5861
9. Adams MM, Damani P, Perl N, Won A, Hong F, Livingston PO, Ragupathi G, Gin DY (2010) Design and synthesis of potent *Quillaja* saponin vaccine adjuvants. J Am Chem Soc 132:1939–1945
10. Chea EK, Fernández-Tejada A, Damani P, Adams MM, Gardner JR, Livingston PO, Ragupathi G, Gin DY (2012) Synthesis and preclinical evaluation of QS-21 variants leading to simplified vaccine adjuvants and mechanistic probes. J Am Chem Soc 134:13448–13457
11. Fernández-Tejada A, Chea EK, George C, Pillarsetty N, Gardner JR, Livingston PO, Ragupathi G, Lewis JS, Tan DS, Gin DY (2014) Development of a minimal saponin vaccine adjuvant based on QS-21. Nat Chem 6:635–643
12. Fernández-Tejada A, Chea EK, George C, Gardner JR, Livingston PO, Ragupathi G, Tan DS, Gin DY (2014) Design, synthesis, and immunologic evaluation of vaccine adjuvant conjugates based on QS-21 and tucaresol. Bioorg Med Chem 22:5917–5923
13. Fernández-Tejada A, Tan DS, Gin DY (2015) Versatile strategy for the divergent synthesis of linear oligosaccharide domain variants of *Quillaja* saponin vaccine adjuvants. Chem Commun 51:13949–13952
14. Walkowicz WE, Fernández-Tejada A, George C, Corzana F, Jiménez-Barbero J, Ragupathi G, Tan DS, Gin DY (2016) *Quillaja* saponin variants with central glycosidic linkage modifications exhibit distinct conformations and adjuvant activities. Chem Sci 7:2371–2380
15. Guo S, Kenne L, Lundgren LN, Rönnberg B, Sundquist BG (1998) Triterpenoid saponins from *Quillaja saponaria*. Phytochemistry 48:175–180

Chapter 5

QS-21 Adjuvant: Laboratory-Scale Purification Method and Formulation Into Liposomes

Livia Brunner, Christophe Barnier-Quer, and Nicolas Collin

Abstract

QS-21, a saponin extracted from the tree *Quillaja saponaria* Molina, is a vaccine adjuvant which has been shown to elicit robust antibody and cell-mediated immune responses in a variety of preclinical and clinical studies [1]. Its purification from the natural source is a lengthy and difficult process. The commercially available saponin mixture Quil-A® is a fraction of the bark extract containing a variety of saponins, including QS-21. In order to facilitate access to QS-21 at laboratory-scale amounts, we propose here a method of purification of QS-21 starting from Quil-A®. In addition, we describe a protocol to appropriately formulate QS-21 into cholesterol-containing, neutral liposomes which are known to decrease QS-21's hemolytic activity while retaining the adjuvant effect. Methods for the physicochemical characterization of purified QS-21 and of the QS-21/liposome formulations are also described.

Key words QS-21, Saponin, Vaccine adjuvant

1 Introduction

The adjuvant effect of extracts of plants from the genus Saponaria has been known for more than 90 years [2]. In particular, bark extracts of the South American tree *Quillaja Saponaria* (QS) Molina have been prepared by Dalsgaard and used as adjuvants in veterinary vaccines [3]. Brenntag Biosector (Frederikssund, Denmark) further developed and validated a process for the preparation of Quil-A®, a fraction of the bark extract containing various saponins. However, Quil-A® has been shown to be too reactogenic for inclusion in human prophylactic vaccines, and subsequent efforts were made to further purify the mixture. In 1991, Kensil et al. [4] described the successful isolation of individual saponin fractions. The saponin fractions named QS-7, QS-17, QS-18, and QS-21 all proved to display strong adjuvanticity. QS-17 and QS-18, the most abundant saponin in Quil-A®, were shown to be highly reactogenic in mice, however QS-7 and QS-21 were both less reactogenic while maintaining adjuvant properties. As QS-21 was more

Christopher B. Fox (ed.), *Vaccine Adjuvants: Methods and Protocols*, Methods in Molecular Biology, vol. 1494,
DOI 10.1007/978-1-4939-6445-1_5, © Springer Science+Business Media New York 2017

concentrated than QS-7 in the *Quillaja Saponaria* extracts, it was selected for further development as vaccine adjuvant.

QS-21 is currently being tested in various clinical studies on adjuvanted vaccines. In July 2015, the European Medicines Agency's Committee for Medicinal Products for Human Use gave a positive scientific opinion for the malaria vaccine Mosquirix® for use in children (6 weeks to 17 months old) in areas where malaria is endemic [5]. Mosquirix™, developed by GlaxoSmithKline, and also known as RTS,S, contains the AS01 adjuvant which is a combination of QS-21 saponin together with monophosphoryl lipid A and liposomes. Other vaccines containing QS-21 are currently being evaluated against cancer, HIV, and Alzheimer's [1].

The use of QS-21 poses certain challenges such as the difficulty of extraction and purification from its natural source and an associated low yield [4, 6, 7], hemolytic properties resulting in a dose-limiting toxicity [4, 8], an instability to hydrolysis at physiological pH [9], and mechanism of action not yet elucidated.

We propose here a laboratory-scale method to isolate QS-21 from the commercially available Quil-A®, with equipment and resources which are accessible by a large number of research groups. The yield of QS-21 resulting from this method, with respect to the starting amount of Quil-A®, is about five times higher than that previously reported in the literature [4, 6]. We also propose a procedure for the preparation of liposomes (containing cholesterol) and their formulation with QS-21 in order to neutralize the hemolytic effect of the saponin. It has been described that saponins bind to cholesterol in membrane lipid bilayers of cells including erythrocytes, resulting in the formation of pores [10–13] and subsequent hemolysis. Liposomes containing cholesterol have the potential to abolish the hemolytic effect of QS-21 while retaining the adjuvant effect [14, 15]. In addition, incorporation of QS-21 in the membrane of liposomes protects the saponin from hydrolysis at physiological pH [15]. Finally, in light of the importance of performing systematic quality control of adjuvant formulations before their use in preclinical models, we provide analytical methods for the characterization of QS-21 and its liposomal formulation.

2 Materials

2.1 Preliminary Purification of QS-21 by Liquid Chromatography (LC) on Silica Gel

1. Rotary evaporator.
2. Nitrogen canister with manometer and pressure regulator.
3. Glass column (30 × 460 mm) with sintered glass filter and two-way plastic stopper at the bottom.
4. Glass adaptor with stopper and tubing to connect the top of the column to the nitrogen bottle.
5. 23-mL glass tubes (13 × 160 mm) to collect fractions (*see* **Note 1**).

6. Quil-A® (Brenntag Biosector).
7. Silica gel (particle size 220–240 mesh).
8. Sand (Merck).
9. Eluent: $CHCl_3/MeOH/H_2O/CH_3COOH$ 270:139:25:1 v/v/v/v; in a 2 L glass cylinder, add 640 mL of methanol (MeOH) to 1240 mL of chloroform ($CHCl_3$), pour into a 2 L glass bottle, close the bottle, and hand shake until homogeneous. In a 200 mL glass cylinder, add 40 mL of ultrapure water (H_2O), then 4.6 mL of acetic acid (CH_3COOH) measured with a graduated glass pipette, add H_2O up to 120 mL, and hand shake. Add the CH_3COOH/H_2O solution to the $MeOH/CHCl_3$ solution, hand shake until homogeneous (*see* **Note 2**).

2.2 Purification of QS-21 by Preparative High Pressure Liquid Chromatography (HPLC)

1. HPLC (Waters) composed of two pumps, pump control module, manual injector, UV absorbance detector, 5 mL injection loop, and Empower™ software.
2. C18 column of 21.2 × 250 mm with particle size 10 μm and pore size 100 A° (Interchim).
3. Eluents: A) 0.1 % trifluoroacetic acid (TFA) in H_2O, B) 0.1 % TFA in HPLC-S gradient grade acetonitrile (CH_3CN).

2.3 Preparation of Neutral Liposomes

1. 10 mL Thermobarrel extruder (Northern Lipids).
2. Heating circulator with water bath (Julabo).
3. Drain disks (Whatman).
4. Polycarbonate filter membranes with pores of 0.4 μm, 0.2 μm and 0.1 μm (Whatman).
5. Rotary evaporator.
6. Nitrogen canister of 200 bar with gas regulator (Linde).
7. 1,2-dioleyl-sn-glycero-3-phosphocholine (DOPC) (Avanti Polar Lipids) stock solution: 40 mg/mL DOPC in $CHCl_3$.
8. Cholesterol stock solution: 10 mg/mL cholesterol in $CHCl_3$.
9. Dulbecco's PBS 1×, without Ca^{2+} and Mg^{2+} pH 7.0–7.3 (DPBS −/−).

2.4 Quality Control

1. Thin Layer Chromatography (TLC) plates (Merck, Kieselgel 60 Alufolien 20 × 20 cm).
2. TLC glass development chamber.
3. Glass capillaries.
4. Hair dryer.
5. Developing agent: $CHCl_3/MeOH/H_2O$ 60/40/10 v/v/v.
6. Revealing agent: 0.1 % orcinol in 5 % concentrated sulfuric acid (H_2SO_4)/EtOH.

7. HPLC (Waters) composed of two pumps, pump control module, manual injector, UV absorbance detector, 50 µL injection loop, and Empower™ software.
8. C18 column of 4.6 × 100 mm with particle size 3.5 µm and pore size 300 A° (Waters, XBridge BEH300).
9. Eluents: (a) 0.1 % TFA in H_2O, (b) 0.1 % TFA in CH_3CN.
10. Micromass QTOF Ultima (Waters), ionization modes: positive and negative electrospray, infusion of 20 µL/min, sample dilution in appropriate eluent to 0.1 mg/ml (just before injection).
11. Positive mode eluent: H_2O/CH_3CN/formic acid (HCOOH) 49.9/50/0.1 v/v/v.
12. Negative mode eluent: H_2O/CH_3CN 59/50 v/v, infusion: 20 µL/min, sample dilution: 0.1 mg/mL (just before injection).
13. Horizontal shaker for 96-well plate.
14. Plate reader for UV-visible detection (TECAN, Sunrise).
15. Minicentrifuge (e.g., VWR Galaxy Ministar, max speed 2000 × *g*).
16. Centrifuge for 96-well plates.
17. U-bottomed 96-well plates.
18. Flat-bottomed 96-well plates.
19. Sheep blood.
20. Water for injection (WFI).
21. Dynamic light scattering particle sizer (e.g., Malvern ZetaSizer® Nano ZS).
22. Disposable microcuvettes (Malvern).
23. Dulbecco's PBS without Ca^{2+} and Mg^{2+} pH 7.0–7.3 (DPBS −/−).
24. Transmission electron microscopy (TEM) microscope (FEI, Tecnai Spirit-Bio).
25. Glow discharge device.
26. Carbon-coated cupper grids 400 mesh (Canemco-Marivac).
27. TEM staining solution: 2 % (w/v) Uranyl acetate dehydrate.
28. Pliers (Dumont).

3 Methods

3.1 Preliminary Purification of QS-21 by Liquid Chromatography (LC) on Silica Gel

1. Weigh 50 g of silica gel in a 500 mL glass beaker, add 100 mL of the $CHCl_3/MeOH/H_2O/CH_3COOH$ eluent (prepared as described in Subheading 2), and hand shake until homogeneous.
2. Pour the suspension into the 30 × 460 mm glass column, leaving the two ways stopper open at the bottom, collect the eluent into a recipient and discard the flow-through.

Recover the rest of silica gel from the 500 mL beaker with about 50 mL of fresh eluent, pour into the column, and discard the flow-through. Wash carefully silica out of the walls of the column with fresh eluent using a Pasteur pipette, then fill column up with fresh eluent.

3. With the two ways bottom stopper always open, apply pressure from the nitrogen bottle until the silica level does not go down any more (*see* **Note 3**). The silica should fill the glass column up to 15.5 cm from the sintered glass filter, and the top of the silica layer should be flat.
4. Having about 10 cm of eluent above the top of the silica layer, add sand slowly to form a layer of about 5–8 mm on top of the silica column (*see* **Note 4**). Using nitrogen pressure, push down the eluent until its level is just above the top of the sand layer. Let about 3–4 mL of eluent flow down by gravity. When the level of the eluent is in the sand layer, close the two ways stopper at the bottom of the glass column. The column is now ready to be loaded with the sample to be purified.
5. Weigh 800 mg of Quil-A® in a glass tube. Add 2 mL of eluent and vortex three times for 10 s, or until obtaining a viscous, dark yellow solution. Add this solution on top of the sand layer with a 5 mL glass pipette by allowing the mixture to flow down along the walls of the column, as close as possible to the top of the sand layer. Open the two ways stopper at the bottom of the glass column and leave it open for the rest of the manipulation.
6. Recover the rest of sample from the glass tube with 0.5 mL of fresh eluent and pour carefully into the column as just described. Let the sample go through the sand layer and adsorb on top of the silica layer. A yellow ring should be visible just under the sand layer.
7. Make sure that there is no sample solution left on the walls of the column by washing these walls twice with 2 mL of eluent, using a long-stem Pasteur pipette. Wait for all the eluent to flow under the sand layer, then add five times 2 mL of eluent with a long-stem Pasteur pipette. Add gently more eluent to fill the column without destroying the sand layer.
8. Collect the first 100 mL in a beaker by gravity (without applying pressure), then 200 mL with pressure from nitrogen bottle at a flow rate of 4–5 mL/min (*see* **Note 5**). After having collected these 300 mL, start collecting fractions of 22 mL using glass tubes, at the same flow rate. QS-21 is expected to be found in fractions 8–14.
9. Spot a QS-21 reference (*see* **Note 6**) and the fractions on the TLC plate, dip the bottom of the plate into the developing agent (prepared as described in Subheading 2), allow the

migration, dry the plate with a hair-dryer at low heat, dip the plate completely in the revealing agent (prepared as described in Subheading 2), retrieve it and dry with the hair dryer at high heat until brown or black spots appear on the plate. Select the fractions that have a similar profile to that of the QS21 and less contaminants (should be fractions 9–13).

10. Pool the fractions containing QS-21 in a 200-mL glass flask (one neck, round bottom) and recover the residues by washing tubes with 2 mL of MeOH. Evaporate using a rotary evaporator at 30 mbar, setting the water bath at 25 °C. Stop evaporation when no more condensation of solvent in the collecting flask is visible. An aqueous residue should remain in the flask (*see* **Note 7**).
11. Transfer the aqueous residue from the flask into a preweighed 15 mL polypropylene tube. Wash the flask twice with 1 mL of ultrapure water and add into the tube. Proceed with the freeze-drying during at least 48 h at –90 °C and 50–100 μbar. Retrieve the tube from the freeze-dryer and weigh. Approximately 55–60 mg of white powder should be recovered (*see* **Note 8**). Store at 2–8 °C until proceeding with next steps.

3.2 Purification of QS-21 by Preparative HPLC

1. Dissolve the freeze-dried product into 1 mL of CH_3CN/H_2O 45/55 v/v and vortex 10 s (*see* **Note 9**).
2. Inject into the preparative HPLC system (with 21.2×250 mm column, as described in Subheading 2), in two injections of 0.5 mL each. Apply the following gradient (using eluent A and B as described in Subheading 2): 5–45% of eluent B in 3 min, then 45–53% in 20 min, then 100% for 6 min, and back to 5%. Apply the following settings during the procedure: flow rate: 10 mL/min, UV detection at 210 or 220 nm, column temperature: 20–22 °C. Start collecting fractions at around 15.5 min and stop at around 18.5 min before appearance of the "shoulder" at the end of the peak (Fig. 1) using preweighed tubes.
3. Pool the fractions collected during both injections. Freeze-dry at least 48 h at -90 °C and 50-100 μbar. Weigh the freeze-dried product. Approximately 15–18 mg of white powder should be recovered (*see* **Note 10**). Store at 2–8 °C.
4. Dissolve the powder into Dulbecco's PBS without Ca^{2+} and Mg^{2+} (pH 7.0–7.3) at 1 mg/mL (*see* **Note 11**) and aliquot into polypropylene tubes of desired volume. Perform quality control analyses (as described in Subheading 3.3 below) and store at –20 °C until use.

3.3 Quality Control of Purified QS-21

1. TLC: spot QuilA®, a QS-21 reference (*see* **Note 6**) and the purified QS-21 (all samples at 1 mg/mL in CH_3CN/H_2O 30/70 v/v) on the TLC plate, dip the bottom of the

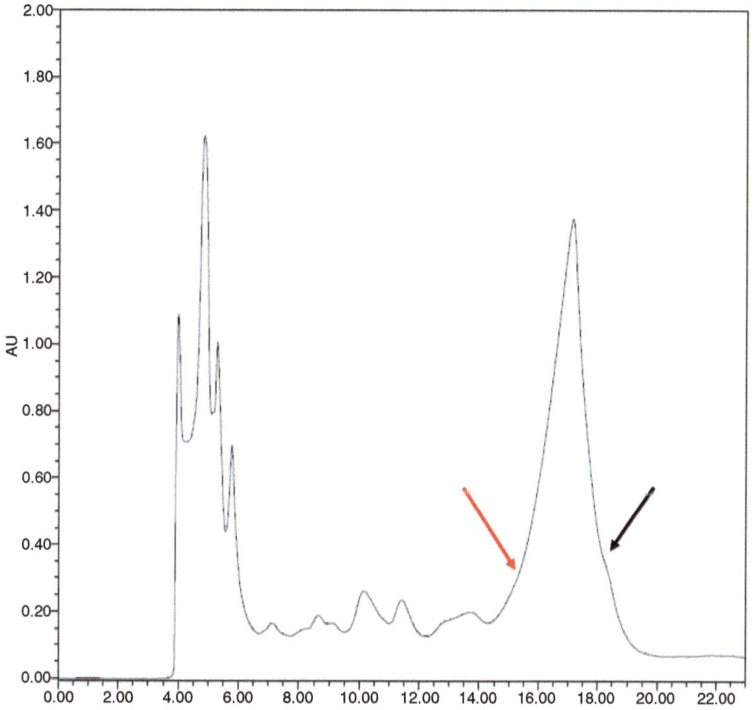

Fig. 1 Preparative HPLC chromatogram of QS-21 after purification on silica gel column. *Red* (left) and *black* (right) *arrows* indicate the time to respectively start and stop the collection of fractions

plate into the developing agent ($CHCl_3$/MeOH/H_2O 60/40/10 v/v/v), allow the migration, dry the plate with a hair-dryer at low heat, dip the plate completely in the revealing agent (0.1 % orcinol in 5 % H_2SO_4-EtOH), retrieve it, and dry with the hair dryer at high heat until brown or black spots appear on the plate.

2. Analytical HPLC: weigh 0.5 mg of freeze-dried product into a polypropylene tube, dissolve with 500 μL of CH_3CN/H_2O (30/70 v/v) and vortex for a few seconds to obtain a clear, foaming solution. Inject 20 μL of the solution and elute with the following gradient of eluent B: 30–55 % in 15 min (flow rate 1 mL/min, UV detection at 210 or 220 nm). QS-21's peak should be detected at around 12 min (*see* **Note 12**) (Fig. 2).

3. Electrospray Ionization Time of Flight Mass Spectrometry (ESI-TOF-MS): weigh about 0.1 mg of freeze-dried product into a polypropylene tube, dissolve with CH_3CN/H_2O (50/50 v/v). Inject immediately into the mass spectrometer with negative mode, infusion at 20 μL/min, source temperature: 80 °C, voltage: 35 V (*see* **Note 13**). An example of a mass spectrum of purified QS-21 is shown in Fig. 3.

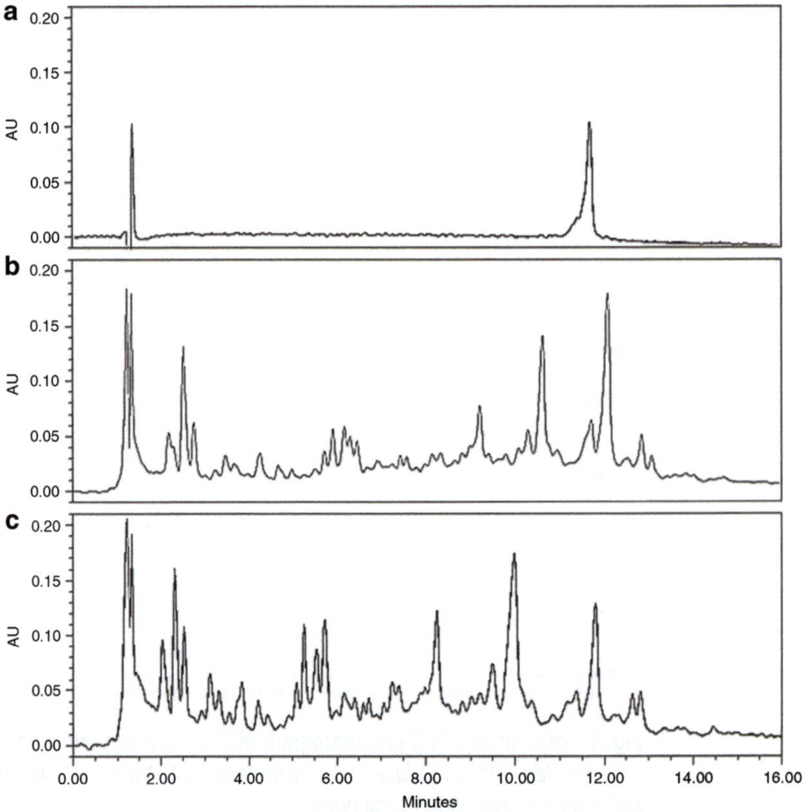

Fig. 2 A: QS-21 after preparative HPLC; B: QuilA®, spiked into the QS-21 sample used to obtain the chromatogram in A; C: QuilA®

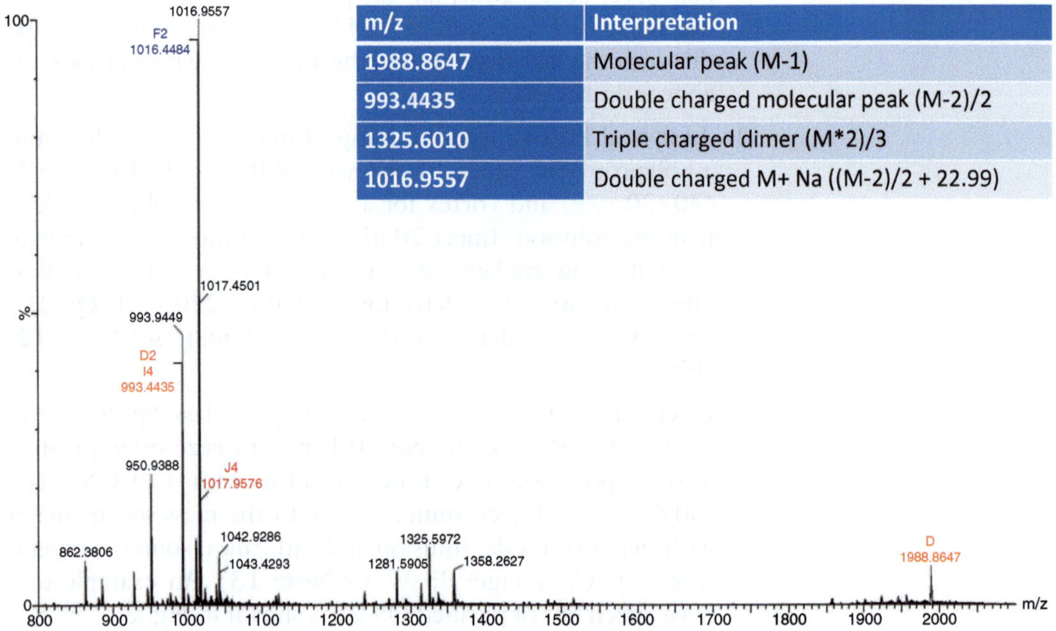

m/z	Interpretation
1988.8647	Molecular peak (M-1)
993.4435	Double charged molecular peak (M-2)/2
1325.6010	Triple charged dimer (M*2)/3
1016.9557	Double charged M+ Na ((M-2)/2 + 22.99)

Fig. 3 ESI-QTOF-MS of QS-21 after preparative HPLC, negative mode

3.4 Preparation of Cholesterol-Containing Neutral Liposomes

1. In a 50 mL glass round-bottomed flask, add 1 mL of the DOPC stock solution, 1 mL of the cholesterol stock solution and 2 mL of $CHCl_3$. Evaporate with the rotary evaporator, setting the water bath at 40 °C: start with a vacuum of 700 mbar and decrease the pressure slowly down to 50 mbar (*see* **Note 14**) to obtain a thin, transparent, homogeneous lipid film on the wall of the flask. The film can be stored at -20 °C up to 72 h before hydration.
2. Prewarm the DPBS -/- buffer at 40 °C. Transfer 4 mL of buffer into the flask containing the lipid film. Vortex 15 min or until all the film is resuspended. Incubate for 30 min at room temperature. During this time, set up the extruder as described in the following step.
3. Assemble the extruder according to the manual instructions [16] and insert a drain disk and a polycarbonate filter of pore size of 0.40 μm. Connect the water bath to the thermobarrel of the extruder and set the temperature at 40 °C.
4. Prewet the filter with one drop of buffer and insert the hydrated lipid film in the thermobarrel and apply pressure slowly and gradually. Stop increasing pressure when the solution starts dropping from the outlet tube, without going over 500 psi as indicated by the manometer on the regulator of the nitrogen bottle. Then adjust the pressure to maintain a dropwise flow and collect the output liquid in a 12-mL polypropylene tube.
5. When all buffer is ejected from the system, reintroduce the collected liposome suspension in the extruder and repeat the manipulation. Perform 10 cycles of extrusion with the 0.4 μm filter, replace the 0.4 μm filter with a 0.2 μm filter and perform 10 cycles of extrusion with the 0.2 μm filter, replace the 0.2 μm filter with a 0.1 μm filter and perform 10 cycles of extrusion with the 0.1 μm filter (*see* **Note 15**).
6. Collect the final suspension into a 12-mL polypropylene tube then filter with a 0.22 μm membrane into another polypropylene tube (*see* **Note 16**). Flush the tube with nitrogen (*see* **Note 17**) and store at 4 °C up to six months. Clean the extruder (*see* **Note 18**).

3.5 Quality Control of Cholesterol-Containing Neutral Liposomes

1. Average particle size and polydispersity index (PdI): add 10 μL of liposomes to 90 μL of DPBS (-/-), vortex and transfer 70 μL of the mix into a micro cuvette for size measurement. Software parameters for the measurement are as follows: material—polystyrene latex, dispersant—water, temperature—25 °C, equilibration time—120 s, backscatter—173°, 3 measurements of 11 runs each. Expected average particle size of liposomes is between 80 and 160 nm and expected PdI lower than 0.2.

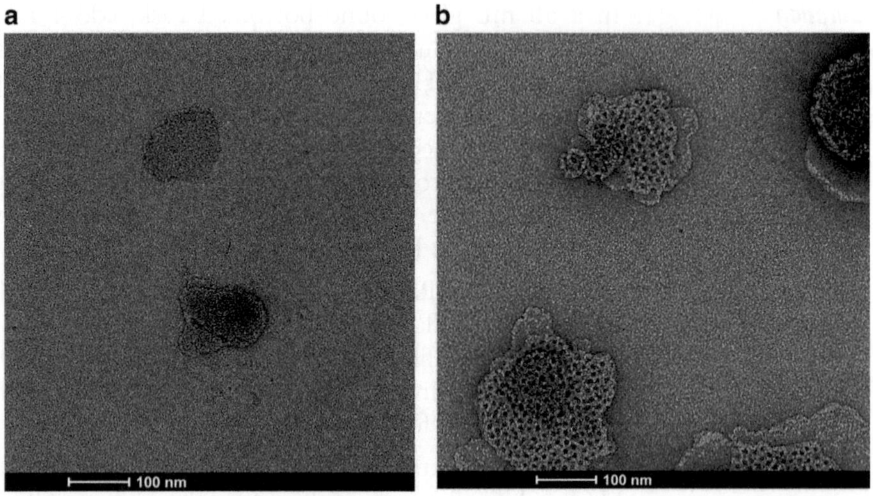

Fig. 4 Transmission Electron Microscopy image of A: liposomes five times diluted in water B: extemporaneous mixture of liposome and QS-21, cholesterol/QS-21 ratio of 1:2 w/w. = 2.6/1 mol/mol. Negative staining with 2 % uranyl acetate

2. Transmission electron microscopy by negative staining with 2 % uranyl acetate: adsorb the sample on glow-discharged, carbon-coated, cupper grids, during 30 s. Rinse the surplus by dipping the grid in Milli-Q water during 1–2 min. Dry the grids with filter paper, then place the grid over a drop of 2 % (w/v) aqueous uranyl acetate for exactly 30 s. Remove the surplus of uranyl acetate solution with a filter paper, and analyze samples at an acceleration voltage of 80 kV under low-dose conditions and a magnification of 43,000. Digital images are recorded on an Eagle CCD camera using FEI TIA software (Fig. 4).

3.6 Formulation of QS-21 with Cholesterol-Containing Neutral Liposomes

1. Bring the liposome suspension (prepared as described in Subheading 3.3) from 4 °C to room temperature and bring the QS-21 solution (1 mg/mL in DPBS −/−, prepared as described in Subheadings 3.1 and 3.2) from −20 °C to room temperature.
2. Add 100 μL of the liposome suspension and 100 μL of the QS-21 solution into a polypropylene tube. Invert the tube gently five times (vortexing is not required).

3.7 Quality Control of QS-21/Liposome Formulation

1. Average particle size and PdI: proceed as described in **step 1** of Subheading 3.5 (*see* **Note 19**).
2. Transmission electron microscopy by negative staining with 2 % uranyl acetate: proceed as described in **step 2** of Subheading 3.5. A cage-like structure should be visible, similar to what is found for ImmunoStimulatory Complex (ISCOM) formulations of liposomes with QuilA® [12]

3. Hemolysis assay: add 200 µL of sheep blood to 1 mL of DPBS (−/−) in a polypropylene tube and invert the tube gently five times. Centrifuge with minicentrifuge at max speed for 10 s and discard the supernatant. Repeat two more times to obtain a clear supernatant.
4. Resuspend the erythrocyte pellet in 1 ml of DPBS (−/−) and transfer the suspension into a tube containing 11 mL DPBS (−/−). Store the suspension at 4 °C while preparing the 96-well plate (*see* below) but use it within 1 h.
5. For preparing plate, use a U-bottomed 96 ell plate, distribute 50 µL of DPBS (−/−) in all wells except for 6 wells (e.g., A7-A12) where 50 µL of WFI per well are added. In one column (e.g., column 1), add 100 µL of QS-21 in DPBS (−/−) solution at 0.2 mg/mL in DPBS −/− (e.g., well B1), 100 µL of one QS-21/liposome formulation to be tested with QS-21 at 0.2 mg/mL (e.g., well C1), 100 µL of a second QS21/ liposome formulation (e.g., in well D1) and so on.
6. Transfer 50 µL from all wells of column 1 (B1-H1) into the next column (B2-H2) with a multipipette, mixing 3 times up and down. Transfer 50 µL from column 2 to column 3 and so on until column 12, then discard the last 50 µL.
7. Shake plate for 10 min at room temperature in order to obtain a homogenous suspension. Add 50 µL per well of sheep erythrocytes suspension and incubate for 30 min at room temperature with shaking.
8. Centrifuge the plate at 1800 g, 20 °C, 5 min. In a flat-bottomed 96-well plate, distribute 250 µL EtOH per well. Transfer 50 µL of supernatant from the centrifuged plate into the plate containing ethanol, mix up and down 7 times with a multipipette and read absorbance of the plate at 412 nm (reference at 700 nm) shaking 30 s.
9. The average absorbance of water is the value for 100% lysis of red blood cells and the average absorbance of PBS is the value of 0% lysis. To calculate the % of lysis for the samples use the following formula: (absorbance of sample—absorbance of PBS)/absorbance of water × 100. Results can be displayed in a graph of % lysis of red blood cells as a function of QS-21 concentration in the formulation (Fig. 5).

3.8 Use of QS-21/ Liposome Formulation in Preclinical Studies

1. Add 300 µL of an antigen solution to 200 µL of the QS-21/ liposome formulation.
2. Use the final formulation within the following 6 h. As an example, 50 µL of formulation are recommended to be used for vaccination per mouse, by intramuscular route (*see* **Note 20**).

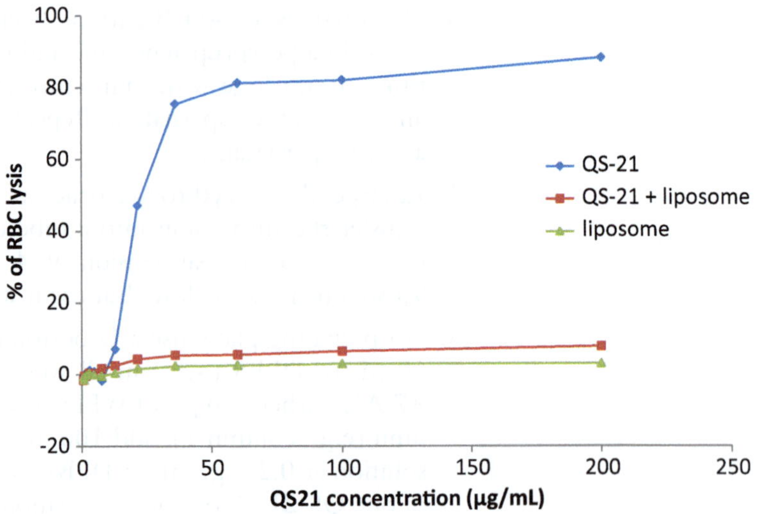

Fig. 5 Percent of red blood cell lysis with respect to water (100 % hemolysis) as a function of the concentration of QS-21 in the sample

4 Notes

1. To minimize the presence of endotoxin, we recommend that all the glassware is kept overnight in an oven at 190 °C before use.
2. Keep the bottle closed to avoid modification of the mixture by evaporation and water intake.
3. Packing of silica in the column may be facilitated by gently tapping on the column with a piece of rubber tube. Make sure that there is always enough eluent above the sedimentation of silica gel during all the manipulation, as the silica should never dry. The eluent will flow through, be collected in a recipient and discarded. It is recommended not to reuse it, as its composition changes during the manipulation.
4. Take care to have a layer of sand of homogeneous thickness. If some sand sticks to the walls of the column, wash it out with some eluent. Never let the level of eluent go below the layer of sand to avoid drying and cracking of the silica.
5. It is important to start the purification slowly, using only gravity, to obtain a good separation. To measure the flow rate, use a tube previously calibrated with 22 ml of water. Flow rate should be 4–5 mL/min.
6. A QS-21 reference can be made available upon request at our laboratory (Vaccine Formulation Laboratory, University of Lausanne, Switzerland).
7. This residue should be frozen with liquid nitrogen as soon as possible to minimize the time of QS-21 in acidic environment which could degrade the product.

8. This intermediate product can be checked by analytical HPLC as described in **step 2** of Subheading 3.3.
9. The freeze-dried product is soluble up to 60 mg/mL in this solvent.
10. The yield of QS-21 is around 2 % with respect to the weight of Quil-A®.
11. This solubilization process is well described in Ref. [17].
12. It is possible to confirm the presence of QS-21, by spiking the product purified as described in this method into a solution of Quil-A® and comparing the HPLC profile of Quil-A® before and after spiking (Fig. 2). An alternative quantification method by HPLC is described in Ref. [17].
13. This analysis can be run also in positive mode. In this case the sample is dissolved into H_2O/CH_3CN/formic acid (49.9:50:0.1 v/v/v). All other parameters are the same as for the analysis in negative mode.
14. During evaporation it is necessary to avoid formation of bubbles that would break the lipid film. If the film is not homogeneous, suspend it in 2 mL of $CHCl_3$ and repeat all the described steps.
15. The correct progress of the extrusion process can be monitored by measuring the average particle size (*see* **step 1** of Subheading 3.5) after each series of cycles on the same filter. Typically, the particle size should be 600–900 nm after 10 cycles on 0.4 μm filter, 140–160 nm after 0.2 μm filter and 80–120 nm after 0.1 μm filter. The extrusion process converts the Multi Lamellar Vesicles (MLVs), obtained by hydration and resuspension of the lipid film, into Small Unilamellar Vesicles (SUVs). Transmission electron microscopy indicates that the shape of these SUVs is not spherical but oblate and sometimes tubular.
16. At the end of the process 3.5 mL of liposome suspension are recovered. The process can be scaled up to obtain 8.5 mL of final suspension, starting with 10 mL of hydrated lipid film suspension. An alternative manufacturing method employs mini-extruders and is described on the web site http://www.avantilipids.com, *see* page about "Avanti Mini-Extruder".
17. Storage under nitrogen is recommended to avoid oxidation of double bonds in DOPC. It is recommended to place a sterile, 1000 μL pipette tip with 0.22 μm filter (e.g., ART 1000E, self-sealing barrier pipette tip) at the exit of the tubing that brings the nitrogen from the bottle to the tube to be flushed.
18. After disassembling the extruder, rinse all the parts with warm water. Rinse all metal parts with ethanol using a syringe. O rings and outlet tube must be immediately rinsed with demineralized water, then with ethanol 70 % (always rinse immediately the O-rings and outlet tube) using a syringe.

Finally, rinse all parts with demineralized water and let dry in a laminar flow hood.

19. No significant difference in the average particle size should be found with respect to the liposome without QS-21.
20. Administration routes other than intramuscular for this formulation have not been tested in our laboratory.

Acknowledgment

The authors thank Maude Marti Favre, Virginie Jakob, and Geraldine Frank for their excellent technical assistance.

References

1. https://clinicaltrials.gov/ ct2/results?term=QS-21&Search=Search.
2. Ragupathi G, Gardner JR, Livingston PO, Gin DY (2011) Natural and synthetic saponin adjuvant QS-21 for vaccines against cancer. Expert Rev Vaccines 10:463–470
3. Dalsgaard (1978) A study of the isolation and characterization of the saponin Quil-A®. Evaluation of its adjuvant activity, with a special reference to the application in the vaccination of cattle against foot-and-mouth disease. Acta Vet Scand Suppl 69:7–40
4. Kensil CR, Patel U, Lennick M, Marciani D (1991) Separation and characterization of saponins with adjuvant activity from *Quillaja Saponaria* Molina cortex. J Immunol 146:431–437
5. http://www.ema.europa.eu/ema/index.jsp?curl=pages/news_and_events/news/2015/07/news_detail_002376.jsp&mid=WC0b01ac058004d5c1.
6. Kensil CR (2001) Saponin adjuvant composition. US Patent 6231859 B1
7. Fernandez-Tejada A, Chea EK, George C, Gardner JR, Livingston PO, Ragupathi G, Tan DS, Gin DY (2014) Design, synthesis, and immunologic evaluation of vaccine adjuvant conjugates based on QS-21 and tucaresol. Bioorg Med Chem 22:5917–5923
8. Kensil CR, Kammer R (1998) QS-21: a water-soluble triterpene glycoside adjuvant. Expert Opin Investig Drugs 7:1475–1482
9. Cleland JL, Kensil CR, Lim A, Jacobsen NE, Basa L, Spellman M, Wheeler DA, Wu JY, Powell MF (1996) Isomerization and formulation stability of the vaccine adjuvant QS-21. J Pharm Sci 85:22–28
10. Lorent JH, Quetin-Leclercq J, Mingeot-Leclercq MP (2014) The amphiphilic nature of saponins and their effects on artificial and biological membranes and potential consequences for red blood and cancer cells. Org Biomol Chem 12:8803–8822
11. Myschik J, Lendemans DG, McBurney WT, Demana PH, Hook S, Rades T (2006) On the preparation, microscopic investigation and application of ISCOMs. Micron 37:724–734
12. Sanders MT, Brown LE, Deliyannis G, Pearse MJ (2005) ISCOM-based vaccines: the second decade. Immunol Cell Biol 83:119–128
13. Seeman P (1974) Ultrastructure of membrane lesions in immune lysis, osmotic lysis and drug-induced lysis. Fed Proc 33:2116–2124
14. Vandepapeliere P (2013) Vaccine composition comprising a saponin adjuvant-Patent EP 2364721 B1.
15. Garçon NM Friede M (2007) Vaccines containing a saponin and a sterol. Patent EP 0 955 059 B1
16. http://www.northernlipids.com/attachments/article/9/LIPEX%201.5%20and%2010%20mL%20Extruder%20Operating%20Manual%20version%201.2.0%20%282011%29.pdf
17. Kensil CR (2000) QS-21 adjuvant. In: Vaccine adjuvants: preparation methods and research protocols, Methods in Molecular Medicine, edited by O'HaganDT, Humana press, New Jersey

Chapter 6

Purification of an Immunoadjuvant Saponin Fraction from *Quillaja brasiliensis* Leaves by Reversed-Phase Silica Gel Chromatography

Anna C.A. Yendo, Fernanda de Costa, Carla Kauffmann, Juliane D. Fleck, Grace Gosmann, and Arthur G. Fett-Neto

Abstract

Saponins include a large variety of molecules that find several applications in pharmacology. The use of *Quillaja saponaria* saponins as immunological adjuvants in vaccines is of interest due to their capacity to stimulate both humoral and cellular responses. The congener species *Q. brasiliensis* has saponins with chemical similarities and adjuvant activity comparable to that of *Q. saponaria* fraction Quil-A®, with additional advantages of showing lower toxicity and reduced hemolytic activity. Here we describe in detail the methods for preparing the aqueous extract from *Q. brasiliensis* leaves, as well as the purification of the bioactive saponin fraction QB-90 using silica reversed-phase chromatography.

Key words Saponin, QB-90, Liquid chromatography, Aqueous extract, *Quillaja brasiliensis*, *Immunoadjuvant*

1 Introduction

Saponins are amphipathic molecules composed of a triterpenic or steroid backbone and glycoside chains, occurring in several families of dicotyledons. The diversity of structures found in plants is associated with several biological activities, including pharmacological applications such as antiplatelet, hypocholesterolemic, hypoglycemic, antibacterial, anti-inflammatory, and immunoadjuvant agents [1–5]. Although they can cause hemolysis by complexing plasma membrane sterols and increasing membrane permeability, the use of certain types of saponins in vaccines is interesting due to their capacity to augment immune responses against both intracellular and extracellular pathogens. In this context, several studies have been carried out in search of saponins with high immunogenicity and low hemolytic capacity.

Christopher B. Fox (ed.), *Vaccine Adjuvants: Methods and Protocols*, Methods in Molecular Biology, vol. 1494,
DOI 10.1007/978-1-4939-6445-1_6, © Springer Science+Business Media New York 2017

Quillaja saponaria Molina saponins are known as immunological adjuvants in vaccines. Quil-A®, a crude preparation extracted from *Q. saponaria* barks, is widely used in veterinary vaccines such as against feline leukemia virus [5]. Aiming at isolating molecules with less toxicity than the crude saponin preparation, an isolated saponin named QS-21 was purified from Quil-A® by high-pressure liquid chromatography (HPLC) and low-pressure silica chromatography [6]. QS-21 has been used as an adjuvant in several promising human vaccine formulations, such as phase 3 clinical trials for malaria and shingles [7, 8].

The congener species, *Quillaja brasiliensis*, has saponins that are chemically similar to those of *Q. saponaria* barks [9], showing a pronounced immunoadjuvant activity. The adjuvant activity is comparable to Quil-A®, being already demonstrated in experimental vaccines against bovine *herpesvirus* type 1 and 5, poliovirus, bovine viral diarrhea virus, and rabies in mice [10–14]. It has been shown that an aqueous extract and a purified saponin fraction, named QB-90, obtained from leaves of *Q. brasiliensis,* can induce both humoral and cellular immune responses in a manner comparable to Quil-A®, presenting significantly less in vivo and in vitro toxicity [11]. Leaves of *Q. brasiliensis* are readily renewable alternative sources of saponins compared to *Q. saponaria* barks. The structural complexity of its molecules is a major challenge for chemical synthesis and development of promising derivatives for commercial applications. However, saponins have been purified for years from *Quillaja saponaria* barks by silica and reverse phase chromatography to attend the large scale demands of the pharmaceutical industry [6]. An alternative procedure for *Q. brasiliensis* saponins purification from leaves was developed using aqueous extraction and liquid chromatography. A detailed protocol on how to prepare aqueous extract from *Q. brasiliensis* leaves, as well as the purification procedure to obtain the immunoadjuvant fraction QB-90, are described herein.

2 Materials

Prepare all solutions using distilled water and analytical grade reagents. Prepare and store all reagents at room temperature. Diligently follow all waste disposal regulations when disposing waste materials.

2.1 Aqueous Extract from Leaves of Q. brasiliensis

1. Circulating air oven.
2. Knife mill.
3. Scale.
4. Beakers (1 L capacity).
5. Graduated cylinder (1 L capacity).
6. Magnetic stirrer plate and magnetic rod.

7. Buchner funnel.
8. Suction flask (1 L capacity).
9. Vacuum pump.
10. Filter paper sheets.
11. Separatory funnel (2 L capacity).
12. Rotary evaporator.
13. Round-bottom flask (250 mL capacity).

2.2 Liquid Chromatography and Thin Layer Chromatography (TLC)

1. C-18 reverse phase silica gel LiChroprep® (40–63 μm) (Merck, Darmstadt, Germany).
2. Glass column with glass frit (2.5 × 40 cm).
3. Graduated cylinders (100 mL capacity).
4. Suction flask (250 mL capacity).
5. Vacuum pump.
6. Rotary evaporator.
7. Round-bottom flask (250 mL capacity).
8. TLC aluminum sheets of silica gel 60 GF_{254}.
9. TLC chamber.
10. Pasteur pipette.
11. Cotton balls.

2.3 Reagents and Solutions

1. 2% Gelatin solution: dissolve 1 g of gelatin U.S.P. in 50 mL of distilled water. Heat to dissolve if necessary.
2. Ethyl acetate p.a.
3. Ethanol p.a.
4. 96% ethanol (v/v).
5. 70% ethanol (v/v).
6. Methanol p.a..
7. TLC mobile phase: butanol p.a.–glacial acetic acid p.a.–distilled water, 5:1:4 v/v/v.
8. ρ-anisaldehyde solution: in a fume hood, homogenize 5 mL of glacial acetic acid in 465 mL of ethanol p.a. Add 12.5 mL of ρ-anisaldehyde 98% and, slowly and carefully, 17.5 mL of sulfuric acid. Store the solution away from light in a closed bottle wrapped in aluminum foil.
9. Quil-A® (Brenntag Biosector, Ballerup, Denmark).

3 Methods

Carry out all procedures at room temperature unless otherwise specified.

3.1 *Q. brasiliensis* Aqueous Extract Preparation

1. Collect leaves from adult *Q. brasiliensis*. Select the fully expanded and healthy leaves, and wash twice with distilled water. Dry the leaves in a circulating air oven at temperature lower than 40 °C for 1 week. Grind the dried leaves in a knife mill and store the powdered leaves away from light and humidity until use.
2. Weigh 100 g of the powdered leaves and transfer to a beaker. Add 800 mL of distilled water. Mix with a magnetic stirrer for 8 h.
3. Filter the extract on a Buchner funnel with two sheets of filter paper using 1 L suction flask under vacuum.
4. Repeat **steps 3–5** with the retained material to improve the extract yield. Combine with the first filtered solution. In order to precipitate condensed tannins, add 50 mL of 2% gelatin solution to the filtered extract solution. Wait for precipitate formation.
5. Filter the extract on a Buchner funnel with three sheets of qualitative filter paper and 1 L suction flask under vacuum. If necessary, repeat the procedure, until precipitation is over and extract is clear.
6. In a 2 L separatory funnel, partition the extract using 200 mL of ethyl acetate. Discard the ethyl acetate phase. Repeat this procedure at least twice (*see* **Note 1**).
7. Using a round-bottom flask, dry the extract in a rotary evaporator at a temperature below 45 °C. Store the residue away from light and humidity.

3.2 QB-90 Purification by Liquid Chromatography

1. Weigh 100 g of C-18 reverse phase silica gel LiChroprep®. Ressuspend silica with approximately 1.5 volumes of 96% ethanol.
2. Transfer the silica to the glass column. Let the stationary phase settle and gently tap the column to remove bubbles, allowing the silica to pack tightly into the column.
3. Rinse the inside of the column by pipetting solvent down the inner edge.
4. Drain the solvent until the solvent level is just even with the surface of the stationary phase.
5. Pass through the column 100 mL of 70% ethanol and repeat **step 4**. Add 100 mL of distilled water. Repeat **step 4**.
6. Weigh 1 g of aqueous extract residue and solubilize in the least volume possible of distilled water.
7. Load the sample onto the silica gel column using a Pasteur pipette.

8. Place a piece of cotton over the loading site to prevent extract leakage.
9. Elute the column with 100 mL of the solvent fractions: start with 100% distilled water and finish with 100% methanol, increasing the methanol gradient 10% at a time. Use a suction flask to collect the fractions under vacuum.
10. Keep fraction eluted with 90% methanol and dry it using a round-bottom flask in a rotary evaporator at a temperature below 45 °C. The expected average yield of QB-90 fraction is 2% (w/w) of aqueous extract residue. Store at room temperature away from humidity. For column cleaning, add 100 mL of 100% ethanol, 100 mL of 70% ethanol and 100 mL of distilled water. Repeat **step 4**.

3.3 Characterization of QB-90 Fraction by TLC

1. Cut the TLC plate, 7 cm long × desired width.
2. Draw with a pencil a parallel line at 0.5 cm above the lower border of the TLC plate. Divide it with separate marks of 1 cm of distance between them, leaving 1 cm of each side of the plate without sample application to prevent border effect on solvent permeation through the silica.
3. Ressuspend fraction QB-90 in 100% methanol p.a. (solution between 0.1 and 10 mg/mL).
4. Spot a small amount of each compound using a capillary tube on top of the pencil parallel line. The spot diameter should be as small as possible. Let the solvent evaporate. Homogenize the TLC mobile phase from **item 7** of Subheading 2.3 and let it settle. Discard the upper organic phase and place the aqueous phase in the chamber (*see* **Note 2**). Place the TLC plate in chamber and let solvent front run up the plate (*see* **Note 3**). When the plate has run far enough (solvent front approx. 1–0.5 cm distance from top of plate), remove it from the TLC chamber. Let the TLC plate dry and proceed with detection.
5. Spray the plate with freshly prepared ρ-anisaldehyde solution (*see* **Note 4**) and heat to 105 °C until maximum visualization of brownish spots, characteristic of terpene compounds. Calculate the retention factor (Rf) for each spot, i.e., the distance migrated by the spot over the total distance covered by the solvent:

$$\mathrm{Rf} = \frac{\text{distance traveled by sample}}{\text{distance traveled by solvent}}.$$

6. The absence of yellow spots, characteristic of phenolic compounds, along with the presence of purple and brownish spots in the same Rf of Quil-A® (positive control) indicate the isolation of QB 90 fraction of saponins (Fig. 1).

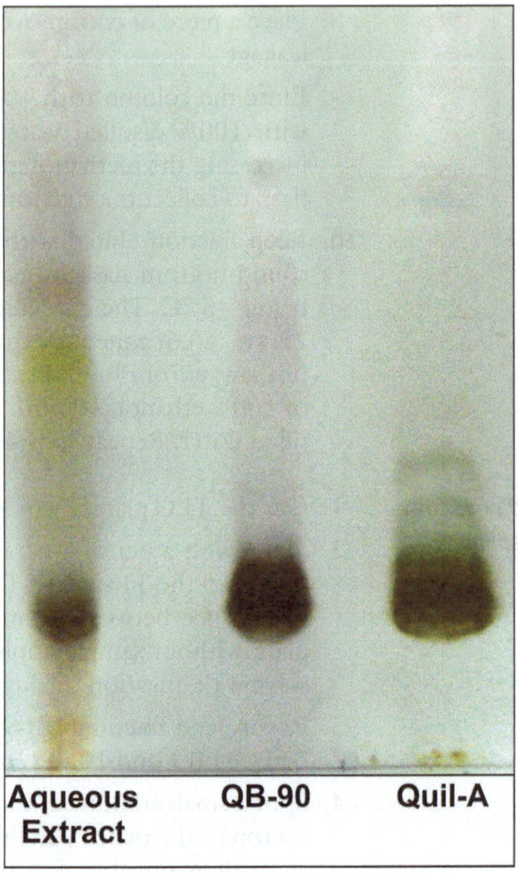

Fig. 1 TLC of aqueous extract, QB-90, and Quil-A

4 Notes

1. Add and mix gently the ethyl acetate solvent in the aqueous extract to prevent emulsion formation.
2. After transfer of the TLC mobile phase to the TLC chamber, wait 1 to 5 min to equilibrate the gas phase inside.
3. Do not place the TLC plate in contact with the TLC chamber wall, this can lead to an inefficient solvent migration by capillarity.
4. The ρ-anisaldehyde solution is toxic by ingestion and inhalation. Use gloves and other individual protection equipment for manipulating and preparing reagents, and spray the solution inside a fume hood.

References

1. Jeon BR, Kim SJ, Hong SB, Park HJ, Cho JY, Rhee MH (2015) The inhibitory mechanism of crude saponin fraction from Korean Red Ginseng in collagen-induced platelet aggregation. J Ginseng Res 39(3):279–285
2. Yu CH, Xie G, He RR, Zhai YJ, Li YF, Tsoi B, Kurihara H, Yang DP (2011) Effects of a purified saponin mixture from alfalfa on plasma lipid metabolism in hyperlipidemic mice. J Health Sci 57(5):401–405
3. Cui J, Xi MM, Li YW, Duan JL, Wang L, Weng Y, Jia N, Cao SS, Li RL, Wang C, Zhao C, Wu Y, Wen AD (2015) Insulinotropic effect of *Chikusetsu* saponin IVa in diabetic rats and pancreatic beta-cells. J Ethnopharmacol 164:334–339
4. Lunga PK, Qin XJ, Yang XW, Kuiate JR, Du ZZ, Gatsing D (2014) Antimicrobial steroidal saponin and oleanane-type triterpenoid saponins from *Paullinia pinnata*. BMC Complement Altern Med 14:369
5. De Costa F, Yendo ACA, Fleck JD, Gosmann G, Fett-Neto AG (2011) Immunoadjuvant and anti-inflammatory plant saponins: characteristics and biotechnological approaches towards sustainable production. Mini Rev Med Chem 11(10):857–880
6. Kensil CR, Patel U, Lennick M, Marciani D (1991) Separation and characterization of saponins with adjuvant activity from *Quillaja saponaria* Molina cortex. J Immunol 146(2): 431–437
7. The RTS,S Clinical Trials Partnership (2014) Efficacy and Safety of the RTS,S/AS01 Malaria vaccine during 18 months after vaccination: a phase 3 randomized, controlled trial in children and young infants at 11 African sites. PLoS Med 11(7):e1001685
8. Lal H, Cunningham AL, Godeaux O, Chlibek R, Diez-Domingo J, Hwang SJ, Levin MJ, McElhaney JE, Poder A, Puig-Barbera J, Vesikari T, Watanabe D, Weckx L, Zahaf T, Heineman TC (2015) Efficacy of an adjuvanted herpes zoster subunit vaccine in older adults. N Engl J Med 372(22):2087–2096
9. Kauffmann C, Machado AM, Fleck JD, Provensi G, Pires VS, Guillaume D, Sonnet P, Reginatto FH, Schenkel EP, Gosmann G (2004) Constituents from leaves of *Quillaja brasiliensis*. Nat Prod Res 18:153–157
10. Fleck JD, Kauffmann C, Spilki F, Lencina CL, Roehe PM, Gosmann G (2006) Adjuvant activity of *Quillaja brasiliensis* saponins on the immune responses to bovine *herpesvirus* type 1 in mice. Vaccine 24:7129–7134
11. Silveira F, Cibulski SP, Varela AP, Marqués JM, Chabalgoity A, De Costa F, Yendo ACA, Gosmann G, Roehe PM, Fernández C, Ferreira F (2011) *Quillaja brasiliensis* saponins are less toxic than Quil A and have similar properties when used as an adjuvant for a viral antigen preparation. Vaccine 29:9177–9182
12. De Costa F, Yendo ACA, Cibulski SP, Fleck JD, Roehe PM, Spilki FR, Gosmann G, Fett-Neto AG (2014) Alternative inactivated poliovirus vaccines adjuvanted with *Quillaja brasiliensis* or Quil-A saponins are equally effective in inducing specific immune responses. PLoS One 9:e105374
13. Cibulski SP, Mourglia-Ettlin G, Teixeira TF, Santos H, Yendo ACA, De Costa F, Fett-Neto AG, Gosmann G, Roehe PM, Silveira F (2016) *Quillaja brasiliensis* saponins induce robust humoral and cellular responses in a bovine viral diarrhea virus vaccine in mice. Comp Immunol Microb 45:1–8
14. Yendo ACA, De Costa F, Cibulski SP, Teixeira TF, Colling LC, Mastrogiovanni M, Soulé S, Roehe PM, Gosmann G, Ferreira FA, Fett-Neto AG (2016) A rabies vaccine adjuvanted with saponins from leaves of the soap tree (*Quillaja brasiliensis*) induces specific immune responses and protects against lethal challenge. Vaccine 34: 2305–2311

Chapter 7

Biosynthetic Approaches to Squalene Production: The Case of Yeast

Martin Valachovič and Ivan Hapala

Abstract

Squalene is a precursor in the eukaryotic sterol biosynthesis. It is a valuable compound with several human health-related applications. Since the traditional natural resources of squalene are limited, alternatives for the production of squalene on industrial scale have been intensively explored during past years. The yeast *Saccharomyces cerevisiae* represents an attractive option due to elaborated techniques of genetic and metabolic engineering that can be applied to improve squalene yields. We discuss in this chapter some theoretical aspects of genetic manipulations of the ergosterol biosynthesis pathway aimed at increased squalene production and describe analytical methods for squalene purification and determination of its content in yeast cells.

Key words Squalene, Yeast, Ergosterol biosynthesis, Squalene monooxygenase, *ERG1* gene, Lipid extraction, Solid phase extraction, Thin-layer chromatography, High-performance liquid chromatography

1 Introduction

Squalene is a linear polyunsaturated triterpenoid with many applications in cosmetic and pharmaceutical industry (e.g., as a vaccine adjuvant component), or as a nutritional supplement. Although it is synthesized in many organisms, its natural sources are limited. The richest available source of squalene is shark liver oil; however, the long-term dependence of squalene production on this oil may not be feasible due to environmental concerns, such as excessive fishing of sharks or increasing contamination by pollutants. Alternative natural sources explored in recent years include plants (e.g., olives or amaranth) or microorganisms [1]. Yeasts represent in this respect a very promising alternative option for squalene production. High levels of squalene have been found in some natural isolates of the genus *Pseudozyma* [2], but the biotechnologically established yeast *Saccharomyces cerevisiae* can be genetically engineered for high production of squalene.

Christopher B. Fox (ed.), *Vaccine Adjuvants: Methods and Protocols*, Methods in Molecular Biology, vol. 1494,
DOI 10.1007/978-1-4939-6445-1_7, © Springer Science+Business Media New York 2017

Squalene is synthesized in *S. cerevisiae* in the mevalonate pathway as the first metabolite dedicated to ergosterol biosynthesis [3]. Its physiological levels are typically very low due to the rapid utilization for ergosterol biosynthesis. Generally, accumulation of squalene can be reached either by increasing the production in the mevalonate pathway, or by reducing the consumption in the post-squalene part of ergosterol biosynthesis. Both approaches have been successfully applied to increase squalene levels in yeast.

There are two enzymes in the mevalonate pathway potentially suitable for increasing squalene levels: HMG-CoA reductase (encoded in two homologous genes *HMG1* and *HMG2*) and squalene synthase (encoded in *ERG9* gene), but only the first one has been proved as an efficient target. HMG-CoA reductase is one of the major control sites of eukaryotic sterol biosynthesis. Yeast *S. cerevisiae* has two isoforms of HMG-CoA reductase: Hmg1p representing the major aerobic activity and Hmg2p expressed preferentially during hypoxia [4]. Simple overexpression of the *HMG1* gene has only limited effect on squalene levels due to the tight control of Hmg1p activity [5] and due to the detrimental effect of the formation of the ER membrane stacks ("carmellae") in cells overproducing Hmg1p [6]. These limitations have been overcome by expressing a truncated form of Hmg1p that lacks ER membrane targeting domain and retains the functional catalytic domain. Expression of this truncated Hmg1p under strong promoters caused significant accumulation of squalene in yeast cells [7–9].

An alternative approach to increase cellular squalene is to limit squalene consumption in the post-squalene part of ergosterol biosynthesis. It must be emphasized that not all enzymes in the pathway are suitable for the genetic modification of squalene levels. Very promising in this respect is squalene monooxygenase catalyzing squalene epoxidation as the first step in squalene metabolic transformation. This enzyme is coded by the *ERG1* gene in *S. cerevisiae* [10] and it is the target for the antimycotic terbinafine commonly used to treat dermatomycoses [11]. Terbinafine at subinhibitory concentrations has been shown to increase very efficiently squalene levels in *Saccharomyces cerevisiae* [12–14] and in *Kluyveromyces lactis* [15]. However, use of this antimycotic for squalene production has several drawbacks, e.g., high economic costs, or loss of yeast cell viability at terbinafine concentrations yielding high squalene levels [14].

During the mutational mapping of the squalene monooxygenase we have engineered a set of single-point mutants in the *ERG1* gene either resistant or hypersensitive to terbinafine [16–18]. The hypersensitive mutants turned out to be very interesting with respect to squalene production. They retained low squalene monoxygenase activity (that was nevertheless sufficient to maintain cell growth) and accumulated high levels of squalene [14, 18]. A spontaneous mutation in the *ERG1* gene isolated as the suppressor of *erg26ts* allele [19] showed similar characteristics as the engineered strains. Moreover, all above mentioned *erg1* mutants accumulated squalene without compromising cell growth and viability. This proves that targeting squalene monooxygenase by mutations of the *ERG1* gene is generally suitable as a tool for the biotechnological production of squalene in yeast.

This chapter describes the basic principles of construction of squalene-accumulating mutants in the *ERG1* gene with reduced activity of squalene monooxygenase. We present here detailed laboratory protocols for the isolation of non-saponifiable lipids (sterols and squalene) from yeast cells, purification of squalene from these lipid extracts by solid phase extraction (SPE) and two chromatographic methods for qualitative and quantitative analysis of squalene and sterols in lipid extracts (thin layer chromatography, TLC, and high-performance liquid chromatography, HPLC) that can be performed in laboratories with standard biochemical equipment. The SPE method described here can be used for the isolation of purified squalene in milligram quantities as well as for the isolation of radiolabeled squalene and ergosterol from yeast cells grown in media supplemented with ^{14}C-acetate.

2 Materials

2.1 Yeast Strains and Isolation of erg1 Mutants

The following *S. cerevisiae* strains were used in the experiments:

1. Wild-type strain W303-1B [genotype *MATα*, *ade2-1 his3-11,15 leu2-3,112 trp1-1 ura3-52 can1-100*].
2. *erg 1* mutant strain [genotype *MATα leu2 ura3 trp1 ERG1::URA3* (transformed with plasmid pNS1 containing the *erg1L37P* allele under own promoter)].

Isolation of erg1 Mutant

erg1L37P mutation causing L37P substitution in the FAD-binding domain of the Erg1p was generated by in vitro random mutagenesis via PCR amplification as described in [18]. Briefly, *ERG1* gene was amplified from a recombinant plasmid carrying the wild-type *ERG1*gene using the forward primer (5′-ACGACGTTGTAAAAC GACGGCCAG-3′) and the reverse primer (5′-TTCACACAGG AAACAGCTATGACC-3′). The amplification was performed with DyNAzyme II DNA polymerase (Finnzymes) in the presence of 5 mM $MgCl_2$ and 0.05 mM $MnCl_2$. PCR fragments were digested with *Pst*I, cloned into the centromere vector pRS315, and transformed into *E. coli* XL1. Plasmid DNA was isolated from *E. coli* by standard procedures [20] and transformed into *S. cerevisiae* KLN1 strain (containing the disruption of chromosomal *ERG1::URA3*, *see* **Note 1**) by the protocol of Gietz et al. [21]. Clones expressing a functional squalene epoxidase were selected by complementation of the aerobic growth defect of KLN1 *ERG1::URA3* on YPD agar plates. Positive clones were tested for terbinafine sensitivity on YPD plates containing 10 μg/ml of terbinafine. Plasmid DNA was isolated from terbinafine-hypersensitive *S. cerevisiae* clones [22], amplified in *E. coli* XL1 and characterized by DNA sequencing.

2.2 Equipment

1. FastPrep®-24 cell homogenizer (MP Biomedicals) with adapter for 15-ml tubes (12 × 15-ml TeenPrep™ adapter).
2. Sample concentrator (Stuart) connected to the source of nitrogen (high purity nitrogen in pressure gas cylinder).
3. Semi-automatic sample applicator Linomat 5 (CAMAG).
4. Glass microsyringes with volumes 25, 100, and 500 μl (Hamilton).
5. Three TLC developing chambers (Twin Trough chamber CAMAG with glass lid, 20 × 20 cm).
6. HPLC instrument (Agilent 1100) equipped with reversed phase C8 column (Eclipse XDB-C8, particle size 5 μm, column size 4.6 × 150 mm, Agilent), diode array detector (Agilent 1100), Corona® Charged Aerosol Detector (ESA/Thermo Scientific), and nitrogen generator (ESA/Thermo Scientific).

2.3 Reagents and Supplies

1. YEPD rich growth medium (1 % yeast extract, 2 % peptone, 2 % dextrose).
2. 15-ml polypropylene tubes.
3. 1.5-ml microcentrifuge tubes.
4. Acid-washed glass beads, diameter 0.4–0.6 mm (Sigma-Aldrich) (*see* **Note 2**).
5. 20 and 12 ml Pyrex® glass tubes with Teflon-lined cups (Corning) (*see* **Note 2**).
6. Methanolic KOH solution with pyrogallol (60% KOH w/v, 50% methanol v/v, 0.5 % pyrogallol w/v) (*see* **Note 3**).
7. Organic solvents: *n*-hexane, methanol, diethylether, petroleum ether (boiling point 60–80 °C), chloroform (all of the highest purity available, *see* **Note 2**).
8. Water (LiChrosolv®, Merck Millipore).
9. Glacial acetic acid (p.a. EMSURE®, Merck Millipore).
10. TLC silica gel 60 aluminum sheets (20 × 20 cm, Merck Millipore).
11. SPE column CHROMABOND® NH2 (3 ml, 500 mg, Macherey-Nagel).
12. TLC solvent developing mixture I: petroleum ether–diethyl ether–acetic acid (35:15:1, v/v).
13. TLC solvent developing mixture II: petroleum ether–diethyl ether (49:1, v/v).

14. TLC charring solution: 0.63 g $MnCl_2.4H_2O$, 60 ml water, 60 ml methanol, 4 ml sulfuric acid (p.a., 96 %).
15. HPLC standard ergosterol (Sigma-Aldrich Fluka, purity ≥95 %); 1 mg/ml stock solution in ethanol.
16. HPLC standard squalene (Sigma-Aldrich, purity ≥98 %); 1 mg/ml stock solution in ethanol.

3 Methods

3.1 Extraction of Non-saponifiable Lipids

1. Grow yeast cells in a rich YEPD medium to late exponential/early stationary phase (16–20 h) (*see* **Note 4**).
2. Harvest the cells by centrifugation at 700 × *g* for 5 min and discard supernatant.
3. Wash the sediment with deionized water and harvest the cells by centrifugation (700 × *g*, 5 min).
4. Resuspend sediment in deionized water to a concentration of 1×10^9 cells/ml. Transfer 1 ml aliquot of cell suspension into a new polypropylene 15-ml tube.
5. Add approx. one volume (1 ml) of glass beads (measured in a calibrated 1.5 ml microcentrifuge tube) to the tube and cool on ice.
6. Break the cells in a FastPrep24 homogenizer 2 × 45 s (6.5 m/s speed) with 5 min cooling on ice between the breaking runs (*see* **Note 5**).
7. Transfer broken cell suspension with a glass Pasteur pipette to 20 ml Pyrex glass tube with Teflon-lined cup. Be careful to avoid the carryover of glass beads.
8. Add three volumes (3 ml) of methanolic KOH with pyrogallol and incubate for 2 h at 70 °C (*see* **Note 6**).
9. Cool the saponification mixture, add three volumes (3 ml) of *n*-hexane and mix well on a vortex mixer.
10. Separate the organic and water phases by centrifugation for 5 min at 1300 × *g*.
11. Transfer the upper organic phase to a clean 12 ml Pyrex glass tube with Teflon-lined cup.
12. Re-extract the water phase with three volumes (3 ml) of *n*-hexane, collect the upper phase separated by centrifugation (as in **step 10** of Subheading 3.1) and join both organic phases.
13. Evaporate *n*-hexane from the joined organic phases in sample concentrator under the stream of nitrogen.
14. Dissolve the lipid residue containing squalene and sterols in desired volume of solvent (e.g., *n*-hexane), and store at −20 °C in 2 ml amber glass vial with Teflon-lined cup.

3.2 Semi-preparative Separation of Squalene and Sterols by Solid Phase Extraction (SPE)

1. Prepare the SPE column by conditioning three times with 3 ml of *n*-hexane (*see* **Note 7**).
2. Load 3 ml of the non-saponifiable lipid extract in *n*-hexane on the top of the column (*see* **Note 8**).
3. Collect the flow-through.
4. Elute squalene from the column two times with 3 ml of *n*-hexane and collect the eluates in the tube with the flow-through.
5. Evaporate the solvent from combined flow-through and two *n*-hexane eluates under the nitrogen stream and dissolve the lipid residue (containing squalene) in desired volume of solvent (e.g., *n*-hexane).

3.3 Two-Step TLC Separation of Squalene and Sterols [23] (See Note 9)

1. Load sample on the TLC plate using sample applicator or manually by glass microsyringe (*see* **Notes 10** and **11**).
2. Put the TLC plate with loaded samples in the preconditioned chamber with the developing solvent mixture I (petroleum ether–diethyl ether–acetic acid, 35:15:1 v/v) and develop until the solvent front reaches 5 cm from the top of the plate (approx. 30 min) (*see* **Note 12**).
3. Take out the TLC plate and evaporate the developing solvent mixture in a fume hood.
4. Transfer the TLC plate to the chamber preconditioned with the developing solvent mixture II (petroleum ether–diethyl ether, 49:1 v/v) and develop until the solvent front reaches about 1 cm from the top of the plate (approx. 45 min).
5. Take out the TLC plate and evaporate the developing solvent mixture in a fume hood.
6. Dip the plate into the charring solution for 0.5–1 min (*see* **Note 13**). Let the TLC plate dry in a fume hood.
7. Incubate the TLC plate at 130 °C in the oven for 10–20 min. Inspect periodically the appearance of dark brown lipid spots during this time period (*see* Fig. 1).

3.4 HPLC Separation of Squalene and Sterols

1. For HPLC analysis of non-saponifiable lipids (squalene and sterols), dry lipid extract equivalent of 1×10^9 cells and dissolve the residue in 300 μl of solvent (e.g., *n*-hexane or acetone) (*see* **Note 10**).
2. Load 10 μl aliquot (equivalent to $3–6 \times 10^7$ cells) on the C8 column using automatic sampler. Lipids are separated with 95 % methanol as the mobile phase. If applicable, column temperature is set to 30 °C (*see* **Note 14**).
3. Lipids are detected using two detectors connected in series. First, lipid peaks are detected based on their UV spectrum in a non-destructive diode array detector (DAD) followed by detection in the Corona Charged Aerosol Detector (CAD) (*see* **Note 15**) (*see* Fig. 2).

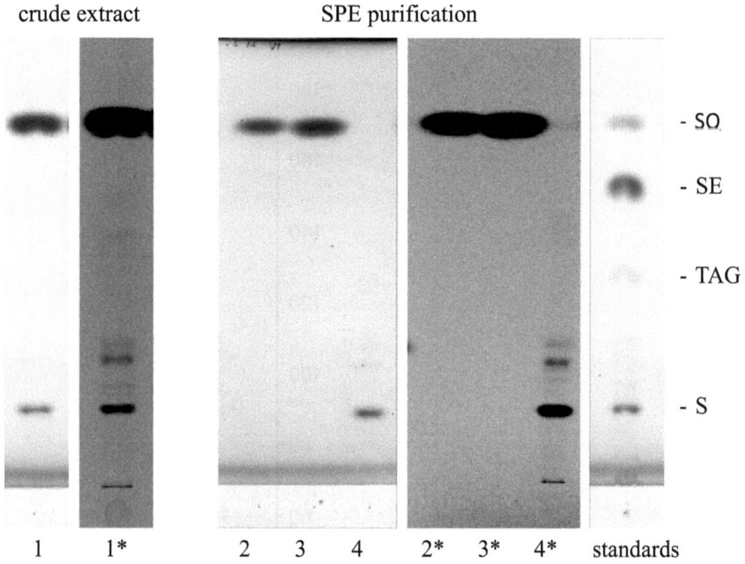

Fig. 1 TLC analysis of squalene purified from the non-saponifiable lipid extract on SPE column. *erg1*^{L37P} cells were grown for 16 h in YPD containing ^{14}C-acetate to label total lipids. Radioactivity on TLC plates was visualized by phosphorimager (*lanes with asterisks*) followed by charring with sulphuric acid (*see* 2.3.3.6) (*lanes w/o asterisks*). *1*: total non-saponifiable lipid extract (equivalent of 3×10^8 cells); *2*: purified squalene (equivalent of 1×10^8 cells); *3*: purified squalene (equivalent of 2×10^8 cells); *4*: methanol eluate of sterols remaining after *n*-hexane elution (equivalent of 3×10^8 cells); Standards: *SQ* squalene, *SE* cholesteryl oleate, *TAG* triolein, *S* sterols

4 Notes

1. Selection of *erg1* mutations with reduced squalene monooxygenase activity is performed in strains with disrupted chromosomal copy of *ERG1* gene. Such disruption is lethal under standard aerobic conditions; however, disruptant strain can be cultivated anaerobically in YPD media supplemented with 20 μg/ml of ergosterol and 0.06 % Tween 80 (as the source of unsaturated fatty acids).
2. All organic solvents used in lipid extraction and chromatographic separation should be of highest purity. Merck LiChrosolv®, EMPLURA®, or EMSURE® quality solvents were tested with satisfactory results and are recommended. Plastic material (tips, containers, etc.) must not be used during the extraction procedure (with exception of the cell breaking step). Organic solvents release additives from the plastics which might interfere with subsequent analysis. Glass and Teflon® materials should be used throughout the procedure.
3. To prepare 10 ml of methanolic KOH solution it is recommended to dissolve 6 g of KOH pellets in 5 ml of 1 % pyrogallol

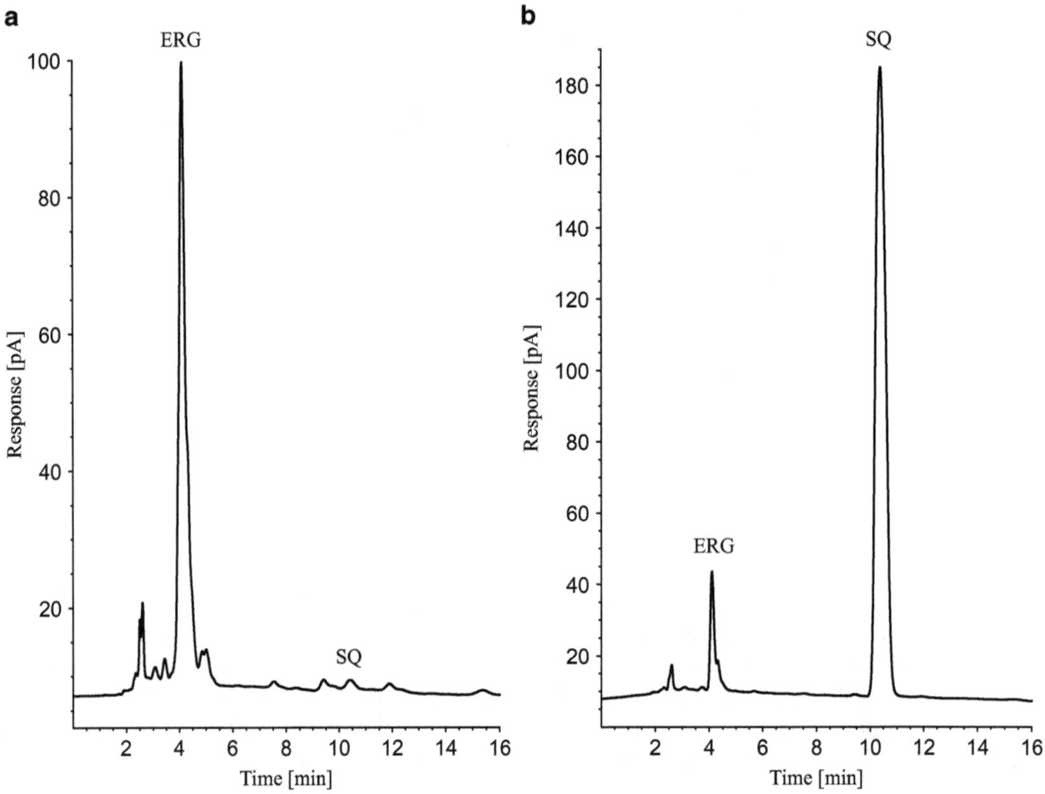

	ERG	SQ
ng/peak	1700	96
µg/10^9 cells	51	3

	ERG	SQ
ng/peak	379	7932
µg/10^9 cells	11	238

Fig. 2 HPLC-CAD chromatogram of non-saponifiable lipid extract from wild-type (**a**) and *erg1*^{L37P} mutant (**b**). Lipids isolated from 1×10^9 cells were resuspended in 300 µl of hexane and 10 µl aliquots were separated by reversed-phase HPLC. Ergosterol (ERG) and squalene (SQ) were quantified as described in **Note 16**. Low amount of ergosterol in *erg1*^{L37P} mutant compared to the wild-type is caused by the absence of steryl esters due to reduced ergosterol biosynthesis

in methanol (w/v) mixed with 2.5 ml of water. When KOH pellets are fully dissolved, final volume should be adjusted to 10 ml with water. The reaction is strongly exothermic thus special care should be taken during preparation of the solution.

4. Start the culture with fresh (up to 24 h old) inoculum. Starting concentration should be in the range 0.5–1×10^6 cells/ml. Squalene levels in *erg1* mutants may decrease in the late stationary phase due to the utilization of accumulated squalene for ergosterol synthesis. It is therefore recommended to collect cells not later than 16–20 h. 40 ml of the culture of *erg1L37P* mutant yields approx. 1 mg of squalene.

5. Due to a rigid cell wall it is essential to break yeast cells for efficient extraction of squalene (and other neutral lipids stored in lipid droplets). If a dedicated homogenizer is not available, cells can be broken in 20 ml Pyrex tubes by vortexing with glass beads on a high-speed vortex. Six one-minute breaking intervals with 1 min cooling on ice between each round are recommended. In such a case **step** 7 of Subheading 3.1 is omitted and methanolic KOH mixture can be added directly to homogenate.
6. Efficiency of neutral lipid hydrolysis depends on the quality of methanolic KOH mixture. It is therefore strongly recommended to use freshly prepared solution and to adhere to the KOH concentration of 60 %. The efficiency of saponification (steryl ester hydrolysis) should be checked on TLC, particularly if isolated lipids will be used for further squalene purification on SPE.
7. Vacuum manifold can be used to speed up the purification process. If the manifold is not available, elution can be driven simply by the gravitation force.
8. Macherey-Nagel claims their silica based CHROMABOND columns has the binding capacity approx. 3–5 % of the amount of the adsorbent. For *erg1L37P* cells the lipid amount equivalent to the cell culture of approx. 500 ml (450–750 ml) can be loaded on the CHROMABOND NH2 (500 mg) column. If other yeast strains or other SPE columns are used, amounts of total isolated non-saponifiable lipids (squalene and sterols) should be determined before loading on SPE column.
9. Separation in a single solvent mixture (petroleum ether–diethyl ether–acetic acid; 35:15:1, v/v) can be used as well; however, it is recommended to perform two-step procedure to achieve good separation of squalene from possible steryl ester contaminants. It is recommended to use separate chambers for each solvent mixture.
10. Due to the high volatility of the solvents, lipid extracts are always dried under the stream of nitrogen and dissolved in an exact volume of the solvent immediately before chromatographic analysis.
11. Set up the sample applicator or load samples manually on the horizontal lines 2 cm from the bottom of the plate. Application spots should be 1.5 cm from the side edges of the plate with 1 cm distance between neighboring spots. Loading spot should be 1 cm long for loading lipids equivalent to 3×10^8 cells (dissolved in organic solvent of volume up to 30 μl). It is recommended to label marks 5 and 1 cm from the top of the plate at both side edges of the plate with soft pencil for the control of the development path in both developing steps.

12. It is essential to precondition the chamber with the developing mixture for at least 30 min with closed lid before putting in the TLC plate. Preconditioning can be improved by lining the walls of the chamber with thick filtration paper. The amount of the solvent used depends on the size of the chamber; however, the level of the solvent should be 1–1.5 cm from the bottom.
13. A developing chamber is used for charring solution. Large Petri dish that will fit 20 × 20 cm TLC plate can be used instead. If the TLC plate will be used for a preparative analysis of lipids, non-destructive staining of lipids with iodine should be used. The developed plate is then exposed to iodine vapors in the desiccator and temporary visible yellow lipid spots are labeled with a soft pencil.
14. Sterols present in the non-saponifiable lipid extracts originate from the free sterol fraction and from hydrolyzed steryl ester fraction. Squalene peak is well separated from sterols and elutes on XDB, C8 column size 4.6 × 150 mm with 5 μm particle size at mobile phase flow rate of 1 ml/min approximately 6 min after sterols. Similar results can be achieved with shorter columns as well as with C18 columns. If HPLC analysis is not used for preparative squalene purification, column temperature can be increased to 40 °C to speed up the separation process.
15. Retention time of squalene standard is used to identify squalene in analyzed samples. In DAD spectral analysis, lipids (including squalene) are detected in the wavelength range 200–220 nm. Some sterol structures have characteristic absorbance peaks outside this range (e.g., ergosterol at 260–300 nm). Be aware of different molar extinction coefficients of individual lipids if you plan to apply UV or DAD detectors for sterol or squalene quantification. If available, Corona CAD detector is highly recommended for lipid analysis. This detector is suitable for absorption spectrum-independent quantification of various analytes, including phospholipids, squalene and sterols. The detector is usually set to sensitivity 200 pA.
16. Ergosterol and squalene quantities were calculated using the following equations:

$$\text{ergosterol}\left[\text{ng}\right] = 2E - 06 \times \mathbf{x}^2 + 0.089 \times \mathbf{x}, \text{where } \mathbf{x} \text{ is the area of the ergosterol peak}$$

$$\text{squalene}\left[\text{ng}\right] = 7E - 07 \times \mathbf{x}^2 + 0.1391 \times \mathbf{x}, \text{where } \mathbf{x} \text{ is the area of the squalene peak.}$$

The equations represent second-order polynomial functions that were derived from the calibration curves for ergosterol and squalene analyzed on the Corona CAD detector. The calibration curves were constructed by measuring three independently weighed ergosterol or squalene standard dilution sets (0.02, 0.05, 0.1, 0.2, 0.4, 1.0 mg/ml.

Acknowledgement

This work was supported by the Slovak Research and Development Agency grant APVV 0785 11 and VEGA 2/0185/14.

References

1. Spanova M, Daum G (2011) Squalene—biochemistry, molecular biology, process biotechnology, and applications. Eur J Lipid Sci Technol 113:1299–1320
2. Chang MH, Kim HJ, Jahng KY, Hong SC (2008) The isolation and characterization of *Pseudozyma* sp. JCC 207, a novel producer of squalene. Appl Microbiol Biotechnol 78:963–972
3. Daum G, Lees N, Bard M, Dickson R (1998) Biochemistry, cell biology and molecular biology of lipids of *Saccharomyces cerevisiae*. Yeast 14:1471–1510
4. Basson ME, Thorsness M, Rine J (1986) *Saccharomyces cerevisiae* contains 2 functional genes encoding 3-hydroxy-3-methylglutaryl coenzyme-A reductase. Proc Natl Acad Sci U S A 83:5563–5567
5. Burg JS, Espenshade PJ (2011) Regulation of HMG-CoA reductase in mammals and yeast. Prog Lipid Res 50:403–410
6. Wright R, Basson M, D'Ari L, Rine J (1988) Increased amounts of HMG-CoA reductase induce "karmellae": a proliferation of stacked membrane pairs surrounding the yeast nucleus. J Cell Biol 107:101–114
7. Donald KA, Hampton RY, Fritz IB (1997) Effects of overproduction of the catalytic domain of 3-hydroxy-3-methylglutaryl coenzyme a reductase on squalene synthesis in *Saccharomyces cerevisiae*. Appl Environ Microbiol 63:3341–3344
8. Polakowski T, Stahl U, Lang C (1998) Overexpression of a cytosolic hydroxymethylglutaryl-CoA reductase leads to squalene accumulation in yeast. Appl Microbiol Biotechnol 49:66–71
9. Asadollahi MA, Maury J, Schalk M, Clark A, Nielsen J (2010) Enhancement of farnesyl diphosphate pool as direct precursor of sesquiterpenes through metabolic engineering of the mevalonate pathway in *Saccharomyces cerevisiae*. Biotechnol Bioeng 106:86–96
10. Jandrositz A, Turnowsky F, Hogenauer G (1991) The gene encoding squalene epoxidase from *Saccharomyces cerevisiae*: cloning and characterization. Gene 107:155–160
11. Ryder NS (1992) Terbinafine: mode of action and properties of the squalene epoxidase inhibition. Br J Dermatol 126(Suppl):2–7
12. Naziri E, Mantzouridou F, Tsimidou MZ (2011) Enhanced squalene production by wild-type *Saccharomyces cerevisiae* strains using safe chemical means. J Agric Food Chem 59:9980–9989
13. Ta MT, Kapterian TS, Fei W, Du X, Brown AJ, Dawes IW, Yang H (2012) Accumulation of squalene is associated with the clustering of lipid droplets. FEBS J 279:4231–4244
14. Garaiová M, Zambojová V, Šimová Z, Griač P, Hapala I (2014) Squalene epoxidase as a target for manipulation of squalene levels in the yeast *Saccharomyces cerevisiae*. FEMS Yeast Res 14:1567–1364
15. Drozdíková E, Garaiová M, Csáky Z, Obernauerová M, Hapala I (2015) Production of squalene by lactose-fermenting yeast *Kluyveromyces lactis* with reduced squalene epoxidase activity. Lett Appl Microbiol 61:77–84
16. Klobučníková V, Kohút P, Leber R, Fuchsbichler S, Schweighofer N, Turnowsky F, Hapala I (2003) Terbinafine resistance in a pleiotropic yeast mutant is caused by a single point mutation in the ERG1 gene. Biochem Biophys Res Commun 309:666–671
17. Leber R, Fuchsbichler S, Klobučníková V, Schweighofer N, Pitters E, Wohlfarter K, Lederer M, Landl K, Hapala I, Turnowsky F (2003) Molecular mechanism of resistance to terbinafine in *Saccharomyces cerevisiae*. Antimicrob Agents Chemother 47:3890–3900
18. Ruckenstuhl C, Lang S, Poschenel A, Eidenberger A, Baral PK, Kohut P, Hapala I, Gruber K, Turnowsky F (2007) Characterization of squalene epoxidase of *Saccharomyces cerevisiae* applying terbinafine sensitive variants. Antimicrob Agents Chemother 51:275–284
19. Germann M, Gallo C, Donahue T, Shirzadi R, Stukey J, Lang S, Ruckenstuhl C, Oliaro-Bosso S, McDonough V, Turnowsky F, Balliano G, Nickels JT Jr (2005) Characterizing

sterol defect suppressors uncovers a novel transcriptional signaling pathway regulating zymosterol biosynthesis. J Biol Chem 280:35904–35913
20. Sambrook J, Fritsch EF, Maniatis T (1989) Molecular cloning: a laboratory manual, 2nd edn. Cold Spring Harbor Laboratory Press, Cold Spring Harbor, NY
21. Gietz RD, Schiestl RH, Willems AR, Woods RA (1995) Studies on the transformation of intact yeast cells by the LiAc/SS-DNA/PEG procedure. Yeast 11:355–360
22. Strathern JN, Higgins DR (1991) Recovery of plasmids from yeast into *Escherichia coli*: shuttle vectors. Methods Enzymol 194:319–329
23. Spanova M, Czabany T, Zellnig G, Leitner E, Hapala I, Daum G (2010) Effect of lipid particle biogenesis on the subcellular distribution of squalene in the yeast *Saccharomyces cerevisiae*. J Biol Chem 285:6127–6133

Chapter 8

In Silico Adjuvant Design and Validation

Matthew N. Davies, Helene Pere, Iris Bosschem, Freddy Haesebrouck, Bram Flahou, Eric Tartour, Darren R. Flower, David F. Tough, and Jagadeesh Bayry

Abstract

Adjuvants are substances that boost the protective immune response to vaccine antigens. The majority of known adjuvants have been identified through the use of empirical approaches. Our aim was to identify novel adjuvants with well-defined cellular and molecular mechanisms by combining a knowledge of immunoregulatory mechanisms with an in silico approach. $CD4^{+}CD25^{+}FoxP3^{+}$ regulatory T cells (Tregs) inhibit the protective immune responses to vaccines by suppressing the activation of antigen presenting cells such as dendritic cells (DCs). In this chapter, we describe the identification and functional validation of small molecule antagonists to CCR4, a chemokine receptor expressed on Tregs. The CCR4 binds the chemokines CCL22 and CCL17 that are produced in large amounts by activated innate cells including DCs. In silico identified small molecule CCR4 antagonists inhibited the migration of Tregs both in vitro and in vivo and when combined with vaccine antigens, significantly enhanced protective immune responses in experimental models.

Key words CCR4, Regulatory T cell, Adjuvant, Small molecule, Vaccine in silico, Dendritic cells

1 Introduction

Vaccines play an indispensible role in the fight against infectious diseases as well as certain types of cancer [1]. Due to their capacity for self-replication, live vaccines to infectious diseases provide sufficient signals to elicit a sustained protective immune response. However, inactivated vaccines, recombinant protein, and subunit vaccines require adjuvants: components that enhance the strength and duration of the immune response to vaccine antigens.

To date, the majority of available adjuvants have been identified by empirical means. Alum that elicits protective humoral immune responses is the most commonly used adjuvant for human vaccines, but is actually a poor inducer of cellular immune response [2]. For this reason, alum is not effective for viral and anti-tumor vaccines. Therefore, identification of molecular adjuvants with

Christopher B. Fox (ed.), *Vaccine Adjuvants: Methods and Protocols*, Methods in Molecular Biology, vol. 1494,
DOI 10.1007/978-1-4939-6445-1_8, © Springer Science+Business Media New York 2017

well-defined cellular and molecular mechanisms that elicit both cellular and humoral immune responses is critical.

We report here the identification of small molecule adjuvants by combining a knowledge of immunoregulatory mechanisms with an in silico approach [3–9]. $CD4^+CD25^+FoxP3^+$ regulatory T cells (Tregs) play a critical role in maintaining immune tolerance and are expanded in the periphery by various signals [10–16]. One of the mechanisms by which Tregs function is by suppressing the activity of innate cells such as dendritic cells (DCs) [17–22]. While such suppression is important for preventing autoimmunity and chronic inflammation [10, 17, 20, 23–25], inhibition of DC functions can also lead to a diminished immune response to vaccines [26, 27]. Of note, depletion of Tregs at the time of vaccination has been shown to lead to significant enhancement of primary and secondary immune responses indicating that Tregs are viable targets to boost the immunogenicity of vaccines [28–30]. As a Treg depletion method has limited translational value due to possible deleterious side effects, we aimed at developing a non-depletion method of targeting Tregs to improve the immune response to vaccines [31].

Tregs express the chemokine receptor CCR4 that is absent on naïve and Th1 cells [28, 32, 33]. CCR4 is a receptor for two chemokines CCL22 and CCL17 that are produced in large amounts by activated innate cells including DCs. By using an in silico approach, we identified small molecule antagonists to CCR4 able to transiently inhibit the recruitment of Tregs both in vitro and in vivo without depletion. Importantly, the use of CCR4 antagonists as "molecular adjuvants" in experimental models in vivo significantly enhanced protective immune responses when injected in combination with various vaccine antigens.

2 Materials

2.1 General Equipment and Reagents

1. Biological safety cabinet for cell culture.
2. A 37 °C incubator with humidity and gas control to maintain >95 % humidity and an atmosphere of 5 % CO_2 in air.
3. Low-speed centrifuge.
4. Vivaspin 20 (cutoff 5000 Mw) (Sartorius).
5. Inverted microscope with 10× and 20× objectives.
6. RPMI 1640 medium.
7. Complete RPMI 1640 medium: RPMI medium with 10% fetal calf serum (FCS), 100 U/mL of penicillin, 100 μg/mL of streptomycin.
8. PBS: 137 mM NaCl, 2.7 mM KCl, 8 mM Na_2HPO_4, 2 mM KH_2PO_4. Dilute 10×PBS to 1×PBS.
9. Sonicator ultrasonic processor XL 2015 (Misonix).

10. Tissue culture flasks (T25, T75).
11. Cell culture grade DMSO.
12. Sterile 6-, 24-, and 96-well plates.
13. Multichannel pipettes.
14. Plastic pipets (1, 5, 10, 25 mL).
15. Micropipettes and tips (20, 200, 1000 μL).
16. 15- and 50-mL conical tubes.
17. Hemocytometer.
18. Flow cytometer.
19. Software for the analysis of FACS data (Flo JO or FACS DIVA).
20. Fluorochrome-conjugated antibodies for the flow cytometry.
21. Fc-receptor blocking reagents.
22. Optical density meter.
23. Ball-tipped gavage needle.
24. Automated slide stainer.
25. Sarstedt tubes.
26. Zirconium/silica beads (Biospec products).
27. Stainless steel beads (Biospec products).
28. MagnaLyser (Roche Applied Science).
29. C1000 Thermal cycler (CFX96 Real-Time System).
30. Software programs and high-speed computers for docking and virtual screening.

2.2 Cell Lines

1. Human Caucasian acute T lymphoblastoid leukemia cell line CCRF-CEM (European collection of cell culture). Culture in RPMI 1640 medium with 10% FCS.
2. Murine T cell hybridoma B9.1. Culture in RPMI 1640 medium with 10% FCS [34].

2.3 Isolation of Human Regulatory T Cells

1. Magnetic cell sorting (MACS) buffer: Degassed PBS, 1% BSA. Always maintain at 4 °C.
2. MACS LD, LS and MS columns (Miltenyi Biotec).
3. MACS magnetic stand and magnet (Miltenyi Biotec).
4. Heparinized blood or buffy bags from healthy donors.
5. Ficoll-Paque ($p = 1.077$ g/mL).
6. Human regulatory T cell isolation kit (Miltenyi Biotec).

2.4 Differentiation of Human Th2 Cells

1. MACS buffer.
2. MACS LS columns.
3. MACS magnetic stand and magnet.

4. Ficoll-Paque ($p = 1.077$ g/mL).
5. Heparinized blood or buffy bags from healthy donors.
6. Human naive $CD4^+$ T cell isolation kit II (Miltenyi Biotec).
7. Neutralizing monoclonal antibodies (mAbs) to human IFN-γ and IL-12.
8. Recombinant human (rh) IL-4 and IL-2.
9. Human anti-CD3 and anti-CD28 mAbs.

2.5 Generation of Murine $CCR4^+$ Regulatory T Cells

1. Mouse anti-CD4-coated magnetic beads (Miltenyi Biotec).
2. Mouse anti-CD3 mAbs.
3. Mouse TGF-β1.
4. Mouse recombinant IL-2.
5. 70 μm cell strainers.

2.6 Chemotaxis Assay for Human $CCR4^+$ Cells

1. rhCCL22 and CCL17.
2. Polycarbonate membrane 24-well Transwell chambers: 5 μm pore (Costar).

2.7 CCR4 Antagonists

Synthesized by chemical laboratories (purity >90%).

2.8 Mice

1. Mice expressing the *neuOT-I/OT-II* transgene in mammary epithelium under the control of the MMTV promoter and a dominant-negative mutant of P53 under the control of the whey acid protein (WAP) promoter (lab of BH Nelson, British Columbia, Canada). The activated rat neu oncogene was tagged at its COOH terminus with $CD8^+$ ($OVA_{257\text{-}264}$) and $CD4^+$ ($OVA_{323\text{-}339}$) T cell epitopes from ovalbumin resulting in $neu^{OT\text{-}I/OT\text{-}II}$ transgenic mice [35].
2. OTII Ly5.2 old females mice with OVA-specific TCR. 6 weeks old.
3. C57 Bl6 Ly5.1 female mice. 6 weeks old.
4. C57 Bl6 mice.
5. BALB/c female mice. 7 weeks old.

2.9 STxB-OVA Vaccine

1. Nontoxic Shiga toxin subunit B.
2. Synthetic OVA-derived peptide $OVA_{257\text{-}264}$ (SIINFEKL).
3. EndoTrap affinity chromatography (Hyglos GmbH).
4. m-maleimidobenzoyl-N-hydroxysulfosuccinimide ester (Thermo Fisher Scientific).
5. Gel filtration and immunoaffinity chromatography.
6. Limulus assay kit (Lonza).
7. Invariant NKT cell ligand α-GalCer (KRN7000) (Funakoshi).

2.10 Evaluation of Adjuvanticity of CCR4 Antagonists in STxB-OVA Vaccine Model

1. Ammonium-Chloride-Potassium (ACK) buffer.
2. Mouse anti-CD8-coated magnetic beads (Miltenyi Biotec).
3. ELISPOT kit (Gen-Probe Diaclone).
4. $OVA_{257-264}/K^b$ tetramer (Beckman-Coulter Immunomics).
5. MACS buffer.
6. MACS LS columns.
7. MACS magnetic stand and magnet.
8. Phorbol myristate acetate (Sigma).
9. Ionomycin (Sigma).
10. Elispot reader, ImmunoSpot (CTL Europe).

2.11 Culture of Helicobacter suis (H. suis)

1. *H. suis* strain (e.g., HS5bLP): isolated from the gastric mucosa of a sow [36, 37].
2. Biphasic culture: Brucella agar (Oxoid) supplemented with 20% of heat inactivated FCS, 5 mg of amphotericin B/l (Fungizone), *Campylobacter* selective supplement (Skirrow, Oxoid; containing 10 mg/L of vancomycin, 5 mg/L of trimethoprim lactate, and 2500 U/L of polymyxin B), and Vitox supplement (Oxoid). Adjust the pH of the agar to 5 by adding HCl to a final concentration of approximately 0.05%. Add Brucella broth (Oxoid) with a pH of 5 on top of the agar to obtain biphasic culture conditions.

2.12 Preparation of H. suis Lysate/ CCR4-Antagonist Vaccine

1. RCDC™ Protein Assay (Bio-Rad).
2. CCR4 antagonist AF-399/42018025: The chemical name of the antagonist is 4-(1-benzofuran-2-ylcarbonyl)-1-{5-[(4-chlorobenzyl)sulfanyl]-1,3,4-thiadiazol-2-yl}-3-hydroxy-5-(2-thienyl)-1,5-dihydro-2H-pyrrol-2-one. Molecular weight 565.93 [3, 4] (*see* Fig. 1).

2.13 Quantification of Colonizing H. suis

1. DNeasy Blood and Tissue kit (Qiagen).
2. iQ SYBR mix (Bio-Rad).
3. *H. suis* Primers: BF_HsuisF1: 5′-AAA ACA MAG GCG ATC GCC CTG TA-3′ (sense) BF_HsuisR1: 5′-TTT CTT CGC CAG GTT CAA AGC G-3′ (antisense).

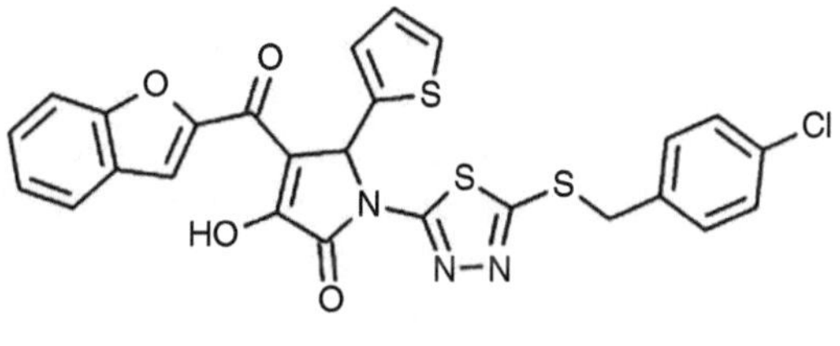

Fig. 1 Structure of CCR4 antagonist AF-399/42018025

2.14 Analysis of Cytokine Expression Profile by RT-PCR

1. RNAlater (Ambion).
2. Tri Reagent.
3. BAN—Phase separation reagent (MRC).
4. RNeasy mini kit (Qiagen).
5. iScript™ cDNA Synthesis kit (Bio-Rad).
6. iQ SYBR mix (Bio-Rad).

3 Methods

3.1 G Protein-Coupled Receptor (GPCR) Model Building

Generate a 3D structure of the CCR4 using an existing crystal structure of a GPCR such as bovine rhodopsin as a scaffold and identify potential agonists and antagonists using virtual screening (*see* **Note 1**).

1. Use the WHATIF program [38] to generate a helical transmembrane section of the desired GPCR structure, CCR4. The program will automatically generate a structure matching the known protein sequence of the desired protein. The orientation of the alpha helices will be calculated with respect to a lipid environment so that hydrophobic faces are orientated into the membrane phase and hydrophilic faces point into the lumen of the protein. The translational and rotational orientation of each helix in the transmembrane bundle is critical to the nature and conformation of the binding site. Hydrophobic areas of the transmembrane bundle will be orientated such that their peak hydrophobicity lies centrally within the lipid plane.
2. With your transmembrane scaffold it is now necessary to model the protein termini (N is extracellular, C is intracellular along with the three intracellular and three extracellular loops in between). In the absence of any definite structural information on the loops, it is necessary to model them in an extended confirmation.
3. Use the structural modeling package to build the loops in an extended confirmation. You now have a coherent protein structure of your GPCR but will need to optimize the structure through simulated annealing in order to create the best possible model for virtual screening.
4. As CCR4 is a transmembrane protein, it is necessary to simulate both the water and lipid bilayer environment. It is possible to combine your structure with a pregenerated lipid bilayer structure such as is available from the Biocomputing Group at the University of Calgary (http://wcm.ucalgary.ca/tieleman/downloads).

5. The two structures can be merged using a structural program such as VMD [39]. The CCR4 structure should be positioned so that it corresponds to the lipid midpoint plane (LMP). Editing of the LMP may be needed to incorporate the CCR4 structure.

3.2 Energy Minimization

1. Using the AMBER program leapi [40], hydrogen atoms must be added to the GPCR structure and the system should be fully solvated using water molecules in the TIP3 model [41]. This creates a solvent box with dimensions of approximately 40 Å by 50 Å by 120 Å and composed of approximately 110,000 atoms. All atoms in the simulation should be explicitly represented.
2. Any known conserved disulfide bonds within the structure should be explicitly represented using leapi.
3. Minimize the energy of the solvated molecular complex using the general AMBER force field with a steepest descent method continued for 50,000 time steps (one time step–one femtosecond) or until the RMSD has fallen below 0.01 Å between successive time steps.
4. In the first stage of minimization, the transmembrane region and lipid region should be frozen in order to allow the loops to order themselves using the transmembrane scaffold. All minimization and annealing steps can be performed using the AMBER sander program.
5. In the second stage, perform simulated annealing on the minimized structure. At this stage, all atoms in the systems can be allowed free movement. The system should be annealed by raising the temperature of the system from 0 K to 500 K over a period of 40,000 time steps and maintaining that temperature for a further 30,000 time steps. The system can then be cooled to 0.2 K over a period of 230,000 time steps before being rested at 1 K for a further 300,000 time steps.
6. Central Processing Unit (CPU) of an individual simulation should be approximately 500 h on a 6-processor High Performance Computing (HPC) cluster.
7. Run the docked small molecules under the same conditions and time period as the initial energy minimization. AMBER antechamber can be used to generate parameters for the small molecules.

3.3 Virtual Screening

1. A database can be generated from structures using a variety of compound suppliers and can be constructed within UNITY [42] and screened for potentially reactive and undesirable molecules.

2. The database can be prescreened using a simple pseudo-pharmacophore derived from properties of known Chemokine antagonists: compounds must have a MW > 500 and contain two or more 5- or 6-membered aromatic rings and one or more nitrogen atoms.
3. Remaining compounds after filtering can be generated in 3D structure built using CORINA [43], and can be tested for their affinity using the GOLD docking program (http://www.ccdc.cam.ac.uk/Solutions/GoldSuite/Pages/GOLD.aspx) and the Goldscore fitness function. Ligands can be docked within a targeted cavity within the CCR4 structure.

3.4 Isolation of Peripheral Blood Mononuclear Cells of Humans

1. Dilute the blood at least two times with RPMI 1640 medium.
2. In a 50-mL conical tube, layer the blood gently on a layer of Ficoll-hypaque using a 25-mL pipette. For every 15 mL of Ficoll-hypaque, add 30 mL of blood. Take extreme care to avoid the mixing of these two layers.
3. Spin the tubes at 400 × *g* for 30 min in a swinging bucket rotor at room temperature without brake. Please check that the brake is off or the acceleration and deceleration of the centrifuge is zero. This ensures that the two layers do not mix.
4. After the spin, using a 10-mL pipette, gently aspirate the intermediate, translucent and white layer containing peripheral blood mononuclear cells (PBMC) into the new tube. Try to take as much as possible. Add large volumes of RPMI 1640 medium to the tube to reduce the toxic effects of Ficoll-hypaque.
5. Wash the PBMC using RPMI 1640 medium at 300 × *g* for 5–10 min at 4 °C. Count the cells and use them for the isolation and the differentiation of various immune cells [44].

3.5 Isolation of Human Regulatory T Cells

1. Add a few mL of MACS buffer to PBMC and wash the cells at 300 × *g* for 5 min at 4 °C.
2. Resuspend the cell pellet in 90 μL of MACS buffer per 10^7 PBMC and add 10 μL of $CD4^+$ T Cell biotin-antibody cocktail per 10^7 PBMC. Mix the cell suspension gently.
3. Incubate the cells at 4 °C (refrigerator) for 5 min (*see* **Note 2**).
4. After 5 min, add 20 μL of anti-Biotin MicroBeads per 10^7 PBMC.
5. Mix the cell suspension gently and incubate the cells at 4 °C (refrigerator) for 10 min.
6. Prepare the LD column by adding recommended volume of buffer. Then apply cell suspension to the column. Collect the unlabelled $CD4^+$ T cells in the flow through (*see* **Note 3**).

7. Then wash the column twice with recommended volume of buffer (Miltenyi Biotec data sheet). Add new buffer only when the column reservoir is empty.
8. Wash the $CD4^+$ T cells at 300×*g* for 10 min at 4 °C and resuspend the cell pellet in 90 μL of MACS buffer per 10^7 PBMC.
9. Add 10 μL of CD25 Microbeads per 10^7 PBMC. Mix the cell suspension gently and incubate the cells at 4 °C (refrigerator) for 15 min.
10. Add 1–2 mL of MACS buffer to the cells, resuspend gently and wash at 300×*g* for 10 min at 4 °C.
11. Add 500 μL of MACS buffer per 10×10^7 PBMC and resuspend the cells gently.
12. Prepare the LS column by adding recommended volume of buffer. Then apply cell suspension to the column. Collect the unlabelled cells in the flow through.
13. Wash the column thrice with recommended volume of buffer (Miltenyi Biotec data sheet). Add new buffer only when the column reservoir is empty.
14. Remove column from the separator and place it on a suitable collection tube. Add suitable volume of buffer to the column as per instructions provided in Miltenyi Biotec data sheet. Quickly flush the contents using the plunger given along with the column.
15. Wash the purified $CD4^+CD25^+$ regulatory T cells in complete RPMI medium. Count the cells and use it for further assays.
16. Confirm the phenotype of Tregs by flow cytometry and validate in functional assays.

3.6 Generation of Human Th2 Cells

1. Add a few mL of MACS buffer to PBMC and wash the cells at 300×*g* for 5 min at 4 °C.
2. Resuspend the cell pellet in 40 μL of MACS buffer per 10^7 PBMC and add 10 μL of naive $CD4^+$ T Cell Biotin-Antibody Cocktail II per 10^7 PBMC. Mix the cell suspension gently.
3. Incubate the cells at 4 °C (refrigerator) for 5 min.
4. After 5 min, add 30 μL of MACS buffer per 10^7 PBMC and 20 μL of naive $CD4^+$ T Cell MicroBead Cocktail II per 10^7 PBMC.
5. Mix the cell suspension gently and incubate the cells at 4 °C (refrigerator) for 10 min.
6. Prepare the LS column by adding recommended volume of buffer. Then apply cell suspension to the column. Collect the unlabelled cells in the flow through that represent naïve $CD4^+$ T cells.

7. Then wash the column thrice with recommended volume of buffer (Miltenyi Biotec data sheet). Add new buffer only when the column reservoir is empty.
8. Wash the purified naïve $CD4^{+}CD45RA^{+}CD25^{-}$ T cells in complete RPMI medium. Count the cells and resuspend in complete RPMI medium.
9. Add naïve $CD4^{+}$ T cells (0.1×10^{6} cells/well) to 24-well tissue culture plates that were precoated with 10 μg/mL of anti-CD3 and anti-CD28 mAbs.
10. Culture the cells in complete RPMI 1640 in the presence of 10 μg/mL of neutralizing anti-IL-12 and IFN-γ mAbs, 10 ng/mL of rhIL-2 and 20 ng/mL of rhIL-4.
11. After 3 days, add 0.5 mL of 4 ng/mL IL-2 to the wells.
12. At day 6, harvest the cells, wash and repeat the stimulation cycle as in **steps 9** and **10**.
13. Harvest the cells, wash and confirm the phenotype (particularly for CCR4 expression) and intracellular cytokine profile of the differentiated Th2 cells.

3.7 Titration Experiments to Establish Optimal Doses of Chemokines for the Chemotaxis of Cell Lines and Primary Cells

1. Place the various concentrations of chemokines (0, 5, 10, 50, 100, and 500 ng/mL) (CCL17 or CCL22) in lower chambers of transwell in a 600 μL volume of RPMI 1640-1 % FCS.
2. Place CCRF-CEM, B9.1, Treg or Th2 cells (1×10^{6} cells/mL) in upper chambers in a 100 μL volume of RPMI 1640-1 % FCS.
3. Incubate the plate for 2 h at 37 °C.
4. Recover the cells in the lower chamber and count.
5. Determine the optimal doses of chemokines for the chemotaxis of cell lines and primary cells.

3.8 Reconstitution of CCR4 Antagonists

1. Reconstitute the CCR4 antagonists in 100 % cell culture grade DMSO (2–4 mg of CCR4 antagonist/mL of DMSO) (*see* **Note 4**).
2. Aliquot in small volumes and store at −20 °C.

3.9 In Vitro Chemotaxis Assay to Measure CCR4 Antagonism

1. Prepare RPMI 1640-1 % FCS-0.5 % DMSO medium for the experiments.
2. Mix the candidate CCR4 antagonists with the determined (*see* Subheading 3.7) concentration of chemokines (CCL17 or CCL22).
3. Place 600 μL of antagonist-chemokine mix in lower chambers of transwell.
4. Place CCRF-CEM, B9.1, Treg or Th2 cells (1×10^{6} cells/mL) in upper chambers in a 100 μL volume of RPMI 1640-1 % FCS-0.5 % DMSO.

5. Incubate the plate for 2 h at 37 °C.
6. Recover the cells in the lower chamber and count.
7. Calculate the percent inhibition of chemotaxis by CCR4 antagonists in relation to controls treated with solvent (DMSO) alone as follows: ([no. cells migrated in the presence of DMSO – no. cells migrated in the presence of antagonist]/ no. cells migrated in the presence of DMSO) × 100.
8. To measure the concentrations required to inhibit 50 % of cell migration in the chemotaxis assay, add graded doses of antagonists to a determined concentration of chemokines.

3.10 Induction of Activated Murine CCR4+ Regulatory T Cells

1. Harvest the lymph nodes of OTII Ly5.2 mice.
2. Homogenize the lymph nodes on 70 μm cell strainers.
3. Wash the cells with 10 mL of RPMI medium in 12 mL conical tubes, centrifuge for 10 min at 300 × *g*.
4. Purify CD4+ T cells from these lymph nodes with anti-CD4 coated magnetic beads (Miltenyi Biotec data sheet).
5. Coat the six wells plates for 2 h at 37 °C with 4 μg of mouse anti-CD3 in 1 mL of sterile PBS.
6. Add 3.3 millions of Ly5.2+ CD4+ T cells in 5 mL of RPMI with TGF-β (5 ng/ml = 30 ng/well) and IL-2 (100 UI/ mL = 600 UI/well).
7. Incubate the plates for 72 h at 37 °C.
8. Confirm the phenotype of cells (CCR4, FoxP3) by flow cytometry.

3.11 In Vivo Inhibition of Migration of Ly5.2+ CCR4+ Regulatory T Cells by CCR4 Antagonists in C57 Bl6 Ly5.1 Mice

1. Incubate 10×10^6 of in vitro induced OTII Ly5.2 CCR4+ regulatory T cells with or without 2 μg of CCR4 antagonist AF-399/42018025.
2. Inject the mixture intravenously in each C57Bl6 Ly5.1 mouse.
3. At the same time, subcutaneously inject each C57Bl6 Ly5.1 mouse with 30 μg of STxB-OVA vaccine and 1 μg of α-galactosyl ceramide to induce local specific immune response against OVA protein.
4. 24 h later harvest the draining lymph nodes of C57Bl6 Ly5.1 mice and homogenize on 70 μm cell strainers.
5. Wash the cells with 10 mL of RPMI medium and centrifuge for 10 min at 300 × *g*.
6. Analyze the Ly5.2+ CCR4+ cells by flow cytometry.

3.12 Reconstitution of STxB-OVA Vaccine

1. Obtain the STxB-OVA vaccine by chemical coupling between the nontoxic Shiga Toxin subunit B and synthetic OVA-derived peptide $OVA_{257\text{-}264}$ (SIINFEKL) [45, 46]. First, activate OVA via amino groups on lysine side chains using the

heterobifunctional cross-linker m-maleimidobenzoyl-N-hydroxysulfosuccinimide ester. Then react OVA with the B-subunit of Shiga toxin modified with a C terminal cysteine (STxB-Cys), and purify the reaction product by gel filtration and immunoaffinity chromatography.

2. Remove the contaminating lipopolysaccharide (LPS) by EndoTrap affinity chromatography.
3. After purification, determine the endotoxin concentration by Limulus assay. Endotoxin level should be < 0.5 EU/mg.

3.13 Evaluation of Adjuvanticity of CCR4 Antagonist in STxB-OVA Vaccine Model

1. Immunize $Neu^{OT\text{-}I/OT\text{-}II}$ mice twice (day 0 and day 14) with STxB-OVA (20 μg)/α-GalCer (1 μg) vaccine combined or not with 1.5 μg of CCR4 antagonist AF-399/42018025 (*see* **Notes 5** and **6**).
2. Harvest the splenocytes 7 days after the last injection.
3. Homogenize the spleen on 70 μm cell strainer.
4. Wash the cells with 35 mL of RPMI medium, centrifuge for 10 min at 300 × *g*.
5. Resuspend the pellet in 500 μL of FCS + 4 ml of ACK buffer (4 mL/spleen)
6. Incubate the cells for 2 min at 20 °C to lyse the red blood cells.
7. Stop the reaction by immersing the tubes in ice.
8. Wash the cells with 30 mL of RPMI and centrifuge at 4 °C for 10 min at 300 × *g*.
9. Resuspend the cells in 2 mL of RPMI medium and count the cells with an optical microscope in trypan blue (1/100 dilution).
10. Purify the $CD8^+$ T cells by using mouse anti-CD8 coated magnetic beads as per Miltenyi Biotec data sheet.
11. Analyze $CD8^+$ T cell specificity by tetramer staining or ELISPOT.
    (a) To detect anti-$OVA_{257\text{-}264}/K^b$ specific $CD8^+$ T cells by tetramer staining, stain the cells with $OVA_{257\text{-}264}/K^b$ tetramer (1 μL/10^6 cells) diluted in 50 μL of PBS BSA 1 % buffer according to the manufacturer's recommendations. Briefly, incubate the cells with PE-labeled tetramer (45 min at 4 °C in the dark). After incubation and washes (2 mL of PBS-BSA 1 %), add labeled anti-CD8 mAbs (1 μL/10^6 cells) diluted in 50 μL of PBS BSA 1 % buffer for 30 min at 4 °C in the dark. After two washes in 2 mL of PBS-BSA1%, fix the cells in 500 μL of PFA. Use irrelevant tetramers recognizing a VSV-derived peptide in the context of K^b in each experiment. Also, include naive non-immunized mice as controls for these experiments.

(b) Determine the functionality of specific anti-$OVA_{257-264}$ $CD8^+$ T cells by ex vivo ELISPOT according to the manufacturer's recommendations [40]. Precoat the ELISPOT plates with anti-mouse IFN-γ mAb overnight. After saturation with PBS-milk 2%, transfer 10^5 $CD8^+$ T cells to precoated wells and culture with 4×10^5 EL4 cells (an $H2^b$ thymoma) or splenocytes previously pulsed or not with specific CD8 peptides derived from OVA and fixed with 1% paraformaldehyde. After 18 h incubation at 37 °C and washings with PBS-Tween-20 0.1% buffer, incubate the plates with biotinylated anti-mouse IFN-γ mAb. Finally, wash the plates again with PBS-Tween20 0.1% and incubate for 30 min at 37 °C with alkaline phosphatase-labeled streptavidin. Develop the spots by adding 5-bromo-4-chloro-3-indolyl-phosphatase/nitroblue tetrazolium. Cells stimulated with phorbol myristate acetate (100 ng/mL) and ionomycin (500 ng/mL) serve as positive controls. Calculate the number of spot-forming cells (spots)/10^5 cells after subtracting negative control values (cells incubated with medium alone). Count the IFN-γ spot-forming cells (SFC) on the CTL ELISPOT reader. A response is considered positive if the number of spots in the wells stimulated with specific peptides is twofold higher than the number of spots in the wells without peptide with a cutoff of 10 spots-forming-cells per 1×10^5 cells [47].

3.14 Preparation of the H. suis Lysate Vaccine

1. After 3 days of incubation at 37 °C under microaerobic conditions (85% N_2, 10% CO_2, 5% O_2), harvest the Brucella broth, containing the *H. suis* bacteria [36].
2. Wash the bacteria 2 times in PBS (centrifugation at 5000×*g*, 10 min, 4 °C) and resuspend in PBS.
3. Sonicate the bacterial suspension 8 times for 30 s with a 50% duty cycle, on ice and with a frequency of 20 kHz, resulting in lysis of the bacteria. After centrifugation (5000×*g*, 10 min, 4 °C), collect the supernatant fluid and store at −70 °C until further use.
4. Determine the protein concentration using the Lowry assay (RCDC™ Protein Assay).
5. Concentrate the lysate using a Vivaspin 20 (centrifuge at 3000×*g*, 15 min). Each vaccine contains 100 μg of protein.

3.15 Evaluation of Adjuvanticity of CCR4 Antagonist in H. suis Lysate Vaccine Model

1. For subcutaneous vaccination, inject a mixture of 100 μg of *H. suis* sonicate and 1.5 μg of CCR4 antagonist AF-399/42018025 in a total volume of 100 μL (*see* **Notes 5** and **6**). Inject this mixture at the lower back of the animals (*see* **Note** 7).
2. For sublingual and intranasal vaccination, use a total volume of 7 μL, containing 100 μg of *H. suis* sonicate mixed with 1.5 μg of CCR4 antagonist AF-399/42018025. Apply the mixture on the external nares of the mice (*see* **Notes 5** and **6**).

3. Prepare *H. suis* strain HS5bLP for the challenge experiments by culturing as described in Subheading 3.14. Determine the final concentration of *H. suis* by counting motile bacteria in an improved Neubauer counting chamber.
4. On day 56 following immunization, inoculate the mice intragastrically with 0.3 mL of the challenge material, containing approximately 2×10^8 of viable *H. suis* bacteria/mL, using a ball-tipped gavage needle (*see* **Note 8**).
5. On day 77, euthanize the mice. Remove the stomachs and preserve in RNAlater at −70 °C until RNA and DNA extraction. Quantify the colonizing bacteria and cytokine response, and analyze the stomach wall by histopathology as described below.

3.16 Quantification of Colonizing H. suis by Quantitative Real-Time PCR (RT-PCR)

1. Extract DNA from the gastric tissue samples with the DNeasy Blood and Tissue kit according to the instructions of the kit manufacturer.
2. Perform RT-PCR using the C1000 Thermal cycler. Each sample contains 5 μL of iQ SYBR Green Supermix, 0.25 μL of each primer, 3.5 μL of distilled water, and 1 μL of DNA.
3. For the enumeration of colonizing bacteria, amplify a fragment of the UreA gene of *H. suis* using the BF_HsuisF1 and BF_HsuisR1 primers. For generation of the external standard, amplify part of the *ureAB* gene cluster (1236 bp) from *H. suis* strain HS5 using primers U430F and U1735R [48].
4. Calculate the copy number concentration based on the length of the amplicon and the mass concentration. The standard consists of tenfold dilutions starting at 10^7 gene copies for each 10 μL of reaction mixture.
5. Perform the data analysis using the Bio-Rad CFX Manager Version 3.0 software.

3.17 Evaluation of Cytokine Response to H. suis Lysate-CCR4 Antagonist Vaccine

1. Place gastric tissue samples in Sarstedt tubes containing 12 Zirconium/silica beads and two Stainless steel beads. Add the appropriate amount of TRI Reagent (1 mL per 50 mg of tissue).
2. Lyse the tissue using the Magnalyser (4 cycles of 30 s at 6000 bpm and 90 s at −20 °C). To ensure complete dissociation of nucleoprotein complexes, allow samples to stand for 5 min at room temperature.
3. Add 50 μL of BAN-phase separation reagent per 50 mg of stomach tissue. Cover the sample tightly, shake vigorously for 15 s, and allow to stand for 5–15 min at room temperature.

4. Centrifuge the resulting mixture at 12,000 ×*g* for 15 min at 2–8 °C. Centrifugation separates the mixture into 3 phases: a red organic phase (containing protein), an interphase (containing DNA), and a colorless upper aqueous phase (containing RNA).
5. Collect the colorless phase and extract the RNA with the RNeasy Mini Kit according to the instructions of the manufacturer.
6. Subsequently convert the RNA into cDNA using the iScript cDNA Synthesis Kit according to the instructions of the manufacturer.
7. Dilute the products 1/5 before use in RT-PCR to determine the messenger RNA expression levels of IL-17, IL-4, IFN-γ, keratinocyte chemoattractant (KC or CXCL1), LPS-induced CXC chemokine (LIX), macrophage inflammatory protein-2 (MIP-2 or CXCL2) and IL-10 (Table 1) [49] in stomach tissue. Perform all reactions in a final volume of 10 μL containing 5 pmole of the sense and 5 pmole of the antisense primer, 5 μL iQ SYBR mix, and 1 μL cDNA.
8. The reaction protocol consists of an initial activation phase at 95 °C for 15 min followed by 40 cycles of 95 °C for 20 s, 60 °C for 30 s, and 73 °C for 30 s. Include a melting curve by increasing the temperature with 0.5 °C every 5 s starting from 65 °C until 95 °C. Include the housekeeping genes H2afz, PPIA, and HPRT as references.
9. Normalize the threshold cycle values (Ct) to the geometric means of the reference genes and calculate the normalized mRNA levels according to 2(−ΔΔCt) method for each individual animal [50].

3.18 Histopathological Analysis of the Stomach Wall of Mice Injected with H. suis Lysate-CCR4 Antagonist Vaccine

1. Cut a longitudinal strip of gastric tissue from the esophagus to the duodenum along the greater curvature. Fix the strip in 4% phosphate buffered formaldehyde, process by standard methods, and embed in paraffin for light microscopy. Cut paraffin sections of 4 μm and leave to dry for 35 min on the heating plate (50 °C).
2. Stain one section with hematoxylin and eosin using an automatic slide stainer to score the intensity of the overall gastritis (infiltration with mononuclear and polymorphonuclear cells), using a visual analog scale similar to the Updated Sydney System [51].
3. On a second section, perform periodic acid-Schiff (PAS) staining to evaluate the presence of pseudo pyloric metaplasia of the fundus, as indicated by replacement of functional gastric epithelial cells by mucus-producing cells.

Table 1
List of genes and sequences of the primers used for RT-PCR gene expression analysis [49]

Gene	Primer	Primer sequence
IFN-γ	Sense	5′-GCG TCA TTG AAT CAC ACC TG-3′
	Antisense	5′-TGA GCT CAT TGA ATG CTT GG-3′
IL-4	Sense	5′-ACT CTT TCG GGC TTT TCG AT-3′
	Antisense	5′-AAA AAT TCA TAA GTT AAA GCA TGG TG-3′
IL-10	Sense	5′-ATC GAT TTC TCC CCT GTG AA-3′
	Antisense	5′-CAC ACT GCA GGT GTT TTA GCT CC-3′
IL-17	Sense	5′-TTT AAC TCC CTT GGC GCA AAA-3′
	Antisense	5′-CTT TCC CTC CGC ATT GAC AC-3′
KC	Sense	5′-GCT GGG ATT CAC CTC AAG AA-3′
	Antisense	5′-TCT CCG TTA CTT GGG GAC AC-3′
MIP-2	Sense	5′-AAA GTT TGC CTT GAC CCT GA-3′
	Antisense	5′-TCC AGG TCA GTT AGC CTT GC-3′
LIX	Sense	5′-CCC TGC AGG TCC ACA GTG CC-3′
	Antisense	5′-TGG CCG TTC TTT CCA CTG CGA-3′
H2afz	Sense	5′-CGT ATC ACC CCT CGT CAC TT-3′
	Antisense	5′-TCA GCG ATT TGT GGA TGT GT-3′
PPIA	Sense	5′-AGC ATA CAG GTC CTG GCA TC-3′
	Antisense	5′-TTC ACC TTC CCA AAG ACC AC-3′
HPRT	Sense	5′-CAG GCC AGA CTT TGT TGG AT-3′
	Antisense	5′-TTG CGC TCA TCT TAG GCT TT-3′

4 Notes

1. We used bovine rhodopsin as a scaffold to build the homology model of human CCR4 (pdb code:1F88). The structure of several chemokine receptors such as CXCR4 (pdb code:3ODU) and CCR5 (pdb code: 4MS) has since been solved and might further improve this model.
2. It is recommended to incubate the cells at 4 °C (refrigerator) for labeling with MicroBeads and not on ice. Incubation on ice reduces the labeling efficiency.
3. Instead of MACS columns and magnets, autoMACS Pro Separator can be used.

4. Since CCR4 antagonists are dissolved in DMSO, experiments should include a group treated with equivalent concentrations of DMSO.
5. The CCR4 antagonist has a short half-life in vivo. For inhibition of Tregs during the priming phase of vaccine administration, one shot of CCR4 antagonist is sufficient. However for long-term inhibition of Tregs, repetitive administration of CCR4 antagonist (every 2 days) is required for sustained Treg inhibition.
6. In contrast to other inhibitors of Tregs (anti-CD25...) [29] that have to be administered before vaccination, the CCR4 antagonist could be injected at the same time as the vaccine, since its effect is very quick. Also, CCR4 antagonists appear to have no effect on the expansion of Tregs at the tumor microenvironment [8].
7. We performed immunizations under light isoflurane anesthesia on days 7, 14, and 35 after arrival.
8. The mice are held in an upright position until they regain consciousness, to minimize the risk of reflux. Alternatively, challenge can be performed without anesthesia by a qualified person.

Acknowledgements

M.N.D., D.R.F., D.F.T., and J.B. were affiliated to Edward Jenner Institute for Vaccine Research, University of Oxford, UK, when the work was initiated. Supported by the Institut National de la Santé et de la Recherche Médicale, Université Pierre et Marie Curie and Université Paris Descartes, Canceropole Ile de France, Agence Nationale de la Recherche, Ligue contre le Cancer, Association pour la Recherche sur le Cancer, Pole de compétitivité Medicen (Immucan) Centre d'investigation Clinique en Biothérapie (CIC-BT505), SIRIC-CARPEM and Labex Immuno-Oncology, France; European Community's Seventh Framework Programme (FP7/2007–2013) under grant agreement HEALTH-2010.2.4.5-2 ALLFUN; and the Indo-French Center for Promotion of Advanced Research (CEFIPRA, Reference No: 4803-1).

References

1. Rappuoli R, Mandl CW, Black S, De Gregorio E (2011) Vaccines for the twenty-first century society. Nat Rev Immunol 11:865–872
2. Aimanianda V, Haensler J, Lacroix-Desmazes S, Kaveri SV, Bayry J (2009) Novel cellular and molecular mechanisms of induction of immune responses by aluminum adjuvants. Trends Pharmacol Sci 30:287–295
3. Bayry J, Tchilian EZ, Davies MN, Forbes EK, Draper SJ et al (2008) In silico identified CCR4 antagonists target regulatory T cells and exert adjuvant activity in vaccination. Proc Natl Acad Sci U S A 105:10221–10226
4. Davies MN, Bayry J, Tchilian EZ, Vani J, Shaila MS, Forbes EK et al (2009) Toward the discovery of vaccine adjuvants: coupling in

silico screening and in vitro analysis of antagonist binding to human and mouse CCR4 receptors. PLoS One 4, e8084. doi:10.1371/journal.pone.0008084
5. Pere H, Montier Y, Bayry J, Quintin-Colonna F, Merillon N, Dransart E et al (2011) A CCR4 antagonist combined with vaccines induce antigen-specific $CD8^+$ T cells and tumor immunity against self antigens. Blood 118:4853–4862
6. Vitali C, Mingozzi F, Broggi A, Barresi S, Zolezzi F, Bayry J et al (2012) Migratory and not lymphoid-resident dendritic cells maintain peripheral self-tolerance and prevent autoimmunity via induction of iTreg cells. Blood 120:1237–1245
7. Othy S, Topçu S, Kaveri SV, Bayry J (2012) Effect of CC chemokine receptor 4 antagonism on the evolution of experimental autoimmune encephalomyelitis. Proc Natl Acad Sci U S A 109:E2412–E2413
8. Shevchenko I, Karakhanova S, Soltek S, Link J, Bayry J, Werner J et al (2013) Low-dose gemcitabine depletes regulatory T cells and improves survival in the orthotopic Panc02 model of pancreatic cancer. Int J Cancer 133:98–107
9. Bosschem I, Bayry J, De Bruyne E, Van Deun K, Smet A, Vercauteren G et al (2015) Effect of different adjuvants on protection and side-effects induced by *Helicobacter suis* whole-cell lysate vaccination. PLoS One 10, e0131364. doi:10.1371/journal.pone.0131364
10. Sakaguchi S, Miyara M, Costantino CM, Hafler DA (2010) FOXP3+ regulatory T cells in the human immune system. Nat Rev Immunol 10:490–500
11. Ohkura N, Kitagawa Y, Sakaguchi S (2013) Development and maintenance of regulatory T cells. Immunity 38:414–423
12. Trinath J, Hegde P, Sharma M, Maddur MS, Rabin M, Vallat JM et al (2013) Intravenous immunoglobulin expands regulatory T cells via induction of cyclooxygenase-2-dependent prostaglandin E2 in human dendritic cells. Blood 122:1419–1427
13. Trinath J, Maddur MS, Kaveri SV, Balaji KN, Bayry J (2012) *Mycobacterium tuberculosis* promotes regulatory T-cell expansion via induction of programmed death-1 ligand 1 (PD-L1, CD274) on dendritic cells. J Infect Dis 205:694–696
14. Gupta N, Hegde P, Lecerf M, Nain M, Kalia M, Vrati S et al (2014) Japanese encephalitis virus expands regulatory T cells by increasing the expression of PD-L1 on dendritic cells. Eur J Immunol 44:1363–1374
15. Maddur MS, Trinath J, Rabin M, Bolgert F, Guy M, Vallat JM et al (2015) Intravenous immunoglobulin-mediated expansion of regulatory T cells in autoimmune patients is associated with increased prostaglandin E2 levels in the circulation. Cell Mol Immunol 12:650–652
16. Stephen-Victor E, Saha C, Sharma M, Holla S, Balaji KN, Kaveri SV et al (2015) Inhibition of programmed death 1 ligand 1 on dendritic cells enhances *Mycobacterium*-mediated interferon γ (IFN-γ) production without modulating the frequencies of IFN-γ-producing $CD4^+$ T cells. J Infect Dis 211:1027–1029
17. Onishi Y, Fehervari Z, Yamaguchi T, Sakaguchi S (2008) Foxp3+ natural regulatory T cells preferentially form aggregates on dendritic cells in vitro and actively inhibit their maturation. Proc Natl Acad Sci U S A 105:10113–10118
18. Bayry J, Triebel F, Kaveri SV, Tough DF (2007) Human dendritic cells acquire a semimature phenotype and lymph node homing potential through interaction with CD4+CD25+ regulatory T cells. J Immunol 178:4184–4193
19. Tang Q, Adams JY, Tooley AJ, Bi M, Fife BT, Serra P et al (2006) Visualizing regulatory T cell control of autoimmune responses in nonobese diabetic mice. Nat Immunol 7:83–92
20. André S, Tough DF, Lacroix-Desmazes S, Kaveri SV, Bayry J (2009) Surveillance of antigen-presenting cells by $CD4^+CD25^+$ regulatory T cells in autoimmunity: immunopathogenesis and therapeutic implications. Am J Pathol 174:1575–1887
21. Navarrete AM, Delignat S, Teillaud JL, Kaveri SV, Lacroix-Desmazes BJ (2011) $CD4^+CD25^+$ regulatory T cell-mediated changes in the expression of endocytic receptors and endocytosis process of human dendritic cells. Vaccine 29:2649–2652
22. Navarrete AM, Meslier Y, Teyssandier M, André S, Delignat S, Triebel S et al (2009) CD4+CD25+ regulatory T cells modulate human dendritic cell chemokines by multiple mechanisms. Arthritis Rheum 60:2848–2849
23. Miyara M, Ito Y, Sakaguchi S (2014) TREG-cell therapies for autoimmune rheumatic diseases. Nat Rev Rheumatol 10:543–551
24. Bayry J, Gautier JF (2016) Regulatory T cell immunotherapy for Type 1 diabetes: a step closer to success? Cell Metab 23:231–233
25. Bayry J, Sibéril S, Triebel F, Tough DF, Kaveri SV (2007) Rescuing the CD4+CD25+ regulatory T cell functions in rheumatoid arthritis by cytokine-targeted monoclonal antibody therapy. Drug Discov Today 12:548–552
26. Maizels RM, Smith KA (2011) Regulatory T cells in infection. Adv Immunol 112:73–136
27. Bayry J (2014) Regulatory T cells as adjuvant target for enhancing the viral disease vaccine efficacy. Virusdisease 25:18–25

28. Sugiyama D, Nishikawa H, Maeda Y, Nishioka M, Tanemura A, Katayama I et al (2013) Anti-CCR4 mAb selectively depletes effector-type FoxP3+CD4+ regulatory T cells, evoking antitumor immune responses in humans. Proc Natl Acad Sci U S A 110:17945–17950
29. Pere H, Tanchot C, Bayry J, Terme M, Taieb J, Badoual C et al (2012) Comprehensive analysis of current approaches to inhibit regulatory T cells in cancer. Oncoimmunology 1:326–333
30. Moore AC, Gallimore A, Draper SJ, Watkins KR, Gilbert SC, Hill AV (2005) Anti-CD25 antibody enhancement of vaccine-induced immunogenicity: increased durable cellular immunity with reduced immunodominance. J Immunol 175:7264–7273
31. Bayry J, Flower DR, Tough DF, Kaveri SV (2008) From 'perfect mix' to '*potion magique*'-regulatory T cells and anti-inflammatory cytokines as adjuvant targets. Nat Rev Microbiol 6:C1
32. Iellem A, Mariani M, Lang R, Recalde H, Panina-Bordignon P, Sinigaglia F et al (2001) Unique chemotactic response profile and specific expression of chemokine receptors CCR4 and CCR8 by CD4(+)CD25(+) regulatory T cells. J Exp Med 194:847–853
33. Bayry J, Tartour E, Tough DF (2014) Targeting CCR4 as an emerging strategy for cancer therapy and vaccines. Trends Pharmacol Sci 35:163–165
34. Cabaniols JP, Cibotti R, Kourilsky P, Kosmatopoulos K, Kanellopoulos JM (1994) Dose-dependent T cell tolerance to an immunodominant self peptide. Eur J Immunol 24:1743–1749
35. Wall EM, Milne K, Martin ML, Watson PH, Theiss P, Nelson BH (2007) Spontaneous mammary tumors differ widely in their inherent sensitivity to adoptively transferred T cells. Cancer Res 67:6442–6450
36. Baele M, Decostere A, Vandamme P, Ceelen L, Hellemans A, Chiers K et al (2008) Isolation and characterization of Helicobacter suis sp. nov. from pig stomachs. Int J Syst Evol Microbiol 58:1350–1358
37. Liang J, De Bruyne E, Ducatelle R, Smet A, Haesebrouck F, Flahou B (2015) Purification of Helicobacter suis strains from biphasic cultures by single colony isolation: influence on strain characteristics. Helicobacter 3:206–216
38. Vriend G (1990) WHAT IF: a molecular modeling and drug design program. J Mol Graph 8:52–56, 29
39. Humphrey W, Dalke A, Schulten K (1996) VMD: visual molecular dynamics. J Mol Graph 14(33-38):27–38
40. Case DA, Cheatham TE 3rd, Darden T, Gohlke H, Luo R, Merz KM Jr et al (2005) The Amber biomolecular simulation programs. J Comput Chem 2005(26):1668–1688
41. Price DJ, Brooks CL 3rd (2004) A modified TIP3P water potential for simulation with Ewald summation. J Chem Phys 121:10096–10103
42. Homer RW, Swanson J, Jilek RJ, Hurst T, Clark RD (2008) SYBYL line notation (SLN): a single notation to represent chemical structures, queries, reactions, and virtual libraries. J Chem Inf Model 48:2294–2307
43. Sadowski J (1997) A hybrid approach for addressing ring flexibility in 3D database searching. J Comput Aided Mol Des 11:53–60
44. Maddur MS, Sharma M, Hegde P, Stephen-Victor E, Pulendran B, Kaveri SV et al (2014) Human B cells induce dendritic cell maturation and favour Th2 polarization by inducing OX-40 ligand. Nat Commun 5:4092. doi:10.1038/ncomms5092
45. Sandoval F, Terme M, Nizard M, Badoual C, Bureau MF, Freyburger L et al (2013) Mucosal imprinting of vaccine-induced CD8(+) T cells is crucial to inhibit the growth of mucosal tumors. Sci Transl Med 5:172ra120
46. Adotevi O, Vingert B, Freyburger L, Shrikant P, Lone YC, Quintin-Colonna F et al (2007) B subunit of Shiga toxin-based vaccines synergize with {alpha} galactosylceramide to break tolerance against self antigen and elicit antiviral immunity. J Immunol 179:3371–3379
47. Bercovici N, Haicheur N, Massicard S, Vernel-Pauillac F, Adotevi O, Landais D et al (2008) Analysis and characterization of antitumor T-cell response after administration of dendritic cells loaded with allogeneic tumor lysate to metastatic melanoma patients. J Immunother 31:101–112
48. O'Rourke JL, Solnick JV, Neilan BA (2004) Description of 'Candidatus Helicobacter heilmannii' based on DNA sequence analysis of 16S rRNA and urease genes. Int J Syst Evol Microbiol 54:2203–2211
49. Flahou B, Van Deun K, Pasmans F, Smet A, Volf J, Rychlik I et al (2012) The local immune response of mice after Helicobacter suis infection: strain differences and distinction with Helicobacter pylori. Vet Res 43:75. doi:10.1186/1297-9716-43-75
50. Livak KJ, Schmittgen TD (2001) Analysis of relative gene expression data using real-time quantitative PCR and the 2–ΔΔCT method. Methods 25:402–408
51. Stolte M, Meining A (2001) The updated Sydney system: classification and grading of gastritis as the basis of diagnosis and treatment. Can J Gastroenterol 15:591–598

Chapter 9

Manufacturing Methods for Liposome Adjuvants

Yvonne Perrie, Elisabeth Kastner, Swapnil Khadke, Carla B. Roces, and Peter Stone

Abstract

A wide range of studies have shown that liposomes can act as suitable adjuvants for a range of vaccine antigens. Properties such as their amphiphilic character and biphasic nature allow them to incorporate antigens within the lipid bilayer, on the surface, or encapsulated within the inner core. However, appropriate methods for the manufacture of liposomes are limited and this has resulted in issues with cost, supply, and wider scale application of these systems. Within this chapter we explore manufacturing processes that can be used for the production of liposomal adjuvants, and we outline new manufacturing methods can that offer fast, scalable, and cost-effective production of liposomal adjuvants.

Key words Liposomes, Manufacturing, Adjuvants, Subunit vaccine, Delivery system, Preparation

1 Introduction

Conventionally, vaccines have been based on live attenuated microorganisms or inactivated/killed pathogens which exhibit high efficacy but are less safe due to the adverse effects that can include mild fever through to reversion of the virulence. Alternatively, modern vaccine technology has led to the development of subunit vaccines, which contain highly purified antigens instead of the whole pathogen. These vaccines offer better side-effect profiles but are poorly immunogenic [1, 2]. Hence, the inclusion of compounds which induce and amplify the protective immune response against an antigen is required in the formulation of subunit vaccines. These adjuvant systems may act in several ways, and can be classified into delivery systems and immunopotentiators albeit they are often a combination of both [3].

Of the particulate drug delivery systems available, liposomes were the first system to have demonstrated adjuvant activity with their immunological role and adjuvant properties being identified by [4]. Liposomes are spherical self-assembled structures, with lipids forming one or several concentric lipid bilayers enclosing

Christopher B. Fox (ed.), *Vaccine Adjuvants: Methods and Protocols*, Methods in Molecular Biology, vol. 1494, DOI 10.1007/978-1-4939-6445-1_9, © Springer Science+Business Media New York 2017

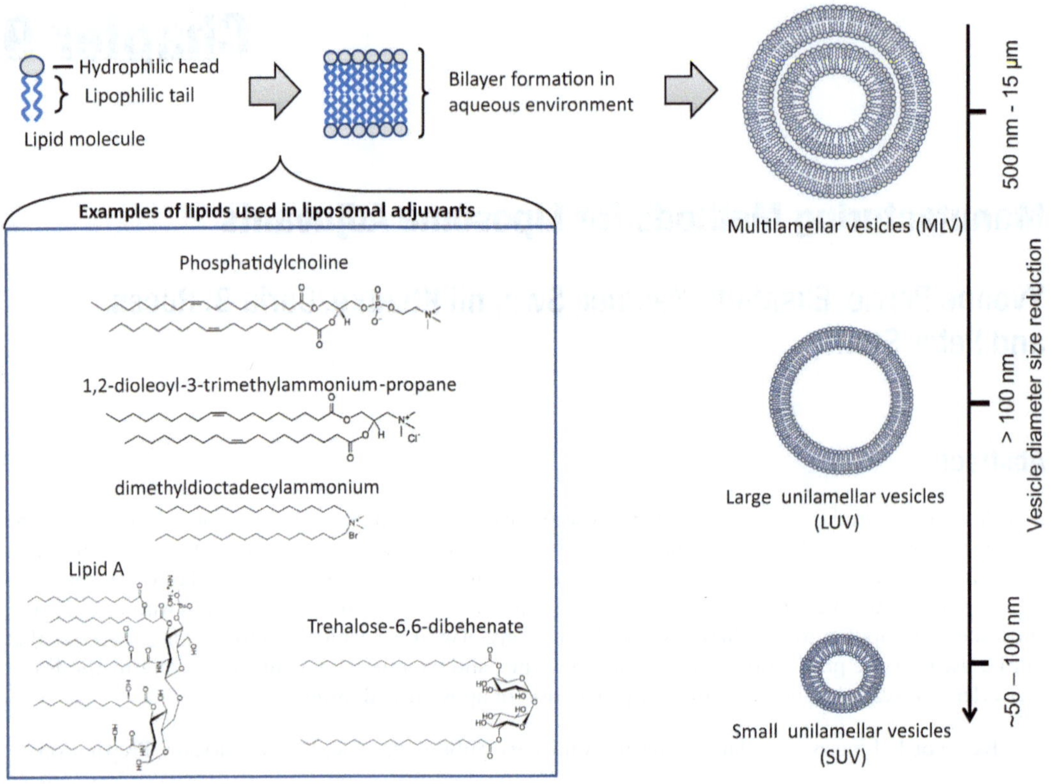

Fig. 1 Schematic of liposomal adjuvant formation

aqueous compartments (Fig. 1). As drug delivery systems, liposomes are well established with around 15 clinically licensed products in use. However, liposomes also offer a range of advantages for the delivery of antigens including versatility in size, bilayer composition, and ability to incorporate and thus protect sub-unit antigens from degradation and facilitate delivery to antigen presenting cells [5]. When liposomes were first investigated as vaccine adjuvants, very little was known of the mechanics of the immune system. However as our understanding of the immune system has expanded, this has fed into the underpinning principles of liposomal adjuvant design with investigations into the impact of their physicochemical attributes (e.g., size [6], charge [7], and bilayer rigidity [8]) and the inclusion of a range of immunological stimulating agents (such as synthetic nucleic acids, lipopeptides, and lipopolysaccharides [9]) on their adjuvant efficacy.

When considering the physicochemical attributes of liposomal adjuvants, it is important to consider that characteristics such as liposome size and surface charge can be modified by variation of the method of preparation and/or changing liposome composition [3, 10]. Given these parameters have been shown to be key performance attributes in the design of liposomal adjuvants (e.g., [11]), controlling these properties is of utmost importance. However, manufacturing, stability, and quality assurance issues are still a major concern for the use of liposome as adjuvants for human use [12]. Therefore, an appropriate manufacturing method should be selected prior to liposome preparation.

1.1 Traditional Top-Down Liposome Manufacturing Methods

Despite all the advances in the application of liposomes they are limited by their manufacturing methods and new systems for reproducible vesicle manufacturing are needed. Furthermore, the method of vesicle manufacture can be a dominating factor on particle size which can in turn impact on adjuvant activity [13]. In the most basic terms, there are two ways of forming liposomes, either top down or bottom up: top-down methods generally rely on size reduction of large multilamellar vesicles, while bottom-up methods result in the formation of small vesicles from individual lipid monomers. Within the lab, top-down methods generally begin with the lipid film hydration method (Fig. 2). The method works by first dissolving the lipid into an organic solvent such as chloroform or methanol to a desired concentration [14]. The lipids are then mixed together to the desired ratio and the solvent removed under reduced pressure to form a film. This film is then hydrated above the transition temperature of the lipids used to ensure efficient hydration. The antigen to be incorporated may be added into

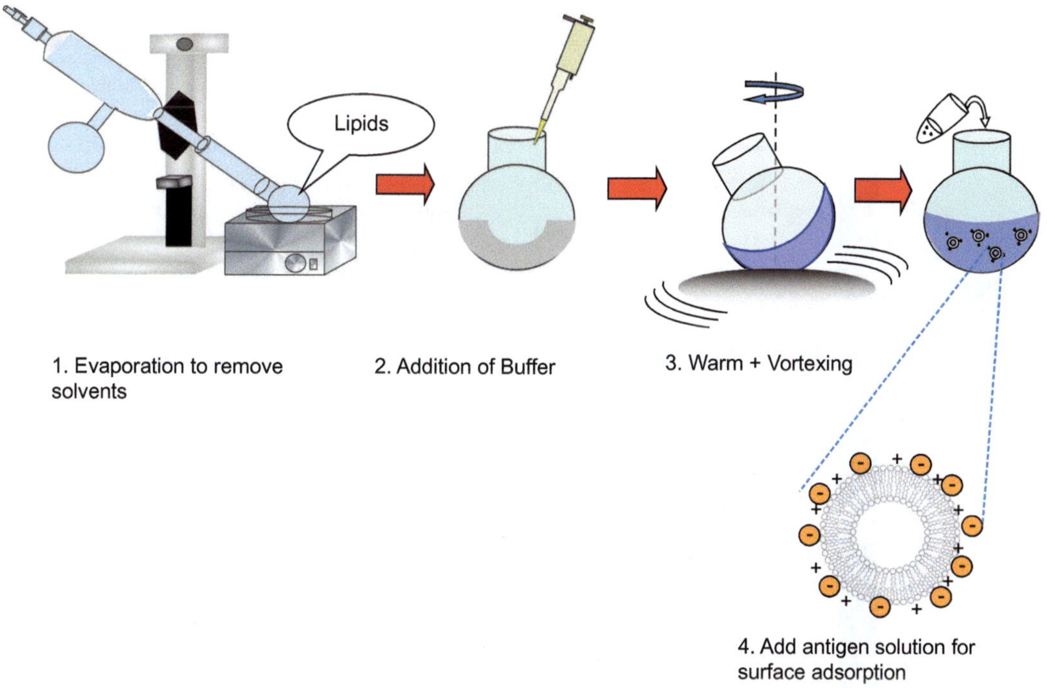

Fig. 2 Schematic of the simple lipid hydration method commonly used for laboratory-scale manufacture of liposomes

the aqueous hydration buffer or in the solvent phase depending on its solubility, leading to encapsulation in the aqueous core or into the lipid bilayer respectively. Once the hydration fluid is added, the film swells and hydrates to form the liposomes. The lipid film hydration method is a quick and simple method for producing large multilamellar vesicles (MLV), but does suffer some drawbacks: the resulting vesicles are generally quite polydisperse and relatively large, ranging up to several microns in size. The resulting size is primarily dictated by the choice of lipids, the aqueous hydration buffer and the temperatures adopted during vesicle formation [15, 16]. Furthermore, encapsulation efficiencies are usually low when this method is employed. Other methods used that result in the formation of large vesicle structures include reverse-phase evaporation and injection methods (Fig. 3).

To reduce vesicle sizes, subsequent mechanical methods are used (Fig. 3). These methods often rely on sonication, shear or pressure forces, including microfluidization, high-pressure homogenization, or other shear force-induced homogenizer [17, 18]. Those methods introduce a high and controlled pressure, disrupting larger multilamellar vesicles and leading to the formation of smaller vesicles in a continuous and scalable process setup [17].

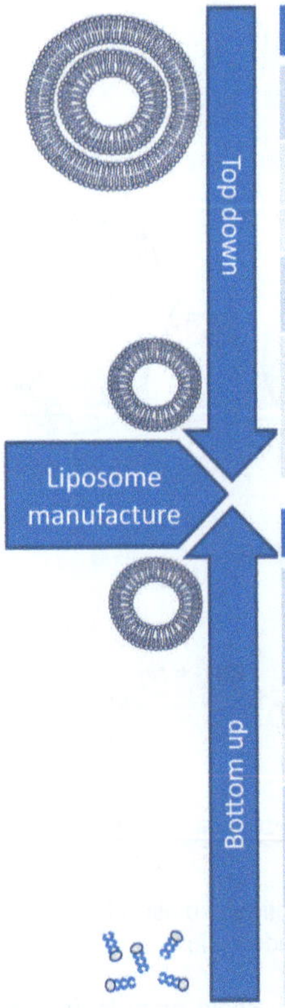

Method	Advantages	Disadvantages	Variables
Homogenisation	Easy. Simple design. Bulk production. Continuous process achievable.	High pressures can damage drug.	Pressure and number of cycles.
Extrusion		Slow, low batch size. Drug degradation. Filter clogging and product loss.	Number of cycle and filter sizes.
High shear mixing		Head generation and shearing can damage drug and lipids	Speed and mixer design.
Sonication	Easy. Relatively quick.	Sterility issues. Degradation. Low encapsulation. Limited scalability.	Bath or probe sonication. Amplitude. Time.

Method	Advantages	Disadvantages	Variables
Solvent injection	Rapid & easy. Non specialist kit. High encapsulation of hydrophobic drugs.	Solvent residue removal. Dilution.	Needle diameter Injection speed Rate of evaporation
Inkjet	Loading in-situ High reproducibility.	Solvent residue. Dilution.	Droplet size & speed Rate of evaporation
Supercritical fluid	Small size range.	High costs. High pressures. Encapsulation lower than with conventional methods.	Injection pressure
Microfluidics	Loading in situ. Scalable and continuous process.	Solvent residue removal.	Mixer design Mixing flow rate

Fig. 3 Summary of some of the commonly used methods for liposome manufacture

Sonication is one of the main methods used to reduce vesicle size with some of the earliest work being carried out by Papahadjopoulos back in 1967 [19, 20]. The sonication method is divided into two approaches: bath and probe sonication, each with their own advantages and disadvantages. Probe sonication is cheap, simple, and well researched but suffers from lipid degradation through overheating and oxidation and contamination both from the probe and larger particles of MLV [21–23]. Bath sonication is a non-contact temperature-controlled method that can run multiple samples at the same time but is not as well researched and can be limited by the ability to provide enough power to reduce the size of the liposomes sufficiently [14, 24]. During sonication, liposomes are subject to ultrasonic energy that shatters the liposome bilayer and allows the fragments to then form smaller vesicles [25]. Along with the lack of industrial scalability and relatively low encapsulation efficiencies [26], using the sonication method has the drawback of difficulty maintaining sterility. Another disadvantage of the sonication method is risk of overheating of the liposome suspension during sonication which can lead to degradation of lipids. This can be avoided by using water/ice baths during sonication to control temperature. During sonication, there is also the problem of the probe tip releasing titanium fragments into the liposomal suspension; this contamination can be removed by centrifugation of the liposome system post-sonication. In contrast, bath sonication can circumvent many of these issues as the liposome suspension does not come in contact with a sonication probe and it can be sonicated as a sealed unit thereby maintaining sterility in the formulation [27]. Other factors including the composition of the lipid membrane, lipid concentration, temperature of hydration, sonication time/frequency, and volume all influence the size and vesicle distribution in both the probe and bath sonication methods [28].

High shear mixing is a method for the production of size-reduced, unilamellar, and uniform liposomes either from preformed liposomes prepared by any known technique or by hydration of lipid powders in an aqueous phase [29]. This technique is built on the rotor-stator principle. The rotational speed produced by the rotor draws the solution inside and then drives it against the stator [29, 30]. Therefore, liposomes collide with the stainless steel of the head of the mixer (stator) shearing off the outer layers of the lipid vesicles and hence, reducing their size [23, 30, 31]. Shearing of the liposomes at high speeds and at temperatures above the transition phase of the lipid system where lipids are in the fluid state (disordered state) guarantees a homogeneous liposomal formulation [29, 30]. Liposomal size and size distribution depend on the time and rotational speed at which the samples are prepared.

Extrusion is another method used for the reduction of vesicle size. Extrusion, like sonication, was one of the earlier methods used for the production of the small liposomes used for drug delivery and is still a common method of size reduction. Extrusion works by using pores of a fixed diameter and forcing preformed liposomes through those pores to generate uniform liposomes with different mean diameters [21]. Most of these filters are formed from polycarbonate [32]. Like sonication and high shear mixing, size reduction via extrusion needs to occur above the transition temperature of the liposome system to ensure efficient and complete size reduction. Because it is a contact method like probe sonication and high shear mixing, it does suffer from possible contamination but can avoid contamination with much larger liposomes or of lipid degradation due to oxidation or overheating.

To reduce vesicle size using microfluidization and high-pressure homogenization pressures as high as 20,000 psi are used to force large vesicles thorough a small gap and collision with a stainless steel wall results in smaller vesicles generated [31, 33]. Often, several cycles are required to yield a homogenous and final size distribution; the option of continuous processing accomplishes this.

1.2 Bottom-Up Methods of Liposome Production

In contrast to the mechanical top down methods described above, methods around fluidic control can be summarized as bottom-up methods (Fig. 3). The ethanol injection method was the first one reported in the 1970s by Batzri and Korn [34]. Within this process, lipids are initially dissolved in a solvent, and then the solvent is rapidly injected into an aqueous buffer stream. The precipitation of the lipids leads to the formation of vesicles. While the method is relatively simple, results are dictated by the solubility of the lipids in the water-miscible solvent. Furthermore, solvent removal post-processing is required and is undertaken by heating. Using this type of method, encapsulation efficiencies within liposomes may be relatively high for hydrophobic drugs, while the encapsulation of a hydrophilic drug is generally relatively low due to the high volumes of aqueous phase and resulting dilution [35]. However, this type of method is scalable, simple, and highly applicable for a large-scale process.

The control of lipid sizes has been reported in an adaptive inkjet method [36]. Within this method, the Inkjet device comprises a glass capillary enclosed by a cylindrical piezoelectric sleeve. By applying a voltage pulse, excitation of the piezoelectric actuator occurs and forces the piezoelectric sleeve to contract and expand around the glass capillary. This causes acoustic compression and rarefaction waves to transmit laterally along the nozzle. Constructive and destructive excitation signals shaped between waves generate a compression wave with sufficient amplitude to overcome the surface tension at outlet and cause the formation of a liposome at the inkjet nozzle [37].

A supercritical fluid method has also been investigated for the production of liposomes. In this method lipids are dissolved after being placed in a cartridge through which repeated cycles of carbon dioxide/ethanol was passed. Lipids with different solubilities in the dense gas phase repetitively dissolve, leading to the formation of a homogeneous liposome suspension. The solution is then rapidly expanded into an aqueous phase containing the hydrophilic compound to be entrapped [38].

A more recent development in the manufacture of liposomes involves the use of rapid microfluidic mixing which enables the bottom-up synthesis of well-defined limited size liposomes with high encapsulation and circumvents the disadvantages of other methods such as sterility issues, degradation, and limited scalability.

1.3 Microfluidics

Microfluidic devices comprise fluid handling in a constrained volume, achieving millisecond mixing at the nanoliter scale [39, 40]. The area of microfluidics and its associated development of novel lab-on-a-chip-based devices gained increasing attention over the past decades [41]. Microfluidics is a complex area; besides the fundamentals of physics and chemistry, mass transport, heat and mass transfer, fluid flow, thermodynamics, elasticity, and electrostatics are important areas incorporated [42]. Characterization of the fluid flow in micromixing is essential for understanding its impact to the mixing performance. It is important to understand that a micromixer is not just a copy of a mixer in a larger size. The design has to control physical characteristics as far as possible [43]. With an increasing number of liposomal products in clinical trials and development [44] the demand for rapid process development tools is rising, emphasised by several microfluidic-based methodologies in drug development [45–48]. Microfluidic-based technologies offer an enhanced control over processing conditions, thus yielding a set-up for reproducible and robust manufacturing, which is required to achieve uniform liposome size distributions. Furthermore, the miniaturisation makes efficient use of materials and by While reducing volumes during development processes, costs can be diminished whereas throughput is increased [49–51].

In order to achieve complete diffusive mixing, devices have been developed to decrease mixing length. Developed micromixers can be classified into active and passive micromixers [43]. Active micromixers require an input from an external energy source; this can be pressure driven, temperature induced, or ultrasonic driven. Active micromixers are categorized by their energy input or disturbance, meaning pressure, electrokinetics, dielectrophoretic, electrowetting, magneto-hydrodynamic, or ultrasound [41]. Despite high mixing efficiencies in active micromixers, their engineering setup can be quite complex. The incorporation of the external power source into the microfluidic mixing chamber or device is cost and time intensive, with resulting restricted application in industry. Besides, high temperatures or ultrasonic applications might lead to damage of biological materials and have to be considered [43].

Table 1
Selection of common passive micromixers

Passive micromixer	Mixing principle	Type	References
T- and Y-shaped	Two streams are guided in one flow path; mixing solely by diffusion and hence generally slow		[68]
Parallel lamination	Split of inlet stream into a number of sub-streams and their rejoining. Enhanced mixing by increased surface area and decreased diffusion length	Bifurcation-type feeds, interdigital-type feeds, chessboard micromixer, circular micromixer	[69]
Sequential lamination	Sequential splitting and recombination and rearrangement of fluid streams	Split-and-recombine micromixer, crossing manifold micromixer	[70]
Flow focusing	Hydrodynamic focusing of the middle inlet stream by two outer fluids, leading to decreased lamination width of the inner stream	Horizontal and vertical flow focusing devices	[71]
Chaotic advection	Increase in interfacial area by altering channel shapes (split, stretch, fold, break) to alter flow direction and induce whirls and chaotic flow, grooved pattern in channel design	Slanted groove micromixer, staggered herringbone micromixer, connected-groove micromixer, circulation disturbance micromixer, 3D serpentine micromixers, zig-zag micromixer	[52]
Droplet	Microdroplet generation by electric fields, micro-injectors, or needles or multiphase flows, droplets lead to reduction in diffusion length and generation of recirculating flow in the droplet	T-junction droplet generator, planar serpentine micromixer	[72]

So-called passive mixers (Table 1) do not require an additional external energy source to achieve mixing, but use the fluid flow and specially designed micro-structures that enhance diffusion and advection processes [41]. In order to maximize diffusion by decreasing the diffusion path and increasing the surface area between different fluids, passive micromixers often undergo extensive channel engineering to modify the flow pattern. Engineering activities, including the splitting of fluid flow streams, introduction of bubbles or gas, and alterations in channel design, width, and shape by introduction of grooves, lead to a number to extensively altered micromixing chambers. Their integration to lab-on-a-chip-based devices is easier as no external power source has to be incorporated [43].

The staggered herringbone micromixer (SHM) is a micromixer based on patterns of grooves in the channel floor (Fig. 4). The design introduces a chaotic flow in a microchannel by subjecting the fluid to repetitive series of a rotational flow profile, which is achieved by alteration of the grooves as a function of the axial position in the channel. Characterization work by Stroock et al. determined the orientation of grooves in the floor changing after a half cycle in the design. This "center of rotation" is hence changed along with the local extensional flow in the transverse flow [52].

The application of microfluidic tools for liposome manufacturing is based on the theory of a nanoprecipitation reaction. Nanoprecipitation produces nanoparticles in a one-step process [61]. The process has been described by Stainmesse as the formation of particles of sub-micron size is possible at the right polymer concentration and if the ratio between aqueous to solvent flow was high enough [53]. This work was taken further, defining the nanoprecipitation process relying on a nucleation process, based on

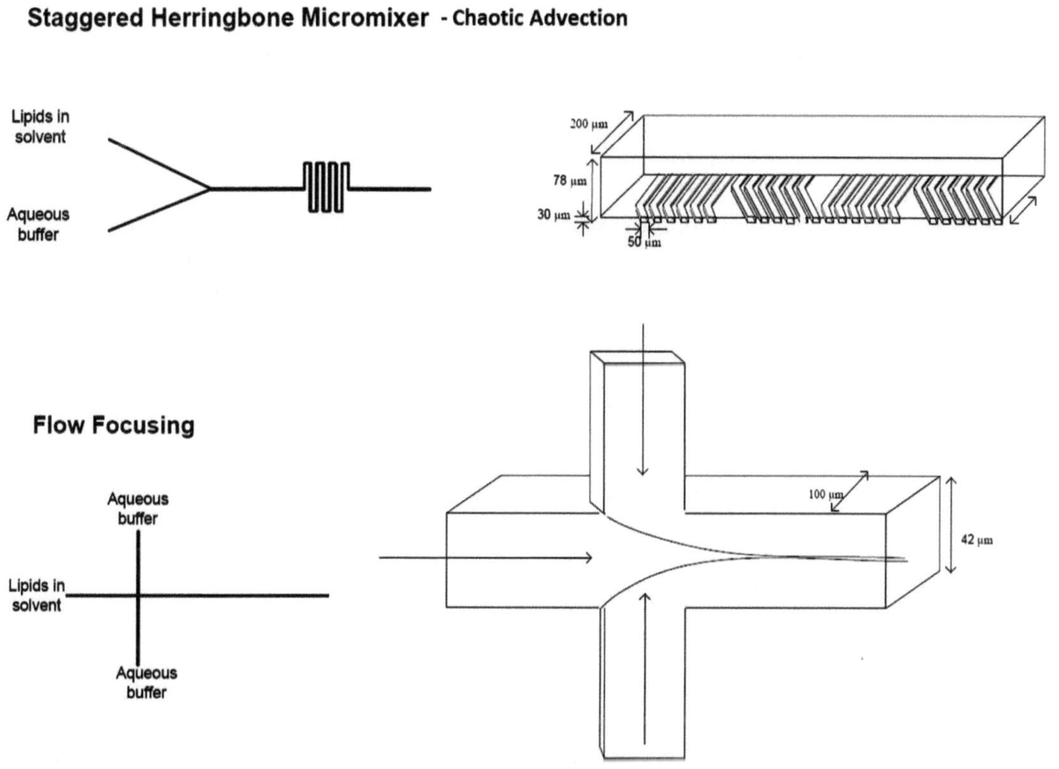

Fig. 4 Overview of the chaotic advection SHM method and the flow focusing method

chemical instability [54]. The solvent needs to be miscible with the non-solvent phase, which is usually a buffer. Opposed to the top-down methods, no further disruption of the resulting nanoparticles is required and the method is categorized as a bottom-up method. Dialysis can be used to drive the nanoprecipitation method [55]. This method was used in a larger scale format (volumes of 20 mL per batch) where solvent phase was added dropwise into an aqueous phase and stirred magnetically, after which evaporation of the solvent was conducted [56].

Recently, the method has been transferred onto microfluidic platforms allowing the high-throughput advantages of microfluidic systems. Opposed to the initial larger scale methods, microfluidics allows for a controlled input of fluid streams in micro-sized flow channels. Given the theory of nanoprecipitation, an aqueous volume is required in order to trigger the precipitation of the amphiphilic molecules. Microfluidic mixing allows for a controlled mixing of solvent and aqueous phase in a rapid process. The alteration of the flow channel, e.g., by aiding the diffusion process in a chaotic advection micromixer, further enhances this mixing process. Using a microfluidic-sized flow channel allows for a tight control of flow rates, as opposed to the ethanol infection method [34], and gives a controlled precipitation method on a small footprint, which is well suited for a high-throughput screening. Compared with process optimization on a larger scale, process development with microfluidic devices allows for a better control of mixing efficiencies, which at this scale is predominantly based on molecular diffusion. The increased surface-to-volume ratios generate fast mixing times by minimizing dimensions and diffusion lengths [57, 58] accompanied with a reduced time for sample handling [45].

Early work focused on the use of a flow-focusing technique on a microfluidic platform. This platform resulted in successful formation of liposomes in size ranges from 35 to 180 nm [59, 60]. Here, the lipid-solvent stream was centered between two streams of aqueous buffer, where mixing occurs at the interfaces primarily dominated by diffusion. The nanoprecipitation method was adapted into a multilamination micromixer for the production of polymer nanoparticles [61]. A chaotic advection micromixer has been initially described for the nanoprecipitation of liposomes, now commercialized by Precision Nanosystems Inc. An SHM mixer resulted in limit-size synthesis of lipid-based nanoparticles. Variations in flow rate and flow rate ratios led to the engineering of liposomes in the range of 20–80 nm for small interfering RNA (siRNA) delivery [62, 63], DNA [64], and low-solubility drugs [65].

1.4 Applications of Microfluidics for Subunit Vaccine Manufacturing

Controllable technologies such as microfluidics represent an attractive method for liposome manufacturing. The ease of formulation, reproducibility, and scalability of this method make it an attractive alternative compared to the bottom-up methods mentioned above [66].

Liposomes with controlled size and a narrow size distribution can be manufactured. Antigen loading can be carried out in three different ways depending on the desired location and characteristics of the antigen (Fig. 5).

- Association of the antigen to the liposome membrane surface
  Antigen can be attached to the surface of preformed liposomes by simple addition after formulation. Appropriate volume of antigen is added to the liposome solution and gently mixed in order to get a homogeneous solution. Care should be taken when selecting the lipid composition of the liposomes, since there must be an adequate interaction between antigen and liposomal surface. Adsorption to the surface may be due to electrostatic or hydrophobic interactions, hydrogen bonding, or van der Waals forces [3]. For example, proteins are commonly negatively charged; therefore, the use of cationic liposomes would favor the association with them [67].
- Encapsulation of the antigen within the liposome aqueous core
  Hydrophilic antigens or proteins can be dissolved in the aqueous phase to the desired concentration and then injected into the microfluidics system. Encapsulation and liposome formation is carried out simultaneously within the microfluidics system.
- Incorporation of the antigen within the liposome lipid bilayer

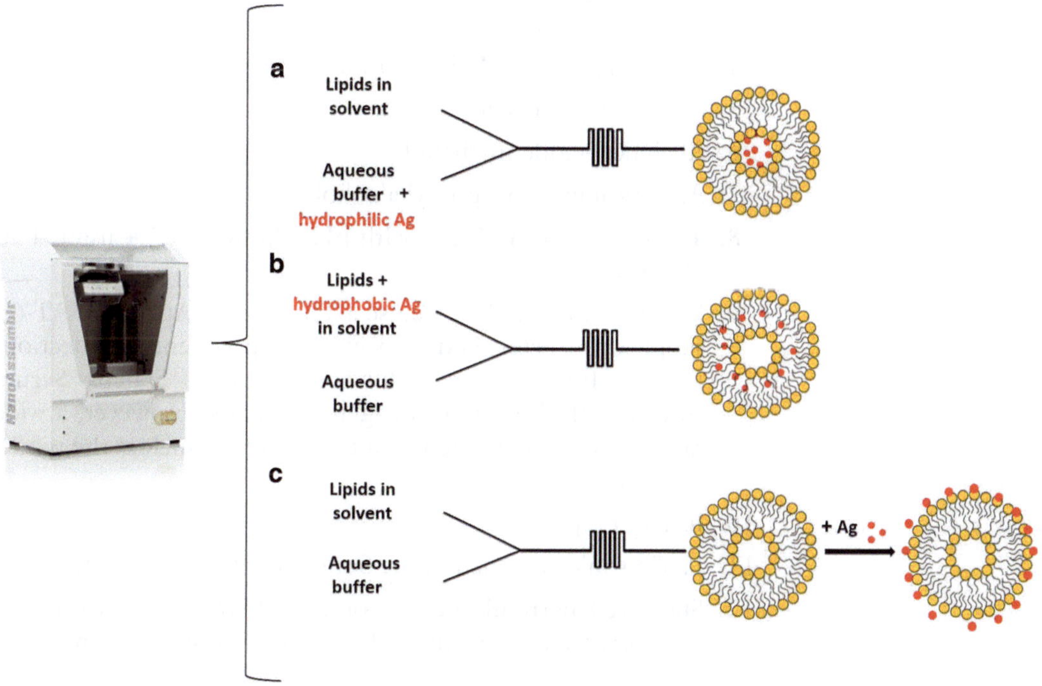

Fig. 5 Manufacture of liposomal adjuvants using microfluidics

On the other hand, hydrophobic antigens may be dissolved in the solvent phase at the desired concentration and then injected into the system. Subsequently, antigen intercalation within the lipid bilayer and liposome formation occur at the same time.

With recent advances in precision manufacturing systems, there is now a range of systems that can be used to produce liposomal vaccine adjuvants in a range of capacities from personalized doses to large continuous throughput production. However, these systems have yet to be exploited in the production of liposomal systems for clinical use.

Within our laboratories we have undertaken a series of investigations and identified a cationic liposome formulation based on dimethyldioctadecylammonium bromide and the immunomodulator α,α′-trehalose 6,6′-dibehenate. We have prepared these vesicles using a range of methods including the lipid hydration, sonication, and microfluidics methods.

2 Materials

1. Cationic surfactant dimethyldioctadecylammonium (DDA) bromide (Avanti Polar Lipids).
2. Immunomodulator α,α′-trehalose 6,6′-dibehenate (TDB) (Avanti Polar Lipids).
3. 2-Amino-2-(hydroximethyl)-1,3.propanediol (Trizma base®) (ICN Biomedicals, Inc.).
4. Ultrapure water (Milli-Q purification system).
5. Analytical grade chloroform.
6. Analytical grade methanol.
7. Analytical grade isopropyl alcohol.
8. Tris buffer: 10 mM Tris with pH adjusted to 7.4 using 1 M HCl solution.
9. Vaccine antigen: Here we use a TB antigen (Ag85B-ESAT-6), supplied by Peter Andersen et al. Department of Infectious Disease Immunology, Adjuvant Research, Statens Serum Institut, DK-2300 Copenhagen, Denmark. However, a wide range of subunit antigens can be employed, such as the model antigen ovalbumin.
10. Rotary evaporator.
11. Probe sonicator, such as the Soniprep150plus (MSE Ltd).
12. Staggered herringbone micromixer (SHM) used within the Nanoassemblr™ Benchtop (Precision Nanosystems, Inc.).

3 Methods

3.1 Manufacture of Cationic Liposomes via Lipid Hydration

MLV are easily prepared by the well-established film technique (i.e., the assembly of phospholipids into closed lipid bilayers within excess water) first observed by Bangham, in the 1960s [15]. A schematic of this process is shown in Fig. 2.

1. Preparation of stock solutions of the lipids: The lipids used in this technique are dissolved in a chloroform:methanol (9:1 v/v) solution at the desired concentrations. DDA is dissolved to a final concentration of 10 mg/mL whereas TDB is dissolved to a final concentration of 2 mg/mL.
2. The required amount of lipid solution is transferred from the stock to a 50 mL round-bottom glass to reach the appropriate concentration and is mixed. DDA/TDB liposomes are commonly prepared in 250/50 μg per vaccine dose (50 μL) (*see* **Note 1**).
3. In order to remove organic solvent, the round bottom flask is placed in a Rotary evaporator under vacuum for 15 min at 200 rpm.
4. Afterwards, the lipid film is further dried for a few minutes with a gentle stream of N_2 in order to remove any trace of organic solvent.
5. The lipid film is hydrated with the appropriate amount of 10 mM Tris buffer (pH 7.4) at temperatures above the lipid transition temperature (*see* **Note 2**). Since the transition temperature of DDA is 47 °C, generally samples are maintained at 60 °C by placing the round bottom flasks in a water bath for 20 min and vortexing for 1 min every 5 min (*see* **Note 3**).
6. Liposomes are allowed to cool down at room temperature and can be stored at 2–8 °C for further experiments (*see* **Note 4**).
7. By this method, multilamellar vesicles of ~500 nm are produced with this lipid combination. The size of the vesicles formed is influenced by the lipid combinations used in the formulation.
8. For these liposomes, any anionic sub-unit antigen can be added to the suspension promoting adsorption of the antigen. The cationic/anionic ratio chosen will impact on antigen loading and high antigen levels can promote aggregation of these vesicle systems. The addition of μg of antigen to 250/50 μg DDA/TDB can normally be easily incorporated without aggregation.

3.2 Manufacture of Cationic Liposomes via Sonication

As mentioned, there are two sonication techniques, bath and probe sonication, where a high-energy input is delivered to the lipid suspension disrupting the vesicles to produce small unilamellar vesicles (SUV). Generally probe sonication is more effective for size reduction and it can be applied as follows:

1. Liposome suspensions prepared by the lipid hydration method are transferred to a flat bottom glass vial and placed on the platform inside the probe sonicator (*see* **Note 5**).
2. The platform is elevated to the right position where the titanium probe is immersed in the liposome suspension.
3. For a 2 mL sample of the DDA/TDB (250/50 μg) formulation, the liposomes are sonicated for 2 min at 10 psi. These parameters will vary with the probe tip diameter, volume, and concentration of your liposome suspension (*see* **Note 6**).
4. The temperature should be maintained above the transition temperature during the process.
5. Liposomes are subsequently cooled to room temperature and stored at 2–8 °C for further experiments. By this method, SUV of 100–150 nm are produced (*see* **Note 7**).

3.3 Manufacture of Cationic Liposomes via Microfluidics

Among the micromixers based on the formation of nanoparticles by chaotic advection, the staggered herringbone micromixer (SHM) used within the Nanoassemblr™ Benchtop (Precision Nanosystems, Inc., Vancouver, Canada) can be used for the manufacturing of liposomes. SHM is based on the mixing of two different fluid streams through the herringbone structures located in the middle of the channel (Fig. 4). Both solutions are injected into the system at selected flow rates and flow ratios as follows:

1. Preparation of stock solutions: Lipids must be dissolved in an adequate solvent compatible with the microfluidics cartridge. Isopropyl alcohol (IPA) is used for DDA and TDB. DDA is dissolved in IPA to a final concentration of 10 mg/mL whereas TDB is dissolved in IPA to a final concentration of 2 mg/mL (*see* **Note 8**). Both stock solutions are heated up at 60 °C until lipids are completely dissolved. Tris buffer is also kept at 60 °C.
2. The Nanoassemblr™ heating block is set at 60 °C (*see* **Note 9**).
3. Microfluidics cartridges are inserted into the Nanoassemblr™ with channel dimensions of 300 μm width and 130 μm height. These dimensions allow the cartridge to use a total flow rate (TFR) from 2 to 20 mL/min.
4. There are two inlets connected to the system: the inlet on the right side is for the lipids dissolved in solvent and the inlet on the left side is for the aqueous buffer. A 1 mL disposable syringe is used for the DDA/TDB mixture in IPA and a 3 mL luer-lok tip syringe was used for the Tris buffer. The microfluidics cartridge block is lifted by hand and syringes are connected into the system.

5. Microfluidics is a software-controlled system. Therefore, the software controls the flow rate ratio (FRR) (ratio between the two stream fluids), the TFR of both streams, and the total amount of sample to be produced.
6. In the preparation of liposomes, a waste volume for all the samples is set at 0.5 mL starting waste and 0.1 mL sample waste in the end of the procedure. Thus, for example a selected sample total volume of 1.6 mL will produce a core sample of 1 mL, and a sample total of 20 mL will produce a core sample of 19.4 mL.
7. A total flow rate of between 2 and 20 mL/min can be used in combination with a flow rate ratio of 1:1, 3:1, or 5:1 to prepare DDA/TDB liposomes in a range of sizes depending on the adopted parameters.

4 Notes

1. It is recommended to use Hamilton syringes to transfer lipid solution into the round-bottom flask. The volume is accurate and since the lipid solutions are dissolved in a mixture of chloroform:methanol it is important to use compatible material such as glass syringes.
2. During hydration of the lipid film it is important to maintain the temperature above the transition temperature of the lipid with the highest Tm within the mixture. DDA has a Tm of 47 °C, so to make sure that the hydration of the film takes place during the lipid fluid state, the water bath is set at ~10 °C above this temperature.
3. When vortexing the solutions, it is important to make sure that the lipid film is completely hydrated and it is not stuck at the bottom of the flask.
4. Allow the liposomes to cool down for 30 min to 1 h at room temperature before further experiments are carried out.
5. Thoroughly clean the titanium probe before and after use in order to avoid cross-contamination.
6. Wear protective headphones to block high-frequency noise.
7. Small amounts of titanium might come off the probe into the sample vials. Therefore, samples must be purified. Samples can be transferred into a Falcon tube and centrifuged at 600 to 800 *g* for 15 min and 25 °C. By this means, the titanium traces will be pelleted and the sample can be pipette out into a new vial. It is necessary to not disturb the titanium pellet and thus be careful when pipetting out the sample to another vial.

8. The choice of solvent is of utmost importance since it must be compatible with the microfluidics cartridge and it also needs to be suitable for lipid dissolution. In addition, the solvent choice might influence the sizes of the liposomes produced.
9. As mentioned for the lipid film hydration, it is necessary to keep the temperature above the lipid transition temperatures throughout the process.

Acknowledgements

This work was part funded by EU Horizon 2020 project TBVAC 2020 (Grant no. 643381) (Y.P. & C.B.R.), the EPSRC Centre for Innovative Manufacturing in Emergent Macromolecular Therapies (E.K.), Aston University (S.K.), and the EPSRC iCASE Scheme (Grant no. BB/L017245/1) (P.S.).

References

1. Leroux-Roels G (2010) Unmet needs in modern vaccinology: adjuvants to improve the immune response. Vaccine 28(Suppl 3): C25–C36
2. Nordly P et al (2009) Status and future prospects of lipid-based particulate delivery systems as vaccine adjuvants and their combination with immunostimulators. Expert Opin Drug Deliv 6(7):657–672
3. Foged C (2011) Subunit vaccines of the future: the need for safe, customized and optimized particulate delivery systems. Ther Deliv 2(8):1057–1077
4. Allison AC, Gregoriadis G (1974) Liposomes as immunological adjuvants. Nature 252:252
5. Korsholm KS et al (2007) The adjuvant mechanism of cationic dimethyldioctadecylammonium liposomes. Immunology 121(2):216–226
6. Henriksen-Lacey M, Devitt A, Perrie Y (2011) The vesicle size of DDA:TDB liposomal adjuvants plays a role in the cell-mediated immune response but has no significant effect on antibody production. J Control Release 154(2): 131–137
7. Henriksen-Lacey M et al (2010) Liposomal cationic charge and antigen adsorption are important properties for the efficient deposition of antigen at the injection site and ability of the vaccine to induce a CMI response. J Control Release 145(2):102–108
8. Christensen D et al (2012) A cationic vaccine adjuvant based on a saturated quaternary ammonium lipid have different in vivo distribution kinetics and display a distinct CD4 T cell-inducing capacity compared to its unsaturated analog. J Control Release 160(3): 468–476
9. Zahringer U et al (2008) TLR2—promiscuous or specific? A critical re-evaluation of a receptor expressing apparent broad specificity. Immunobiology 213(3-4):205–224
10. Torchilin VP (2005) Recent advances with liposomes as pharmaceutical carriers. Nat Rev Drug Discov 4(2):145–160
11. Perrie Y et al (2013) A case-study investigating the physicochemical characteristics that dictate the function of a liposomal adjuvant. Hum Vaccin Immunother 9(6):1374–1381
12. Aguilar JC, Rodriguez EG (2007) Vaccine adjuvants revisited. Vaccine 25(19):3752–3762
13. Brewer JM et al (2004) Vesicle size influences the trafficking, processing, and presentation of antigens in lipid vesicles. J Immunol 173(10):6143–6150
14. Dua JS, Rana AC, Bhandari AK (2012) Liposome: methods of preparation and applications. Int J Pharm Stud Res 3(2):14–20
15. Bangham A, Standish M, Watkins J (1965) Diffusion of univalent ions across the lamellae of swollen phospholipids. J Mol Biol 13(1): 238–252
16. Gregoriadis G et al (2002) A role for liposomes in genetic vaccination. Vaccine 20:B1–B9
17. Wagner A, Vorauer-Uhl K (2011) Liposome Technology for Industrial Purposes. J Drug

Deliv 2011, 591325. doi:10.1155/2011/591325
18. Szoka F Jr, Papahadjopoulos D (1980) Comparative properties and methods of preparation of lipid vesicles (liposomes). Annu Rev Biophys Bioeng 9(1):467–508
19. Papahadjopoulos D, Miller N (1967) Phospholipid model membranes. I. Structural characteristics of hydrated liquid crystals. Biochim Biophys Acta 135(4):624–638
20. Papahadjopoulos D, Watkins JC (1967) Phospholipid model membranes. II. Permeability properties of hydrated liquid crystals. Biochim Biophys Acta 135(4):639–652
21. Uchegbu IF et al (2013) Fundamentals of pharmaceutical nanoscience. Springer, New York
22. Lapinski MM et al (2007) Comparison of liposomes formed by sonication and extrusion: rotational and translational diffusion of an embedded chromophore. Langmuir 23(23): 11677–11683
23. Foged C et al (2014) Subunit vaccine delivery. Springer, New York
24. Liu R (2008) Water-insoluble drug formulation, 2nd edn. CRC Press, Boca Raton, FL
25. Richardson ES, Pitt WG, Woodbury DJ (2007) The role of cavitation in liposome formation. Biophys J 93(12):4100–4107
26. Riaz M (1996) Liposomes preparation methods. Pak J Pharm Sci 9(1):65–77
27. Kataria S et al (2011) Stealth liposomes: a review. Int J Res Ayurveda Pharm 2(5):1534–1538
28. Lasic DD (1988) The mechanism of vesicle formation. Biochem J 256(1):1
29. Andreasen LV, Wood G, Christensen D (2012) Methods for producing liposomes. Google Patents
30. Brandl M et al (1990) Liposome preparation by a new high pressure homogenizer Gaulin Micron Lab 40. Drug Dev Ind Pharm 16(14):2167–2191
31. Barnadas-Rodŕiguez R, Sabés M (2001) Factors involved in the production of liposomes with a high-pressure homogenizer. Int J Pharm 213(1):175–186
32. Olson F et al (1979) Preparation of liposomes of defined size distribution by extrusion through polycarbonate membranes. Biochim Biophys Acta 557(1):9–23
33. Bergstrand N et al (2003) Interactions between pH-sensitive liposomes and model membranes. Biophys Chem 104(1):361–379
34. Batzri S, Korn ED (1973) Single bilayer liposomes prepared without sonication. Biochim Biophys Acta 298(4):1015–1019
35. Jaafar-Maalej C et al (2010) Ethanol injection method for hydrophilic and lipophilic drug-loaded liposome preparation. J Liposome Res 20(3):228–243
36. Hauschild S et al (2005) Direct preparation and loading of lipid and polymer vesicles using inkjets. Small 1(12):1177–1180
37. Bogy D, Talke FE (1984) Experimental and theoretical study of wave propagation phenomena in drop-on-demand ink jet devices. IBM J Res Dev 28(3):314–321
38. Frederiksen L et al (1997) Preparation of liposomes encapsulating water-soluble compounds using supercritical carbon dioxide. J Pharm Sci 86(8):921–928
39. Song Y, Hormes J, Kumar CS (2008) Microfluidic synthesis of nanomaterials. Small 4(6):698–711
40. Demello AJ (2006) Control and detection of chemical reactions in microfluidic systems. Nature 442(7101):394–402
41. Nguyen N-T, Wu Z (2005) Micromixers—a review. J Micromech Microeng 15(2):R1
42. Squires TM, Quake SR (2005) Microfluidics: fluid physics at the nanoliter scale. Rev Mod Phys 77(3):977
43. Capretto L et al (2011) Micromixing within microfluidic devices. Top Curr Chem 304: 27–68
44. Chang H-I, Yeh M-K (2012) Clinical development of liposome-based drugs: formulation, characterization, and therapeutic efficacy. Int J Nanomedicine 7:49
45. Weigl BH, Bardell RL, Cabrera CR (2003) Lab-on-a-chip for drug development. Adv Drug Deliv Rev 55(3):349–377
46. Whitesides GM (2006) The origins and the future of microfluidics. Nature 442(7101):368–373
47. Dittrich PS, Manz A (2006) Lab-on-a-chip: microfluidics in drug discovery. Nat Rev Drug Discov 5(3):210–218
48. Hood R, Vreeland W, DeVoe D (2014) Microfluidic remote loading for rapid single-step liposomal drug preparation. Lab Chip 14(17):3359–3367
49. van Swaay D (2013) Microfluidic methods for forming liposomes. Lab Chip 13(5):752–767
50. Weibel DB, Whitesides GM (2006) Applications of microfluidics in chemical biology. Curr Opin Chem Biol 10(6):584–591
51. Jensen KF (2001) Microreaction engineering—is small better? Chem Eng Sci 56(2):293–303
52. Stroock AD et al (2002) Chaotic mixer for microchannels. Science 295(5555):647–651
53. Stainmesse S et al (1995) Formation and stabilization of a biodegradable polymeric colloidal

suspension of nanoparticles. Colloid Polymer Sci 273(5):505–511

54. Mora-Huertas C, Fessi H, Elaissari A (2011) Influence of process and formulation parameters on the formation of submicron particles by solvent displacement and emulsification–diffusion methods: critical comparison. Adv Colloid Interface Sci 163(2):90–122
55. RemziáBecer C (2009) Synthetic polymeric nanoparticles by nanoprecipitation. J Mater Chem 19(23):3838–3840
56. Govender T et al (1999) PLGA nanoparticles prepared by nanoprecipitation: drug loading and release studies of a water soluble drug. J Control Release 57(2):171–185
57. Lee C-Y et al (2011) Microfluidic mixing: a review. Int J Mol Sci 12(5):3263–3287
58. Mengeaud V, Josserand J, Girault HH (2002) Mixing processes in a zigzag microchannel: finite element simulations and optical study. Anal Chem 74(16):4279–4286
59. Jahn A et al (2007) Microfluidic directed formation of liposomes of controlled size. Langmuir 23(11):6289–6293
60. Valencia PM et al (2010) Single-step assembly of homogenous lipid–polymeric and lipid–quantum dot nanoparticles enabled by microfluidic rapid mixing. ACS Nano 4(3):1671–1679
61. Bally F et al (2012) Improved size-tunable preparation of polymeric nanoparticles by microfluidic nanoprecipitation. Polymer 53(22): 5045–5051
62. Zhigaltsev IV et al (2012) Bottom-up design and synthesis of limit size lipid nanoparticle systems with aqueous and triglyceride cores using millisecond microfluidic mixing. Langmuir 28(7):3633–3640
63. Belliveau NM et al (2012) Microfluidic synthesis of highly potent limit-size lipid nanoparticles for in vivo delivery of siRNA. Mol Ther Nucleic Acids 1(8), e37
64. Kastner E et al (2014) High-throughput manufacturing of size-tuned liposomes by a new microfluidics method using enhanced statistical tools for characterization. Int J Pharm 477(1-2):361–368
65. Kastner E et al (2015) Microfluidic-controlled manufacture of liposomes for the solubilisation of a poorly water soluble drug. Int J Pharm 485(1):122–130
66. Yu B, Lee RJ, Lee LJ (2009) Microfluidic methods for production of liposomes. Methods Enzymol 465:129–141
67. Schwendener RA (2014) Liposomes as vaccine delivery systems: a review of the recent advances. Ther Adv Vaccines 2(6):159–182
68. Gobby D, Angeli P, Gavriilidis A (2001) Mixing characteristics of T-type microfluidic mixers. J Micromech Microeng 11(2):126
69. Erbacher C et al (1999) Towards integrated continuous-flow chemical reactors. Microchim Acta 131(1-2):19–24
70. Lee JN, Park C, Whitesides GM (2003) Solvent compatibility of poly (dimethylsiloxane)-based microfluidic devices. Anal Chem 75(23):6544–6554
71. Wu Z, Nguyen N-T (2005) Rapid mixing using two-phase hydraulic focusing in microchannels. Biomed Microdevices 7(1):13–20
72. Quevedo E, Steinbacher J, McQuade DT (2005) Interfacial polymerization within a simplified microfluidic device: capturing capsules. J Am Chem Soc 127(30): 10498–10499

Chapter 10

Synthesis of Lymph Node-Targeting Adjuvants

Melissa C. Hanson and Darrell J. Irvine

Abstract

Molecular adjuvants based off of pattern recognition receptor agonists are capable of potently stimulating innate immunity and inducing protective immune responses to subunit antigens. One significant disadvantage to these small molecule adjuvants is their pharmacokinetic profile of entering the blood stream rather than the lymphatics after parental injection. In order to target molecular adjuvants to lymph nodes, we have developed nanoparticle carriers whose size has been optimized to avoid the blood and efficiently drain to lymph nodes (Hanson et al. Vaccine 33:861–8,2015; Hanson et al. J Clin Invest 125:2532–2546, 2015). This chapter describes in detail the materials and procedures necessary to synthesize liposome nanoparticle carriers of either hydrophobic or hydrophilic adjuvants, including synthesis tips, alternative equipment options, and pitfalls to avoid.

Key words Nanoparticles, Adjuvant carriers, Liposomes, Lymph node targeting, Cyclic dinucleotides, Cyclic di-GMP, MPLA

1 Introduction

The identification of pattern recognition receptors (PRRs) and their agonists has revolutionized the vaccine adjuvant field [1]. The development of molecular adjuvants that can stimulate PRRs offers the vaccine field a "toolbox" with which it is possible to induce efficacious immune responses to poorly immunogenic subunit antigens. Unfortunately, when administered parentally, small molecule adjuvants such as cyclic dinucleotides, resiquimod (R848) and related imidazoquinoline TLR7/8 agonist compounds, muramyl dipeptides that trigger NLRs, and RNA oligonucleotide ligands of RIG-I [2–4] suffer from very poor lymphatic uptake. Instead, these small molecules directly disseminate into the blood. This biodistribution issue is a property of molecular size: because the blood absorbs ~ tenfold more fluid from tissues than lymph, molecules small enough to permeate blood vessels (< ~1 kDa) tend to show predominant clearance to the blood [5]. As a consequence of this, systemic inflammatory toxicity occurs [6–8].

Christopher B. Fox (ed.), *Vaccine Adjuvants: Methods and Protocols*, Methods in Molecular Biology, vol. 1494,
DOI 10.1007/978-1-4939-6445-1_10, © Springer Science+Business Media New York 2017

We have developed lipid nanoparticles (liposomes) as carriers of hydrophilic or hydrophobic adjuvants which efficiently drain to the lymphatic system—in a size-dependent manner—after parental administration [9,10]. We demonstrated that lymph node targeted delivery of a small molecule adjuvant (cyclic di-GMP) minimizes systemic inflammation and simultaneously induces widespread activation of antigen presenting cells (APCs) in lymph nodes, elicits strong and durable humoral responses and also promotes strong antigen-specific CD4$^+$ and CD8$^+$ T-cell priming. This protocol details the synthesis of small unilamellar liposomes as carriers for hydrophobic or hydrophilic adjuvants. Liposomes are particularly useful as adjuvant carriers due to their ease of synthesis, ability to simultaneously carry both hydrophobic adjuvants (embedded in the lipid bilayer) and hydrophilic adjuvants (encapsulated in the liposome interior), and the possibility of covalently linking peptides or proteins to the surface of liposomes using chemically reactive phospholipids [9]. While this protocol uses the cyclic dinucleotide cyclic di-GMP and the TLR-4 agonist monophosphoryl A as examples of hydrophilic and hydrophobic adjuvants, respectively, it is easily adaptable to any molecular adjuvant. In general, during synthesis, include hydrophobic adjuvants in the organic solvent in **step 2** of Subheading 3.1 and include hydrophilic adjuvants in the rehydration buffer in **step 6** of Subheading 3.1. For highly soluble adjuvants, where the volume to be added is less than 100 μL, the adjuvant may be included in **step 4** of Subheading 3.1. A strategy to synthesize liposomes containing both hydrophobic and hydrophilic adjuvants is outlined in Subheading 3.3. The main steps detailed here are dehydration of lipids into a thin film, rehydration of these lipids in aqueous buffer, the processing steps of vortexation, freeze–thaw cycles, and extrusion, and lastly purification and quantification of liposomes containing hydrophilic adjuvants. Rehydration of lipids in aqueous buffer results in the formation of large multilamellar vesicles and the subsequent processing steps are necessary to transform these large vesicles into small unilamellar vesicles. A list of required equipment is included in Subheading 2 and possible alternative equipment is listed in the notes, where relevant.

2 Materials

Prepare and store all reagents at room temperature (unless indicated otherwise).

1. Gas nitrogen line in a chemical fume hood (*see* **Note 1**).
2. Vacuum oven (*see* **Note 2**).
3. Air-driven ultracentrifuge (Beckman Coulter Airfuge) (*see* **Note 3**).

4. Laminar Flow Hood/Biosafety Cabinet.
5. Mini-extruder (1-mL syringe volume) with filter supports (Avanti Polar Lipids).
6. Polycarbonate membranes, 19 mm diameter, 0.2 μm pore size (Whatman).
7. Extruder cleaning solution: 70% v/v ethanol, 30% v/v water.
8. Phosphate buffered saline (PBS): 137 mM NaCl, 2.7 mM KCl, 10 mM Na_2HPO_4, 1.8 mM KH_2PO_4, pH 7.4.
9. 1,2-dioleoyl-*sn*-glycero-3-phosphocholine (DOPC) stock solution: DOPC (Avanti Polar Lipids) dissolved in chloroform at 54.5 mg/mL and stored at −80 °C after nitrogen purge (*see* **Note 4**).
10. 1,2-dioleoyl-*sn*-glycero-3-phoshpo-(1'-rac-gylcerol) (DOPG) stock solution: DOPG (Avanti Polar Lipids) dissolved in chloroform at 14.5 mg/mL and stored at −80 °C after nitrogen purge (*see* **Note 4**).
11. 1,2-dimyristoyl-*sn*-glycero-3-phosphocholine (DMPC) stock solution: DMPC (Avanti Polar Lipids) dissolved in chloroform at 25 mg/mL and stored at −80 °C after nitrogen purge (*see* **Note 4**).
12. 1,2-distearoyl-*sn*-glycero-3-phosphoethanolamine-*N*-[methoxy(polyethylene glycol)-2000] (DSPE-PEG) stock solution: DSPE-PEG (Avanti Polar Lipids) dissolved in chloroform at 25 mg/mL and stored at −80 °C after nitrogen purge (*see* **Note 4**).
13. Monophosphoryl lipid A (MPLA) from *Salmonella enterica* serotype minnesota Re 595 (Sigma-Aldrich), stock solutions: For **step 2** of Subheading 3.1, dissolve in 1 part methanol, 3 parts chloroform at 5 mg/mL. Store at −80 °C after nitrogen purge. For **step 3** of Subheading 3.3, dissolve in sterile dimethyl sulfoxide (DMSO) at 20 mg/mL. Store at 4 °C.
14. Cyclic di-GMP (cdGMP) stock solution: Dissolve cdGMP (Invivogen) in distilled water at 2 mg/mL. Store at −20 °C.

3 Methods

3.1 Synthesis of MPLA and cdGMP Liposomes

Perform these steps in the order outlined below. If a break in the process is required, this can be done at **step 5** of Subheading 3.1 where the lipid film can remain under vacuum at room temperature for up to 1 week.

1. Mixing of Lipids: Aliquot lipids into a 20 mL scintillation vial using glass pipettes according to Table 1 (*see* **Note 5**).
2. If making MPLA liposomes, add 20 μL of MPLA to the lipid solution. Upon synthesis, this results in a final concentration of 0.2 μg MPLA/μL of liposomes.

Table 1
Lipid composition

Lipid	Molar %	Stock conc. (mg/mL)	µL to aliquot
DOPC	38	54.5	100
DOPG	19	14.5	185
DMPC	38	25	185
DSPE-PEG2K	5	25	100

3. Evaporate the organic solvent by gently blowing nitrogen gas onto the solution. The flow should be gentle enough that no bubbling or backsplash of the solution occurs (*see* **Notes 1 and 6**).
4. Add 60 µL of cdGMP on top of the dried lipid film (*see* **Note 7**). Evaporate the water by once again gently blowing nitrogen gas onto the solution.
5. Solvent evaporation: After the lipids have dried down into a thin film and no liquid remains, transfer the vial (uncapped) to a vacuum oven. Incubate overnight (6–15 h) at room temperature (*see* **Note 2**).
6. Lipid rehydration: Remove scintillation vial from vacuum oven, replace the cap, and transfer to a laminar flow hood. Rehydrate lipids with 500 µL of sterile PBS and vortex for 30 s every 10 min for 1 h at room temperature (*see* **Note 8**).
7. Freeze–thaw cycles: Transfer rehydrated lipids into a 1.5-mL plastic Eppendorf tube. Conduct six freeze–thaw cycles by submerging the tube in liquid nitrogen for 1 min then transfer immediately to a 37 °C water bath for 3 min and repeating these two steps an additional five times (*see* **Note 9**).
8. Vesicle extrusion: Assemble the mini-extruder following the manufacturer's instructions. Thoroughly clean all components prior to assembly with the extruder cleaning solution from **step 7** of Subheading 2. Before extrusion of liposomes, test the water-tightness of the extruder by passing 1 mL of PBS through the extruder (*see* **Note 10**). After confirming there is no leakage of PBS from the extruder, empty the 1 mL of PBS and load one of the syringes with the vesicle solution and reattach the syringes to the extruder. Extrude the vesicles by passing 21 times through the extruder. A reduction in the opacity of the solution should be observed as small unilamellar liposomes are formed (*see* **Note 11**). The diameter of the liposomes should be in the range of 150 ± 12 nm [9]. Liposomes can now be stored in 1.5-mL plastic tubes at 4 °C for 3–5 days post-synthesis. Deconstruct the extruder and clean and dry all of its components prior to storage (*see* **Note 12**).

3.2 Purification of Liposomes Containing Aqueous Adjuvants

1. As aqueous adjuvants are encapsulated in the core of liposomes, the unencapsulated material must be removed from the preparation. The following steps detail our method to do this for cdGMP liposomes using an Airfuge centrifuge (*see* **Note 3**).
2. Load each Airfuge tube with 150 μL of liposome solution. Spin tubes in the Airfuge at top speed for 90 min. Carefully remove the supernatant from each tube and save for quantification.
3. Add 150 μL sterile PBS to each tube and let sit for 30 min at room temperature. Then gently resuspend the liposomes using a 200 μL pipette. Collect all of the liposomes into a 1.5 mL tube, and store at 4 °C until further use.
4. Calculate the amount of cdGMP encapsulated from the amount of unencapsulated cdGMP measured in the supernatant. cdGMP presence can be detected by UV spectroscopy at 254 nm, using a tenfold dilution in PBS of the cdGMP liposome supernatant. Trace amounts of lipid may interfere with this signal due to turbidity; therefore, determine the amount of lipid present in the supernatant by detection of the lipid-induced turbidity signal at 350 nm and then generate a cdGMP standard curve adjusted to contain the same amount of lipid as the supernatant (*see* **Note 13**). Using this protocol, encapsulation efficiencies of 25–30 % of cdGMP are typical.

3.3 Synthesis of Liposomes Carrying MPLA and cdGMP

1. It is possible to synthesize liposomes which carry multiple adjuvants. To synthesize liposomes carrying two hydrophobic adjuvants, simply include both adjuvants in **step 2** of Subheading 3.1 (*see* **Note 14**).
2. To synthesize liposomes carrying both hydrophobic and hydrophilic adjuvants (such as MPLA and cdGMP), follow the procedure listed above for synthesizing and purifying cdGMP liposomes (*see* **Note 15**). Once the amount of encapsulated aqueous adjuvant has been quantified, dilute the liposomes to the final desired concentration of aqueous adjuvant.
3. Calculate the volume of MPLA required to add to the cdGMP liposomes to achieve the correct dose of MPLA per volume of liposomes. Ideally, the volume of MPLA in DMSO to add should be at a 1:200 ratio to the total volume of liposomes. A ratio of 1:100–1:400 is acceptable. Make an additional dilution of MPLA in DMSO if necessary to achieve this volumetric ratio.
4. Add the desired amount of MPLA in DMSO to the cdGMP liposome solution. Immediately mix thoroughly with a 1 mL pipette. As MPLA is a very hydrophobic adjuvant, it will directly incorporate into the lipid bilayer of the liposomes (*see* **Note 16**).

4 Notes

1. An alternative to using nitrogen gas is to instead aliquot the lipids into a round bottom flask and then use a rotary evaporator to remove the organic solvent.
2. If you do not have access to a vacuum oven, a lyophilizer is a good alternative. Be sure to completely evaporate all organic solvent from the lipid compositions before adding to the lyophilizer.
3. If you do not have an Airfuge, there are several alternative methods for purifying liposomes from unencapsulated materials. We suggest traditional ultracentrifugation or size-exclusion chromatography.
4. Lipids must be stored in glass vials with Teflon-coated caps, with the vial–cap junction wrapped in Parafilm.
5. If you plan to scale up this production, the amount of lipid per scintillation vial may be doubled. For larger production volumes, use multiple scintillation vials.
6. Restrict the flow of the nitrogen gas by attaching the gas line to a 1-mL syringe. Add a 200-μL plastic pipette tip to the end of the syringe and adjust this tip to rest directly above the 20-mL scintillation vial of lipid.
7. While the encapsulation efficiency is greatest via this method, it is most appropriate for highly soluble molecules, since there is a limit to the amount of aqueous buffer that should be added on the dry lipid film that can be immediately dried off rather than resuspending the lipids in the water.
8. From this point onwards in the protocol, maintain sterility by only exposing the sample to air when under a laminar flow hood.
9. We highly recommend evaluating tubes to determine suitable suppliers. We have experienced breakage of tubes from some suppliers when transferring the tubes between liquid nitrogen and the 37 °C water bath. Tubes supplied by Eppendorf work well.
10. For the water-tightness test: it is expected to lose ~50–100 μL of volume upon the first passage of buffer through the extruder. However, after this first passage, no more additional volume should be lost. If this is the case, deconstruct and reassemble the extruder.
11. While extruding the liposomes, it should require a moderate amount of force to push the liposomes through the extruder. If extreme force is required, there is most likely a blockage due to lipid buildup. Flush the syringes with the extruder cleaning solution and rebuild the extruder with new filter supports and filter if this occurs. If a sudden decrease in required force

occurs, a torn filter is the most probably cause. Deconstruct and rebuild the extruder with new filter supports and filter if this occurs.

12. It is very important to remove the screw cap, needle, and plunger from the syringe and clean and dry all of the components separately. We also recommend that the syringes be stored in a disassembled state. These measures ensure that there is no rust accumulation in the syringes which could contaminate the liposome samples.
13. A simple method to quantify the amount of lipid present in the cdGMP liposome supernatant is detailed here. First synthesize plain liposomes containing no adjuvants. Centrifuge these liposomes at top speed in the Airfuge for 90 min and collect the supernatant. Make a serial dilution of this supernatant, detect the UV signal at 350 nm, and calculate a standard curve. Next, read the UV signal at 350 nm of the whole cdGMP liposome supernatant. Use the standard curve to convert this signal into the equivalent concentration relative to the plain liposome supernatant. Multiply this concentration number by the total volume of the cdGMP standard curve samples to calculate the amount of plain liposome supernatant to add to each of the cdGMP standard curve samples. Since the cdGMP signal is read at a tenfold dilution, the amount of plain liposome supernatant required to add to the cdGMP standard curve is roughly 10% of the total volume of each sample. However, this varies based off of the exact speed and time of the centrifugation step and thus we recommend this calculation step.
14. A good rule of thumb is to keep the total mole % of adjuvant to less than 1% of the total lipid mole %.
15. In this case, MPLA is not included in the organic solvent lipid mixture because there is a small inherent loss of lipid material during each centrifugation step depending on the centrifugation speed, time, resuspension step, etc.
16. While this technique works well for other hydrophobic agents, incubation at 37 °C after mixing may be required to fully incorporate the hydrophobic adjuvant; testing with each specific adjuvant is required.

References

1. Kanzler H, Barrat FJ, Hessel EM, Coffman RL (2007) Therapeutic targeting of innate immunity with Toll-like receptor agonists and antagonists. Nat Med 13:552–559. doi:10.1038/nm1589
2. Harrison LI, Astry C, Kumar S, Yunis C (2007) Pharmacokinetics of 852A, an imidazoquinoline Toll-like receptor 7-specific agonist, following intravenous, subcutaneous, and oral administrations in humans. J Clin Pharmacol 47:962–969. doi:10.1177/0091270007303766
3. Kulkarni RR, Rasheed MAU, Bhaumik SK et al (2014) Activation of RIG-I pathway

during influenza vaccination enhances germinal center reactions, T follicular helper cell induction, and provides dose-sparing effect and protective immunity. J Virol. doi:10.1128/JVI.02273-14

4. Walder P, Buchar E, Machková Z et al (1991) Pharmacokinetic profile of the immunomodulating compound adamantylamide dipeptide (AdDP), a muramyl dipeptide derivative in mice. Immunopharmacol Immunotoxicol 13:101–119. doi:10.3109/08923979109019694
5. McLennan DN, Porter CJH, Charman SA (2005) Subcutaneous drug delivery and the role of the lymphatics. Drug Discov Today Technol 2:89–96. doi:10.1016/j.ddtec.2005.05.006
6. Gray PM, Forrest G, Wisniewski T et al (2012) Evidence for cyclic diguanylate as a vaccine adjuvant with novel immunostimulatory activities. Cell Immunol 278:113–119. doi:10.1016/j.cellimm.2012.07.006
7. Ilyinskii PO, Roy CJ, O'Neil CP et al (2014) Adjuvant-carrying synthetic vaccine particles augment the immune response to encapsulated antigen and exhibit strong local immune activation without inducing systemic cytokine release. Vaccine 32:2882–2895. doi:10.1016/j.vaccine.2014.02.027
8. Smirnov D, Schmidt JJ, Capecchi JT, Wightman PD (2011) Vaccine adjuvant activity of 3M-052: an imidazoquinoline designed for local activity without systemic cytokine induction. Vaccine 29:5434–5442. doi:10.1016/j.vaccine.2011.05.061
9. Hanson MC, Abraham W, Crespo MP et al (2015) Liposomal vaccines incorporating molecular adjuvants and intrastructural T-cell help promote the immunogenicity of HIV membrane-proximal external region peptides. Vaccine 33:861–868. doi:10.1016/j.vaccine.2014.12.045
10. Hanson MC, Crespo MP, Abraham W et al (2015) Nanoparticulate STING agonists are potent lymph node-targeted vaccine adjuvants. J Clin Invest 125:2532–2546. doi:10.1172/JCI79915

Chapter 11

Preparing an Adjuvanted Thermoresponsive Gel Formulation for Sublingual Vaccination

Manjari Lal, Jessica White, and Changcheng Zhu

Abstract

Thermoresponsive gels have unique physicochemical properties that may enable more effective mucosal delivery of active compounds. The thermoresponsive gel (TRG) formulation developed by our group for sublingual delivery maintains fluid-like liquid properties at 2 °C–8 °C and forms a gel at the physiological temperature (~37 °C) within a few seconds. Here, we describe the preparation of a thermoresponsive gel vaccine formulation. Our preclinical studies with various antigens suggest that the mucoadhesive, adjuvanted TRG formulation enabled increased contact of the vaccine antigen with the mucosa, resulting in increased mucosal response(s) with a potential for antigen dose reduction.

Key words Mucosal, Sublingual, Gel, Thermoresponsive, Vaccination, Pluronics, Immunization

1 Introduction

Although most vaccines today are liquid formulations for parenteral administration, this approach has some significant drawbacks. One is that injectable vaccines, which mainly induce systemic immune responses, are usually ineffective at generating a protective mucosal immune response. For protection against infections at mucosal surfaces, such as those in the gastrointestinal tract, mucosal vaccination is a promising option. Vaccine administration via a mucosal surface stimulates the mucosal immune system, which protects various mucosal surfaces and thereby the body interior. Mucosal vaccines also have other advantages over injectable vaccines, including better patient compliance in many disease areas [1].

When designing mucosal vaccines, it is important to consider crucial formulation properties in relation to the required functionality and efficacy of the dosage form. Current approaches to sublingual delivery typically require that the vaccine antigen be administered as a solution without any adjuvant or formulation and then held under the tongue for 1–2 minutes before being swallowed. Under those conditions, no significant systemic

Christopher B. Fox (ed.), *Vaccine Adjuvants: Methods and Protocols*, Methods in Molecular Biology, vol. 1494, DOI 10.1007/978-1-4939-6445-1_11, © Springer Science+Business Media New York 2017

absorption occurs through the sublingual mucosa, and only a small fraction (<10%) remains in contact with the mucosa [2].

Gels are semisolid dispersal systems with properties falling between those of a liquid and a solid. Their viscoelastic properties can be exploited to optimize the delivery of drugs and biologicals for improved retention at the site of administration. For example, the thermoresponsive property of pluronics—non-ionic block co-polymers that form gel upon heating—is due to the surfactant nature of these polymers. These block co-polymers consist of two different (hydrophilic and hydrophobic) polymer chains repeated in long sequences or blocks. At low temperatures in aqueous solutions, the polyethylene hydrophilic portion of the molecule is hydrated. When the temperature rises above the lower critical solution temperature (LCST), there is a reduction in the hydrogen bonding associated with the hydrophilic segment of the molecule and the hydrophilic chains become dehydrated. Because of this dehydration, the hydroxyl groups on adjacent chains become more accessible and interact with one another, forming a gel. The LCST for poloxamers is around physiological or body temperature, where sol-gel conversion occurs (Fig. 1) (*see* **Note 1**). This behavior of poloxamers makes them interesting formulation systems for mucosal delivery, where the formulation enables easy delivery as a liquid that instantaneously becomes a gel at the site of administration [3] (*see* **Note 1**).

1.1 Formulation Considerations for Sublingual Immunization

Although the sublingual route is promising for delivery of vaccine antigens, there are challenges in developing an optimal dosage form that prolongs retention at the site of administration in the presence of saliva (*see* **Note 2**) while increasing permeability and uptake of

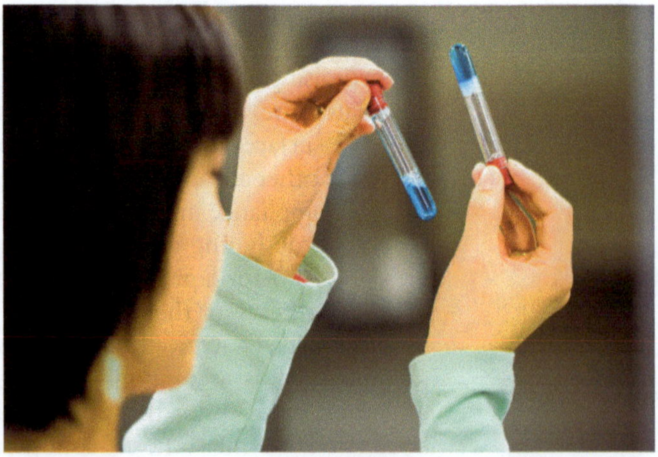

Fig. 1 TRG formulation as a liquid at room temperature (*left*) and a gel immediately after removal from 37 °C ± 2 °C (*right*). Photo: PATH/Areman

antigen at the mucosal site. An ideal dosage form for sublingual delivery should maintain antigen stability, be easy to administer, and be retained long enough to allow antigen permeability and uptake (*see* **Notes 3** and **4**).

Rheology studies on the thermoresponsive gel (TRG) developed by our group showed a gradual increase in viscosity beginning at about 20 °C and plateauing between 35 °C and 40 °C, associated with the formation of a gel in this temperature range (*see* **Note 5**). The transepithelial electrical resistance (TER) data using human oral tissues showed that the TRG formulation could lower mucosal epithelial resistance with a potential for improving antigen uptake (*see* **Note 5**).

1.2 Scale-Up Considerations with TRG Formulation

During the manufacturing of a thermoresponsive formulation containing multiple polymers and thermosensitive surfactant and vaccine antigen(s), the difference between mixing conditions in a beaker at the laboratory bench and in massive production tanks can cause profound differences in antigen stability, formulation viscosity, and formulation properties as a whole. Whereas TRG can be prepared on a laboratory scale using a standard mixer in a glass beaker or vials, for scale-up of mucosal gel formulations, several different vessels are employed during manufacturing. For example, the polymer phases are heated separately in jacketed vessels along with the surfactant while the aqueous phase containing the antigen and the adjuvant is dissolved separately and introduced in multiple steps into the homogenizer mixer. During mixing, excessive heat and shear must be avoided to prevent damage and degradation of the vaccine components. Often the homogenizer is built into a jacketed tank to continuously cool down the process during mixing to ensure homogeneity and stability of the final gel formulation. This is not only critical for temperature-sensitive, labile vaccines, but also for the TRG, which may undergo gelation during the manufacturing process due to fluctuations in temperature (elevated temperatures cause gelation). After manufacturing, the TRG is transferred into storage tanks that can be transported and connected to filling lines for the final product. Again, low temperatures must be maintained during the pumping process to avoid clogging filling lines due to liquid-to-gel formation (*see* **Note 6**).

2 Materials

1. 0.22 μm cellulose acetate (CA) filter flasks.
2. Magnetic stirrer.
3. Erlenmeyer flask (100, 125 mL).

4. Sterile 60 mL PETG media bottle.
5. Sterile 125 mL PETG media bottle.
6. Analytical balance with readability to four decimal places to the right of decimal point.
7. Benchtop vortex.
8. Repeating pipette and tip.
9. Ultrasonic bath.
10. Volumetric flask for formulation preparation (100 mL).
11. Milli-pure water, 18.2 MΩ·cm resistivity.
12. Pluronic F127 (*see* **Note** 7).
13. Carbopol 971P (carbomer) (*see* **Note 8**).
14. Hydroxypropyl methylcellulose (HPMC), (*see* **Note 9**).
15. Double-mutant LT toxin (lyophilized dmLT, Walter Reid Army Institute of Research [WRAIR]) (*see* **Note 10**).
16. Phosphate-buffered saline (PBS): 0.01 M phosphate-buffered saline, NaCl 0.138 M; KCl 0.0027 M; and pH of 7.4 at 25 °C.
17. Pooled human saliva (multiple donors, Lee Biosolutions Inc.).

3 Methods

The formulations were developed on a laboratory scale. The largest batch size prepared was 5 mL. Care must be exercised in scaling up from laboratory scale to production scale (*see* **Note 6**).

3.1 Preparation of 30% (w/v) PF-127 Stock Solution. The 30% PF-127 Solution Is Prepared by the Cold Method as Described Below (See Note 7)

1. Cool 100 mL of sterile water and glassware in the refrigerator 1 day before use.
2. Using an analytical balance, weigh out 30 g of Pluronic F127 in a 100 mL Erlenmeyer flask.
3. Place the flask with Pluronic F127 in the refrigerator in a salt ice bath on a magnetic stirrer.
4. Stir the powder with a magnetic stir bar and slowly add about 60 mL cold water to the Erlenmeyer flask.
5. Allow the mixture to stir overnight in the refrigerator until the Pluronic F127 is completely dissolved.
6. Next day, transfer the resulting solution to a 100 mL pre-chilled volumetric flask.
7. Measure 10 mL of cold water using a volumetric flask and wash the original remaining contents in the Erlenmeyer flask and combine into the 100 mL volumetric flask.
8. Add additional cold water to reach the 100 mL fill line of the volumetric flask.

9. After mixing, store the solution at 2 °C–8 °C for 1 hour and then filter using a disposable sterile filter system (150 mL, 0.22 μm CA membrane) set up on ice.
10. Store the final sterile filtered stock solution at 2 °C–8 °C until use.

3.2 Preparation of 3 % (w/v) Hypromellose (HPMC) Stock Solution (See Note 9)

1. Move an analytical balance into a biosafety hood and clean with 75 % isopropyl alcohol (IPA).
2. Sterilize a magnetic stirring bar with 75 % IPA and place it into the Erlenmeyer flask.
3. Using a measuring cylinder, measure 75 mL of sterile water into a 100 ml Erlenmeyer flask and heat the water to 90 °C on a hot plate.
4. Using an analytical balance, weigh out 2.5 g of HPMC and transfer to an Erlenmeyer flask.
5. Add about 40 mL of hot water to the HPMC contained in an Erlenmeyer flask with stirring.
6. After dissolution of HPMC in the hot water, add about 40 mL of cold water and stir for 0.5 hour (*see* **Note 11**).
7. Place the resulting solution in an ultrasonic bath to remove bubbles in the solution, followed by transfer to a 100 mL volumetric flask.
8. Measure 10 mL sterile water and wash the original flask and then combine into 100 mL volumetric flask.
9. Add additional sterile water to reach the fill line to achieve the final stock concentration.
10. Transfer the final stock solution to a sterile square media bottle (125 mL) in a biosafety hood and then store at 2 °C–8 °C until use.

3.3 Preparation of 1 % (w/w) Carbomer Stock Solution (See Note 8)

1. Move an analytical balance to the biosafety hood and clean with 75 % IPA.
2. Open a square media bottle (125 mL) in a biosafety hood.
3. Set the container on the balance and weigh out 1 g of Carbopol 971P.
4. Sterilize a magnetic stirring bar with 75 % IPA and place it into the container.
5. Add about 100 g of sterile water into the container.
6. Seal the container with a cap in the biosafety hood.
7. Stir the mixture at 800 rpm for 1 hour to dissolve the Carbopol 971P and then change to 250 rpm and stir overnight to remove bubbles.
8. On the next day, remove the magnetic stir bar in the biosafety hood.
9. Store the resulting carbomer stock solution at 2 °C–8 °C.

3.4 Preparation of 1 mg/mL dmLT Solution: Lyophilized Vial of dmLT Is Stored at −20 °C (See Note 10)

1. Reconstitute a single vial containing 0.7 mg lyophilized dmLT with 0.7 mL milli-pure water and mix gently by inverting the vial several times to obtain 1 mg/ml concentration.

3.5 Preparation of PBS

1. Prepare PBS ahead of time by the standard method provided by the supplier (one packet per liter of milli-pure water).
2. Sterilize the PBS either through 0.22 μm filtration or autoclaving at 121 °C for 20 minutes.

3.6 Preparation of TRG Vaccine Formulation

Using the stock excipients prepared above:

1. Cool all reagents, containers, and pipette tips in the refrigerator 1 day prior to the preparation of formulation.
2. Open a 60 mL square media bottle in a biosafety hood and place a sterilized magnetic stir bar with 75 % IPA.
3. Use a repeating pipette to pipette 25 mL of 30 % PF-127 stock solution into the square media bottle and start to stir.
4. Pipette 15 mL of 3 % HPMC stock solution.
5. Pipette 5 mL of the 1 % carbomer stock solution.
6. Stir for 5 minutes and then move the bottle to the freezer and continue to stir for 1 hour (*see* **Note 12**).
7. Store the TRG placebo stock (if prepared under aseptic/sterile conditions) at 2 °C–8 °C for up to 6 months prior to addition of the antigen and dmLT.
8. To formulate a 0.5 mL batch size of TRG vaccine, take a pre-sterilized 5 mL glass vial and using a positive displacement pipette add 0.275 mL of TRG placebo stock, followed by 0.1 mL vaccine antigen in PBS into the vial (*see* **Note 13**).
9. Mix gently by inverting the vial several times.
10. Pipette 0.125 mL of the reconstituted dmLT solution into the vial from **step 9** to achieve a final dmLT concentration in the TRG of 0.25 mg/mL.
11. Vortex for 5 seconds to obtain a clear, particulate-free solution (*see* **Note 12**).
12. The final volume of the TRG vaccine formulation volume should be 0.5 mL.
13. Store at 2 °C–8 °C and use within 24 hours of preparation.

4 Notes

1. The gelation temperatures (Tsol/gel) of in situ-forming gels were measured using oscillatory rheometry. The samples were subjected to a constant shear stress value and frequency

(chosen in the linear viscoelastic region, previously determined). The temperature was increased in a stepwise manner from 4 °C to 40 °C (heating rate: 1 °C/min) and the elastic modulus (G′) was measured. The phase transition from liquid to gel (Tsol/gel) was inferred from the inflexion point of G′.

2. Thermo-reversible gelation in pooled human saliva: the human sublingual tissue is covered by a thin layer of saliva that lubricates the underlying tissue and is the first barrier encountered during sublingual administration. The normal or resting level of saliva is reported to be less than 0.1 mL/min [4, 5]. In this testing, 200 μL of pooled human saliva was maintained at 37 °C and then 50 μL of TRG vaccine formulation containing FDC-blue dye was added. Timing for the gel formation (as a colored gel drop) in pooled saliva was monitored. The same volume (50 μL) of dyed PBS was added to pooled saliva as a control. The control sample showed uniform diffusion of the dye throughout the saliva solution.
3. The TRG formulations were not cytotoxic to baby hamster kidney fibroblast cells (BHK-21) based on cytolytic and metabolic activity assays. Gelation studies in guinea pigs showed that the formulations formed a gel when delivered to the sublingual mucosa of guinea pigs and were retained at the administration site for at least 10 minutes.
4. Sublingual immunization using dmLT-adjuvanted TRG vaccine formulation in a tetanus toxoid proof of concept study: mice were used to test the immunogenicity of TRG with 20 μg of antigen given via three different administration routes: sublingual, rectal, and vaginal, with an IM control group. TRG was administered to anesthetized mice on days 0, 14, and 28. On day 42, serum, saliva, vaginal washes, and fecal pellets were collected. Antibody titer results by ELISA for animals immunized sublingually are shown below. Tetanus toxoid adjuvanted with dmLT in a TRG formulation helped to elicit strong serum antibody responses higher than elicited by intramuscular injection. In addition, the TRG vaccine formulation also helped to induced high levels of IgA antibodies in the mucosal (saliva, vaginal, and fecal) samples. In contrast, intramuscular injection of these antigens did not elicit detectable IgA antibodies in the mucosal samples tested (Table 1). Similar results were observed with dmLT-adjuvanted TRG with IPV in a published study [6].
5. Tight junctions between epithelial cells serve as a paracellular barrier to regulate the passage of water, ions, macromolecules, and pathogens [7]. Tight junctions also inhibit the ability of electric current to flow across tissues, generating a measurable electrical resistance known as transepithelial electrical resistance (TER). Measurement of TER provides a method to monitor tight junction development and barrier function.

Table 1
Results from sublingual vaccination in mice using TRG formulation

	Sublingual immunization		IM	
Sample	**IgG**	**IgA**	**IgG**	**IgA**
Serum	15821	6259	1602	10
Saliva	290	15345	11	11
Vaginal wash	1038	16043	20	20
Fecal pellets		4646		5

Abbreviations: IM, intramuscular; IgG, immunoglobulin G; IgA, immunoglobulin A

Table 2
TER results on human buccal tissue treated with TRG

Sample	TER after 2 h of treatment (Ω) Average ± SD
PBS	389 ± 39
TRG	268 ± 14

Abbreviations: TER, transepithelial electrical resistance; SD standard deviation; PBS phosphate-buffered saline; TRG thermoresponsive gel

In this study, TER measurements were performed on human buccal tissue samples (MatTek EpiOral™ tissues) [8] after exposure to selected mucosal gel formulations. Tissues were washed with sterile water prior to measuring resting TER after the addition of pre-warmed PBS (100 μL). Tissues were then treated with mucosal gel formulations (100 μL) and placed at 37 °C for 2 hours. After incubation, tissues were washed with pre-warmed PBS, and measurements were recorded after treatment. The reduction in the TER indicates the increased permeability of the oral tissue after treatment with the selected TRG formulation (Table 2). EndOhm tissue resistance measurement chambers (World Precision Instruments) were used for TER measurements. All treatments were performed in duplicate on separate tissue samples.

6. During scale-up, processing conditions must be considered at every step, and gel viscosity and antigen content/properties must be measured at various stages of the process. Because the TRG vaccine formulation is thermosensitive, it is important to ensure that the temperature is always maintained between 2 and 8 °C while handling the formulation. Since gel formation is reversible, the formulation can be immediately cooled to bring it back to its liquid form. Since the TRG formulation is

slightly viscous, a positive displacement pipette must be used with the TRG vaccine formulation to reduce errors arising from trapped air pockets while using a standard pipette.

7. Poloxamer—also known as polyethylene-propylene glycol copolymer and by trade names such as Supronic, Pluronic, or Tetronic—was introduced in 1950 as a non-ionic triblock copolymer. Since then, poloxamer has been used in diverse pharmaceutical applications. Chemically, poloxamer is α-hydro-ω-hydroxypoly (oxyethylene)$_a$ poly (oxypropylene)$_b$ poly (oxyethylene)$_a$, a block copolymer. It consists of two hydrophilic chains of ethylene oxide chains (PEO) that sandwich one hydrophobic propylene oxide chain (PPO). It has the chemical formula HO(C2H4O)a(C3H6O)b(C2H4O)aH, where a and b have the values ranging anywhere from 10 to 100. The varying length of polymer blocks gives rise to different polymers identified as 124, 188, 237, 338, and 407, which show slight differences in their properties. The common representation of a poloxamer is "P" followed by three digits. Multiplying the first two digits by 100 gives the molecular mass of the hydrophobic propylene oxide and multiplying the last digit by 10 gives the content of hydrophilic ethylene oxide as a percentage. The common trade name used is Pluronic, and the usual copolymer representation denotes its physical appearance (L—Liquid, P—Paste, and F—Flake). The trade name coding is given as Pluronic, followed by a single letter representing the physical form and then by two digits. The first digit is multiplied by 300 to give the molecular mass of propylene oxide, and the next digit is multiplied by 10 to obtain the ethylene oxide as a percentage [9]. PF-127 is more soluble in cold water than in hot water as a result of increased solvation and hydrogen bonding at lower temperatures [10].
8. Carbopol 971P is a lightly cross-linked polymer from the acrylic acid family. Carbopols have been used as thickening and viscosity agents to modify flow characteristics. Because of their mucoadhesive properties and bioadhesive potentials, these polymers have been increasingly applied in ophthalmic, rectal, buccal, nasal, intestinal, vaginal, and topical drug delivery [11]. For preparing large batch carbomer dispersions, add the polymer very slowly under vigorous agitation using a propeller for good vortex. Allow 15 min for the polymer to become hydrated. Using a heat-based sterilization approach for carbomer dispersions changes the polymer viscosity; hence during the preparation of TRG formulations using carbomer, aseptic conditions must be employed.
9. HPMC has the official name of hypromellose in the USP and the European Pharmacopoeia. It is typically prepared by reaction of cellulose with propylene oxide and methyl chloride to obtain hydroxypropyl substitution on the anhydroglucose

units. The varying ratios of hydroxypropyl and methyl substitution result in products with different organic solubility, thermal gelation temperature of aqueous solutions, and other performance characteristics. Dow Chemical provided a series of HPMC products (METHOCEL™ E, F, J, and K brand products) for use in our work to develop thermoresponsive gels [12].

10. Bacteria-derived enterotoxins such as cholera toxin (CT) produced by *Vibrio cholera* and the closely related heat-labile toxin (LT) produced by *Escherichia coli* can increase the immunogenicity of co-administered antigens given orally [13], making them effective adjuvants. However, even low doses can induce side effects when given to human volunteers. To reduce the toxicity but maintain the adjuvant activity, amino acid substitutions were introduced into LT. A single mutant form of LT (mLT) contains one amino acid substitution at site 192, where a glycine was substituted for an arginine. This substitution prevents the separation of the A-subunit into A1 and A2 by proteolytic cleavage. Reduced toxicity was observed in both animal and human studies while maintaining the same adjuvant activity of LT. However, mild toxicity was still observed with mLT in human volunteers. To further reduce the toxicity of mLT, a second amino acid substitution was introduced at site 211, where a leucine was substituted with an alanine. The resulting double mutant has demonstrated little to no toxicity while maintaining similar adjuvanticity [14].
11. While preparing a stock solution of HPMC, at the beginning the HPMC may "float" on the surface of the water. The HPMC will eventually disperse in the water and form a slurry. Clear solution will be obtained only after the addition of cold water. HPMC typically agglomerates when directly added to water (cold), forming clumps that result in slow dissolution.
12. During the preparation of TRG on a laboratory scale, moderate stirring is better than vigorous stirring because the latter may result in "foam" that may be difficult to remove. When using vortex keep the setting high (8 or 9) and vortex for 5 seconds to minimize the formation of fine bubbles.
13. For vaccine antigens, the addition of salts such as sodium chloride is acceptable at low concentrations (0.1–0.2 M), though this will lead to a slight change in consistency of the gel.

Acknowledgement

This work was funded by grants from the Bill & Melinda Gates Foundation. The views expressed herein are solely those of the authors and do not necessarily reflect the views of the Gates Foundation.

References

1. Holmgren J, Svennerholm AM (2012) Vaccines against mucosal infections. Curr Opin Immunol 24(3):343–353
2. Kraan H, Vrieling H, Czerkinsky C, Jiskoot W et al (2014) Buccal and sublingual vaccine delivery. J Control Release 190(28): 580–592
3. (2010) The Indian Pharmacopoeia. Ghaziabad, India: Ministry of Health and Public Welfare, Government of India, New Delhi
4. Mestecky J (1993) Saliva as a manifestation of the common mucosal immune system. Ann N Y Acad Sci 694:184–194
5. Ekstrom J, Khosravani N, Castagnola M, Messana I (2012) Saliva and the control of its secretion. In: Dysphagia, medical radiology. diagnostic imaging. Berlin: Springer.
6. White JA, Blum JS, Hosken NA, Marshak JO, Duncan L, Zhu C et al (2014) Serum and mucosal antibody responses to inactivated polio vaccine after sublingual immunization using a thermoresponsive gel delivery system. Hum Vaccin Immunother 10:3611–3621
7. Gonzalez-Mariscal L, Betanzos A, Nava P, Jaramillo BE (2003) Tight junction proteins. Progr Biophys Mol Biol 81:1–44
8. MatTek corporation (2012) Measurement of Transepithelial Electrical Resistance (TEER) and potential difference. MK-24-007-0051. Ashland, MA
9. Raymond CR, Paul JS, Sian CO (2006) Handbook of pharmaceutical excipients, 5th edn. American Pharmacists Association, Washington
10. Schmolka IR (1977) A review of block polymer surfactants. J Am Oil Chem Soc 54:110–116
11. Bonacucina G, Martelli S, Palmieri GF (2004) Rheological, mucoadhesive and release properties of Carbopol gels in hydrophilic cosolvents. Int J Pharm 282:115–130
12. Dow Chemical (1998) METHOCEL cellulose ethers. Technical handbook. Midland, MI
13. Norton EB, Lawson LB, Freytag LC, Clements JD (2011) Characterization of a mutant Escherichia coli heat-labile toxin, LT(R192G/L211A), as a safe and effective oral adjuvant. Clin Vaccine Immunol 18(4):546–551
14. El-Kamary SS, Cohen MB, Bourgeois AL, Van De Verg L, Bauers N et al (2013) Safety and immunogenicity of a single oral dose of recombinant double mutant heat-labile toxin derived from enterotoxigenic Escherichia coli. Clin Vaccine Immunol 20(11):1764–1770

Chapter 12

Manufacture of Oil-in-Water Emulsion Adjuvants

Jean Haensler

Abstract

Emulsion adjuvants for human vaccines have evolved gradually over the last century. Current formulations are the result of many refinements to their composition and manufacturing, as well as optimization for safety and efficacy. Squalene has emerged as being particularly suitable for the manufacturing of safe oil-in-water (O/W) adjuvants for parenteral applications due to its biocompatibility and ability to be metabolized. Emulsion particle size has been identified as an important parameter affecting the pharmaceutical performance of O/W emulsion adjuvants. Submicronic emulsions with sizes in the 80–200 nm range are preferred for potency, manufacturing consistency, and stability reasons. Two manufacturing processes, high pressure homogenization (HPH or microfluidization) and a phase inversion temperature method (PIT), are described to yield such fine and long-term stable emulsion adjuvants.

Key words Emulsion, Adjuvant, Squalene, Microfluidization, PIT, MF59, AS03, SE, AF03

1 Introduction

Oil-in-water (O/W) emulsions are oil dispersions in water in the form of small droplets stabilized with one or several surfactants i.e., emulsifiers. Surfactants act to reduce tension at the interface between the oil and water phases which is necessary to provide long-term stability to the dispersed oil droplets. O/W emulsion adjuvants are generally used in injectable vaccines, although some examples of their use in mucosal vaccines can be found [1]. Emulsion adjuvants have evolved gradually from Le Moinic's and Pinoy's first observations on adjuvant effects of oil suspensions in 1916, and from Freund's pioneering work on water-in-oil (W/O) emulsions in the 1930s. In the 1970s, scientists at Syntex and Chiron identified submicronic O/W emulsions, and in particular those made of low amounts of squalene (shark liver oil) or squalane (hydrogenated derivative of squalene), as safe and efficacious alternatives to the more reactogenic W/O emulsions, such as Freund's adjuvants [2–4]. In 1997, the submicronic O/W emulsion MF59 became the first O/W adjuvant approved for human use in Europe,

Christopher B. Fox (ed.), *Vaccine Adjuvants: Methods and Protocols*, Methods in Molecular Biology, vol. 1494, DOI 10.1007/978-1-4939-6445-1_12, © Springer Science+Business Media New York 2017

as a component of the Novartis seasonal influenza vaccine, FluAd® [5]. Since then, squalene-in-water nano-emulsion adjuvants were administered to almost 200 Million people worldwide especially in the context of the adjuvanted influenza vaccines developed and used during the 2009–2010 H1N1*v* influenza pandemic [6] and, in 2015, the MF59-adjuvanted seasonal influenza vaccine, FluAd®, was approved in Canada for infants from 6 months to 2 years of age [7] and in the USA for elderly aged 65 and older [8]. During clinical development of adjuvanted influenza vaccines, the squalene-in-water emulsion adjuvants were shown to increase immunogenicity, to enable antigen dose-sparing, and to induce epitope spreading and influenza cross-strain reactive antibodies [6]. From a mechanistic point of view, published work on MF59 indicates that O/W emulsions function as "reverse targeting systems" meaning they create a local chemokine/cytokine environment responsible for enhanced immune cell recruitment and antigen uptake at the intramuscular injection site [9, 10]. The pharmaceutical emulsion adjuvants all have small particle sizes generally in the 80–200 nm range, as this facilitates consistent manufacturing, terminal sterile filtration, and may improve efficacy through more efficient lymph node delivery [11–13]. Two manufacturing methods, that are described in this chapter, have emerged for the consistent manufacturing of emulsion adjuvants with such small particle sizes: High Pressure Homogenization (HPH) or microfluidization, as used for MF59, AS03, and SE, and the Phase Inversion Temperature (PIT) method, as used for AF03 (Table 1). The pharmaceutical emulsions described in Table 1, except AS03 [14, 15], are plain squalene-in-water emulsions, meaning without added immunostimulant, but any of these emulsions could be formulated with additional immunostimulants (e.g., Toll-like receptors (TLR) agonists) to increase adjuvant activity as shown in many preclinical models [6]. In this case, depending on its lipophilic/hydrophilic properties, the immunostimulatory molecule will partition between the oil and water phases or migrate at the oil/water interface of the emulsion. Note, however, that when an additional immunostimulant is incorporated, this requires careful selection and formulation as increased immunostimulation generally comes with a potential risk of increased reactogenicity [5, 16]. For antigen incorporation O/W emulsion adjuvants are simply mixed with antigen solutions without any further processing. This enables the adjuvant and antigen to be prepared and stored separately which is advantageous in situations where single vial formulations are unstable long term, and in the context of influenza pandemic preparedness plans where large amounts of adjuvant are prepared and stockpiled before the actual antigen becomes available. In addition, antigen and adjuvant mixing at point of use (i.e., "bedside mixing") facilitates preclinical and clinical dose finding studies. Note that antigens do not need to associate with the dispersed oil droplets for the O/W emulsion to be adjuvant active [11].

Table 1
Detailed composition of different pharmaceutical squalene-in-water emulsion adjuvants

Name	Squalene	Dil. prior admin.	Surfactant 1	Surfactant 2	Aqueous phase	Comment references
MF59 Novartis	4.5 % (v/v)	2× with antigen	Span 85 (0.47 %; w/v)	Tween 80 (0.47 %; w/v)	10 mM Na^+ Citrate, pH 6.0	Citrate helps limiting squalene oxidation [11, 36]
AS03[a] (GSK)	4.3 % (w/v)	2× with antigen	N/A	Tween 80 (1.94 %; w/v)	8.5 mM Na^+/K^+ Phosphate, 121 mM NaCl, 2.4 mM KCl, pH 6.8	Contains also α-tocopherol oil (4.7 % w/v) as immunostimulant [14, 15]
SE[b] (IDRI)	4 % (v/v)	2× with antigen	Synthetic phosphatidylcholine (0.76 %; w/v)	Pluronic F68 (0.036 %; w/v)	25 mM $NH4^+$ phosphate, 2.3 % glycerol, pH 5.7	May contain also α-tocopherol oil (0.05 % w/v) as antioxidant [25, 30, 37]
AF03 (Sanofi)	32.5 % (w/w)	6.5× with buffer and 2× with antigen	Montane 80 (0.74 %; w/w)	Eumulgin B1 PH (0.95 %; w/w)	9.6 mM Na^+/K^+ Phosphate, 137 mM NaCl, 2.7 mM KCl, pH 7.2	Contains also mannitol (0.92 % w/w) to decrease the PIT [32]

The two most widely injected squalene emulsion adjuvants are AS03 comprised in GSK's influenza pandemic vaccines Pandemrix®, Arepanrix®, and Pumarix® and MF59 in Novartis' seasonal influenza vaccine, FluAd®, and pandemic vaccines Focetria®, Celtura®, and Aflunov®. Other squalene emulsions in clinical development are AF03 (component of Sanofi's adjuvanted H1N1 influenza vaccine Humenza®) and SE of IDRI (Infectious Disease Research Institute, Seattle, WA). MF59, AS03, and SE are produced by microfluidization whereas AF03 is produced by PIT. The two processes result in fine and long-term stable squalene-in-water emulsions for these adjuvants [6]

[a]AS03 may be considered as an adjuvant system with α-tocopherol as the additional immunostimulant. In the manufacturing of AS03, the α-tocopherol oil is mixed with squalene prior to emulsification [14, 15]

[b]SE is generally used as a vehicle for the synthetic TLR4 agonist Glucopyranosyl Lipid A (GLA) in an adjuvant system termed GLA-SE. In the manufacturing of GLA-SE, GLA is generally dispersed into the oil phase prior to emulsification [37]

2 Materials

2.1 Excipients

1. Oils: Squalene and its hydrogenated homolog squalane can be obtained from different sources and suppliers (SAFC, Wilshire, etc.) at a purity > 98 % (*see* **Note 1**).
2. Surfactants: Pharmaceutical grade surfactants distributed under the brand Tween® (Croda), Span® (Croda), Pluronic® (BASF), Montane® (Seppic), Eumulgin® (Cognis/BASF), and lecithin or synthetic phosphatidylcholine (Avanti Polar Lipids, Lipoid, Merck KGaA, etc.) can be used as emulsifiers for the preparation of stable O/W emulsions (*see* **Note 2**).
3. Buffers (emulsion aqueous phase): Most commonly used buffers for the preparation of O/W adjuvants are citrate, phosphate, and Tris buffers in a pH 5.5–7.5 range with or without sodium chloride or glycerol to adjust solution tonicity (*see* **Note 3**). Sodium citrate buffer in "MF59-like emulsion" is 10 mM sodium citrate, pH 6.5 ± 0.1 prepared from citric acid monohydrate and trisodium citrate dihydrate. PBS in AF03 is 9.6 mM Na/K phosphate prepared from disodium phosphate dihydrate and monopotassium phosphate; 137 mM NaCl; 2.7 mM KCl, pH 7.0 ± 0.2.

2.2 Equipment

1. IKA T25 Ultra-Turrax (IKA, Wilmington, NC) or Silverson Heavy Duty laboratory Mixer Emulsifier-Model L4R (Silverson, East Longmeadow, MA) or reactor equipped with a helix impeller for primary emulsion formulation.
2. High Pressure Homogenizer or microfluidizer: e.g., Microfluidizer M110P (Microfluidics Corporation, Newton, MA) and EmulsiFlex-C50 (Avestin, Ottawa, Canada) or other high pressure homogenizer such as Panda 2K NS1001L (Niro Soavi, Parma, Italy) may be used.
3. Glass or stainless steel reactor compatible with stirring and heating/cooling. For PIT method, the reactor is typically equipped with a thermometer and a conductivity probe (e.g., Tacussel CD60; Radiometer Analytical, Villeurbanne, France) for process monitoring.
4. Magnetic stirrer.
5. Heated circulating water bath.
6. Filters for sterile filtration: commonly used filters for the sterilization of squalene-in-water emulsions are made of polyethersulfone (PES) and are available from different suppliers such as Millipore, Pall, and Sartorius (e.g., Opticap XL150 capsule with Millipore Express SHC membrane).

3 Methods

3.1 General Process for Manufacture of O/W Nano-emulsion by High Pressure Homogenization

During HPH a primary O/W emulsion is forced under high pressure through a small orifice. During this process, several forces, such as hydraulic shear, intense turbulence, and cavitation, act together to yield nano-emulsions with very small droplet size. Microfluidization employs high pressure to accelerate the primary emulsion through a series of microchannels to create high velocity liquid streams that collide and impinge onto a wear-resistant surface (interaction chamber) breaking the primary emulsion into a very fine nano-emulsion. For both HPH and microfluidization, the nano-emulsions with the desired size range can be obtained by varying the operating pressure of the equipment and number of cycles through the interaction chamber (*see* **Note 4**). The following section describes the manufacture of 100 g (ca. 100 ml) of a squalene/Tween80/Span85 emulsion ("MF59-like emulsion") using microfluidization (*see* Fig. 1).

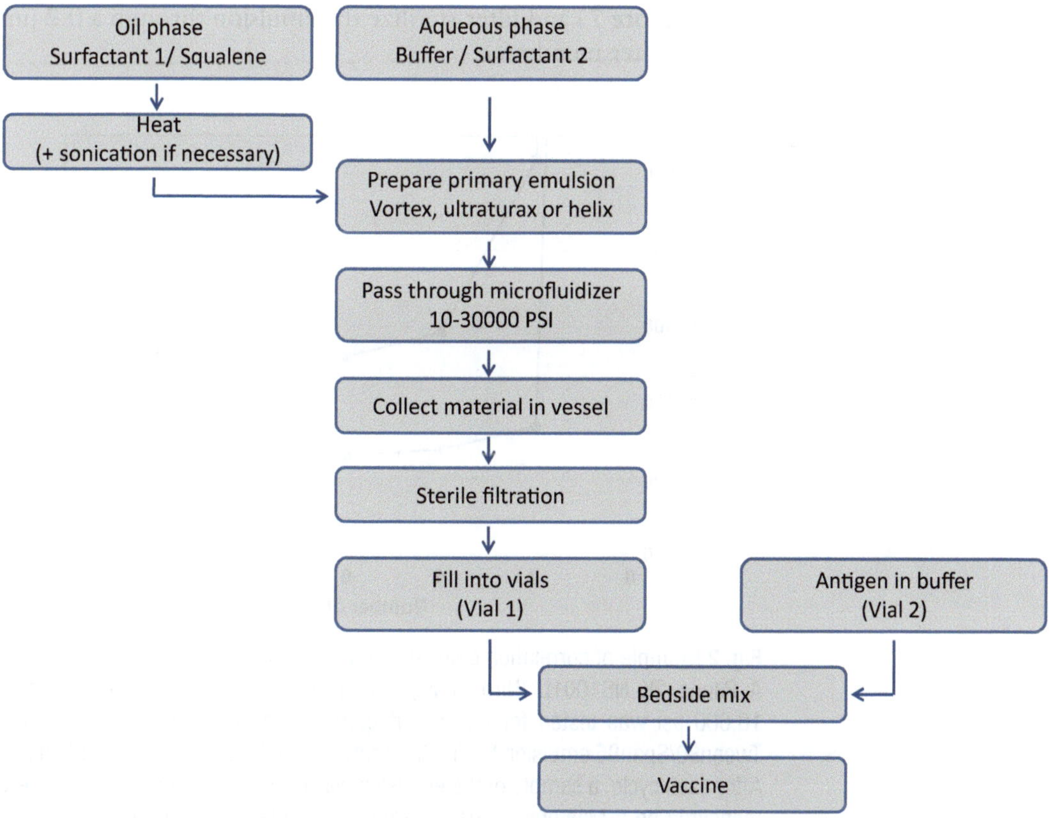

Fig. 1 Outline of squalene in water emulsion adjuvant manufacturing process by microfluidization or HPH

3.2 Manufacture of "MF59-like Emulsion" by Microfluidization

1. Aqueous phase preparation: Dissolve 0.5 g of Polyoxyethylene Sorbitan Monooleate (Tween®80) into 95.1 g of sodium citrate buffer stirring at 40 °C.
2. Oil phase preparation: Dissolve 0.5 g of Sorbitan trioleate (Span®85) into 3.9 g of squalene under stirring at 40 °C (*see* **Note 5**).
3. Primary O/W emulsion preparation: Mix the oil and aqueous phases prepared above in a beaker or glass flask and pre-emulsify the mixture using a T25 Ultra-Turrax device with a 13.4 mm diameter rotor at 24,000 rpm or equivalent high shear homogenizer.
4. High Pressure Homogenization: Process primary O/W emulsion prepared above with M110P Microfluidizer with an ice bath cooling coil or equivalent HPH equipment. Eight to twelve cycles at 25–30,000 psi are generally required to obtain a homogeneous nano-emulsion in the 100–160 nm range. Quality of emulsion should be controlled by particle sizing (*see* **Note 6** and Fig. 2). Note the pressure and number of cycles for batch record.
5. At the end of process, collect the emulsion in a cooled vessel (*see* **Note 7**) and filter-sterilize the emulsion through a 0.2 μm PES filter membrane.

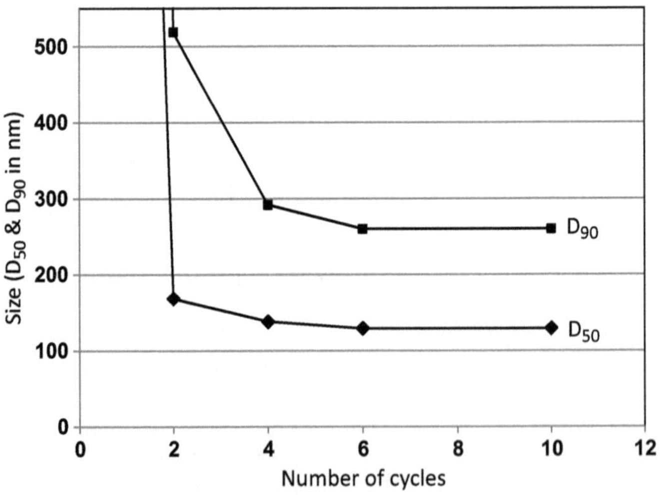

Fig. 2 Example of correlation between emulsion size and number of HPH cycles. A Panda 2K NS1001L (Niro Soavi) high pressure homogenizer operated at 10,000 psi was tested for the manufacturing of a 500 g batch of squalene/Tween80/Span85 emulsion having the composition described in Subheading 3.2. After each cycle, a sample of the emulsion was collected and particle sizes were measured on a Mastersizer 2000 particle sizer (Malvern instruments). D_{50} and D_{90} values are shown. Prior to HPH treatment, the size of the primary emulsion was $D_{50} = 3850$ nm and $D_{90} = 14{,}240$ nm

3.3 General Process for Manufacture of O/W Emulsion by the Phase Inversion Temperature (PIT) Method

The PIT manufacturing process is based on a unique property of ethoxylated nonionic surfactants that undergo a phase transition in aqueous solutions, from a classical micellar phase to an inverted micellar phase upon heating. When present in adequate proportion with water and oil, such surfactants will be able to stabilize O/W emulsions at low temperatures and drive the inversion of the O/W emulsion into a water-in-oil (W/O) emulsion as the temperature increases above a critical threshold referred to as "phase inversion temperature (PIT)." Conversely, when the temperature is decreased below the PIT, the system reverts into an O/W emulsion [17]. It has been shown that heating and cooling a coarse primary O/W emulsion comprising an adequate amount of polyethoxylated surfactant could yield a fine and long-term stable O/W emulsion [18]. With the PIT process O/W emulsions are usually manufactured as concentrated bulks as to facilitate the O/W to W/O inversion process, which are then diluted with water for injection or antigen buffer to the final oil concentration. The following section describes the procedure for manufacturing 100 g (ca. 100 ml) of AF03 concentrated bulk squalene emulsion (32.5 % w/w squalene) by the PIT method, followed by dilution to achieve ca. 650 ml of AF03 emulsion at 5 % w/w squalene (*see* Fig. 3).

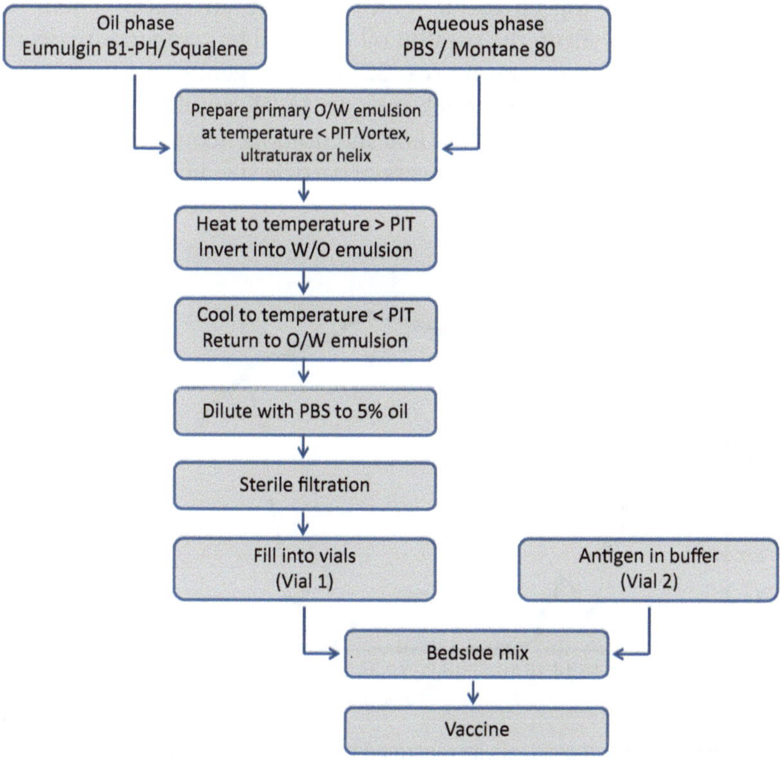

Fig. 3 Outline of squalene-in-water emulsion adjuvant manufacturing process by PIT method

3.4 Manufacture of AF03 Squalene Emulsion by PIT Method

1. Aqueous phase preparation: Dissolve 6.18 g of Polyoxyethylene(12)-ceto-stearylether (Eumulgin®B1 PH) and 6 g of mannitol (*see* **Note 8**) into 50.5 g of PBS under stirring at 40 °C.
2. Oil phase preparation: Dissolve 4.82 g of Sorbitan monooleate (Montane®80 PPI) into 32.5 g of squalene under stirring at 40 °C (*see* **Note 9**).
3. Primary O/W emulsion preparation: Mix the oil and aqueous phases prepared above in a beaker or glass flask and pre-emulsify the mixture by vigorous stirring using a magnetic stirrer or a high shear mixing device (Silverson L4R or T25 Ultra-Turrax) as described in **step 3** of Subheading 3.2.
4. Nano-emulsion formation: Equip vessel containing the primary emulsion with thermometer and conductivity probe and place the vessel under argon or nitrogen into a heating paraffin oil bath (*see* **Note 10**). Progressively increase the temperature of the primary O/W emulsion (ca. 1 °C/min from 40 °C to 70 °C) under moderate stirring until conductivity of the medium drops to zero, which indicates complete inversion into W/O emulsion (*see* **Note 11**). Note the inversion temperature for batch record. Normally, the selected composition has an inversion temperature of around 60 °C and may require heating up to 70 °C for complete inversion. Then, remove vessel from the paraffin oil bath and let temperature decrease to room temperature (ca. 22 °C) with gentle stirring as to inverse W/O emulsion back into an O/W emulsion (Fig. 4). This should now be a very fine and homogeneous concentrated O/W emulsion with an average particle size in the range of 80–100 nm; if

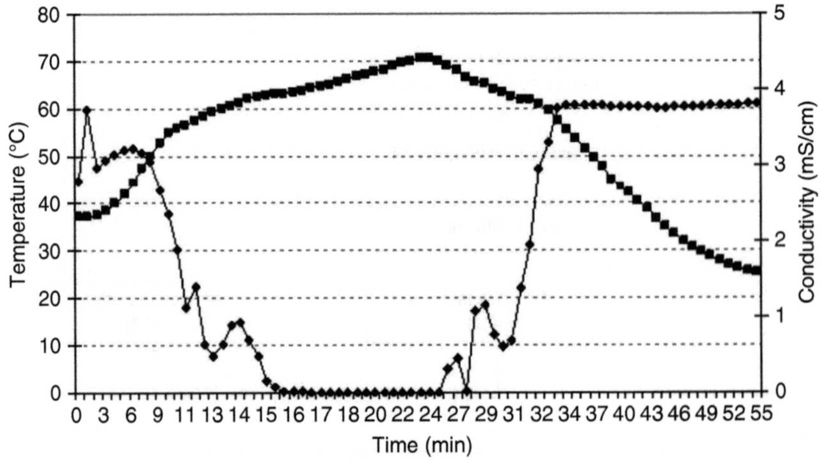

Fig. 4 In-process temperature and conductivity recording during AF03 manufacturing. The temperature (*filled square*) and conductivity (*filled diamond*) were recorded throughout an AF03 batch manufacturing process and plotted against time

not the case the heating/cooling cycle may be repeated. Quality of emulsion should be controlled by particle sizing.

5. Dilute concentrated emulsion 6.5-fold with PBS (or antigen buffer) as to adjust the squalene concentration to 5 % (w/w) and filter-sterilize as described in **step 5** of Subheading 3.2.

3.5 Characterization and Quality Control of O/W Emulsions

Appropriate analytical methods are important for the documentation of the quality and stability of O/W emulsions. Typical test methods are listed in Table 2 with reference to the EU and US Pharmacopeia when available.

Besides the characterization of appearance, pH, osmolality, endotoxin content, and sterility, O/W adjuvants should also be controlled for their oil and surfactant contents, particle size and size distribution and zeta potential (particle surface charge) when containing a charged surfactant. The presence of degradation products such as those resulting from the oxidation of squalene in case of squalene-in-water emulsions and fatty acids or fatty alcohols resulting from the decomposition of surfactants may also be characterized. Note that the viscosity of such diluted O/W emulsion adjuvants is essentially that of water which facilitates injection through needle and syringe.

Table 2
Typical analytical methods for the characterization of O/W emulsion adjuvants

Test	Method	Comments
Appearance	Visual inspection (Eur. Pharm. 2.9.20 and USP <787>/<788>)	Primary quality check in stability testing
pH	Amperometry (Eur. Pharm. 2.2.3 and USP <791>)	
Osmolality	Osmometry (Eur. Pharm. 2.2.35 and USP <785>)	
Endotoxin content	LAL test (Eur. Pharm. 2.6.14 and USP <85>)	
Bioburden	Bacterial and fungal sterility (Eur. Pharm. 2.6.1 and USP <71>)	
Oil and surfactant content	Specific RP-HPLC	
Particle size and size distribution	Laser light scattering	
Particle surface charge	Zetametry	When charged surfactants are used
Phase inversion temperature	Conductivity/temperature recording	For PIT emulsion only
Acetone content	Gas chromatography	For squalene emulsions only
Peroxide content	Merckoquant® test strips	

Note also that some vaccine antigens become unstable when stored formulated in a squalene emulsion adjuvant [19]. In this case the antigen and adjuvant need to be packaged in separate vials. Conversely, for antigens that have demonstrated long-term stability in the presence of squalene adjuvant, the antigen-adjuvant mixture can be sterile filtered and packaged as a single vial formulation. For long-term storage, filling in amber glass vials under nitrogen or argon is recommended.

1. Oil and surfactant content is generally analyzed by specific HPLC techniques. RP-HPLC with UV, evaporating light scattering, charged aerosol (Corona) or mass spectrometry (MS) detection is often used as a method of choice [20, 21]. An ideal HPLC method would detect not only the oil and surfactants used in the formulation but also the major degradation products generated upon potential chemical decomposition of these materials. Note that surfactant integrity can also be assessed indirectly as surfactant decomposition would inevitably affect the emulsion colloidal stability (phase separation, coalescence, and creaming easily evidenced by visual inspection or particle sizing).
2. Particle sizing is generally performed by laser light scattering techniques. Nano-emulsion particle sizing can be performed by dynamic light scattering (DLS) also known as photon correlation spectroscopy (PCS) or quasi-elastic light scattering (QELS) and by static light scattering. The PCS instrument (e.g., Zetasizer Nano-S or Nano-ZS from Malvern instruments) analyzes the fluctuations in the intensity of light scattered by droplets/particles due to their Brownian motion upon illumination of the sample by a laser beam. Instrument software calculates particle diameter (d) of equivalent spheres, using the translational diffusion, D, according to the Stokes-Einstein equation:

$$d = k_B T / (3\pi\mu D),$$

where T is the temperature, μ the viscosity of the medium (set at 1.332 for water), and k_B is Boltzmann's constant.

The PCS instrument gives the "z-average" and "polydispersity index" of the droplet population, corresponding respectively to the mean particle size and to the broadness of the size distribution derived from the cumulants analysis of the dynamic light scattering experiment. The polydispersity index indicates the quality or homogeneity of the dispersion. Equipment based on laser light diffraction, i.e., static light scattering, (e.g., Malvern Mastersizer 2000 or 3000), afford the detection of a wide range of particles in the 20 nm to 2 mm range, enabling the detection of larger droplets that may appear upon emulsion coalescence. The instrument calculates the size of droplets/particles in suspension from light scattering patterns obtained by recording the intensity of the light scattered by the particles at different angles (large, medium, and small angles) upon illumination of the sample by a laser beam. The Mie scattering model taking into account the refractive index of the particle (1.495 for squalene) and of its medium (1.332 for water) is applied by the equipment software to correlate the light scattering to an equivalent spherical particle size distribution. The fundamental particle size distribution, *DN*, derived by this technique is volume based and *DN* means that the volume percentage of particles with diameters up to *D* equals to *N*%. The polydispersity of the particle population can be assessed by two factors/values, namely uniformity (how symmetrical the distribution is around the median point) and span (the width of the distribution). The span value is defined by the expression:

$$\text{Span} = \left(D_{90} - D_{10}\right) / D_{50}$$

The smaller the span value the narrower the particle size distribution.

3. Other techniques useful for O/W emulsion particle analysis are cryo-transmission electron microscopy [22], nanoparticle tracking analysis (NTA) using the NanoSight (Malvern instruments, Malvern, UK), and particle counting with a Qnano counter from Izon Science (Oxford, UK).
4. Zeta potential, i.e., particle surface charge at a given pH, is a useful measure to characterize O/W emulsions comprising charged surfactants. Zetameters used for the determination of O/W emulsion zeta potentials (e.g., Malvern Zetasizer Nano-ZS) operate by measuring the electrophoretic mobility of the charged oil droplets.
5. Oxidation which is potentially occurring in some O/W emulsions, especially those containing squalene, can be characterized by the detection of peroxides (using for instance Merckoquant® analytical test strips from Merck Millipore) and by head space gas chromatography detection of the acetone formed by oxidative decomposition of squalene [23].

4 Notes

1. The nature of the oil is critical for the safety and efficacy of emulsion adjuvants. Preferred oils are fully biocompatible and metabolizable. In this regard, squalene and squalane have emerged as particularly suitable oils. Indeed, squalene is a natural constituent of the human body, an intermediate of human steroid hormone biosynthesis, a precursor of cholesterol, and a major component of human sebum. Squalane, the hydrogenated

homologue of squalene, can also be used but it is not as metabolizable as squalene [3, 24]. Squalene can be prepared from different sources such as shark liver, olive oil, or fermentation in yeast but the most common source is shark liver [25–29]. As the oil component of an O/W emulsion adjuvant, squalene has also been reported to outperform a series of vegetable oils in terms of consistency, safety, and adjuvanticity [25, 30]. In addition, since squalene is essentially insoluble in water (water solubility is 0.124 mg/L), the coalescence of the dispersed squalene droplets in water by Ostwald ripening is expected to be minimal [24]. However, since squalene is susceptible to oxidation, it is recommended to use raw material with low peroxide value, typically <2 meq/kg. Note that squalene needs to be emulsified to be adjuvant active [31].

2. Nature and concentration of surfactants are critical in emulsion manufacturing. Surfactants reduce the interfacial tension at the oil water interface. For the manufacturing of long-term stable O/W nano-emulsions, the surfactant molecules need to be flexible enough to accommodate the high surface curvature of the dispersed oil droplets and the concentration must be high enough to provide enough surfactant molecules to cover the totality of the oil droplets surface. Surfactants are selected according to their hydrophilic/lipophilic balance (HLB). The HLB scale has been created to classify surfactant emulsification properties. This scale ranges from 1 (more lipophilic surfactants) to 20 (more hydrophilic surfactants). For optimal emulsification and stability of O/W emulsions, the surfactant's HLB needs to match the oil's required HLB which is usually defined experimentally through a phase diagram approach (e.g., required HLB for squalene is around 9.2). In some cases, low and high HLB surfactants are combined as to better match the oil's required HLB (e.g., in MF59 and AF03). The HLB of a combination of surfactant A and B is calculated by the following formula:

$$\text{HLB}_{\text{A+B}} = \text{HLB}_{\text{A}}^{*}[\text{A}] + \text{HLB}_{\text{B}}^{*}[\text{B}] / [\text{A}] + [\text{B}],$$

where HLB_A and [A] are respectively the HLB and concentration of surfactant A and HLB_B and [B] are respectively the HLB and concentration of surfactant B.

While different kinds of surfactants can be used as emulsifiers in high shear emulsification processes [25], PIT emulsions require at least one of a particular type of surfactant, such as a polyoxyethylene alkyl ether, to drive the phase inversion process [32]. In pharmaceutical emulsions, nonionic surfactants are often preferred over charged surfactants due to their generally better tolerability and lower propensity to bind to other formulation additives or containers. However, O/W emulsions with cationic surfactants have been proposed for the adjuvantation/delivery of mucosal vaccines [1, 33] and for nucleic acid-based vaccines [34, 35].

3. Saline has been reported to decrease stability in phospholipid emulsified O/W emulsions such as SE (Table 1). In this case glycerol can be used as an alternative isotonic agent [27].
4. Emulsions such as MF59, AS03, and SE (Table 1) are produced by such a method as twofold concentrates and final concentration is achieved upon vol/vol dilution with the antigen solution [36]. Another approach is to produce concentrated emulsion and dilute after manufacture; for instance, SE (Table 1) can also be produced by microfluidization as a fivefold concentrate which is then diluted with buffer prior to sterile filtration and mixing with the antigen to achieve final concentration. Production of the emulsion as a concentrated bulk is advantageous in terms of time and energy savings, as this reduces the volumes to be processed. SE is generally used as a vehicle for the synthetic Toll-like receptor (TLR)-4 agonist, Glucopyranosyl Lipid A (GLA) [37].
5. The speed of dissolution/dispersion of surfactants into squalene depends on the nature of the surfactant. Some phospholipid surfactants as used in SE (Table 1) may require heating and sonication to achieve complete dispersion/dissolution. In this case, the heating temperature should be kept as low as possible to prevent or limit squalene oxidation. The addition of α-tocopherol (ca. 5–6 mg/ml squalene) as an antioxidant, and preparing the oil phase under nitrogen or argon, can help prevent squalene and phospholipid oxidation.
6. The emulsion size depends on its composition and on several homogenization parameters such as pressure, geometry of the interaction chamber, and number of cycles. Design or geometry of the interaction chamber will depend on HPH supplier/model. The number of cycles (at a given pressure) is defined empirically when the desired particle size is reached (Fig. 2). When the HPH equipment is operated in a continuous re-circulation mode, the number of cycles is calculated for a given pressure by the ratio between the volume of product to be treated and HPH flow rate. A pressure/flow rate calibration is usually established beforehand on the equipment. To help reduce the size further, in particular with high flow rate devices, a back-pressure valve can be installed at the outlet of the interaction chamber. The gain in particle size reduction is then around 20 nm [38, 39].
7. During HPH treatment a particular attention must be given to the product temperature. Up to 1 °C per 500 psi can be transferred to the product at every cycle. Besides the cooling system of the interaction chamber, collecting the product in a cooled vessel helps reduce the temperature more effectively.

8. In the AF03 composition, mannitol is introduced to decrease the PIT by assisting the subtraction of water molecules from the polyethoxylated surfactant, Eumulgin B1 PH, as temperature increases. Mannitol at a final concentration of 6 % (w/w) was found to decrease the PIT in AF03 by around 10 °C without affecting the emulsion particle size [32].
9. The composition described in the example is that of AF03. This process was since developed with other compositions starting for instance with an aqueous phase composed of 45 g PBS plus 6.05 g Polyoxyethylene(10)-oleylether (Brij®O10; Croda, East Yorkshire, UK) and an oil phase composed of 45 g squalene plus 3.95 g Sorbitan monooleate (Montane® 80PPI, Seppic). This yielded a concentrated bulk emulsion at 45 % (w/w) squalene that was diluted ninefold with PBS to 5 % (w/w) squalene and sterilized by 0.2 μm filtration prior to mixing vol/vol with the antigen solution.
10. Alternatively, a jacketed glass or stainless steel reactor equipped with a helix impeller, a thermometer, and a conductivity probe can be used. Heating is achieved by circulating water from a heated circulating water bath.
11. Emulsion inversion is accurately monitored in-process by using a conductivity probe (or a pH meter) since O/W emulsions conduct electric current while W/O emulsions do not (Fig. 4).

Acknowledgements

The author would like to thank Alexis Parisot (Merial R&D, Lyon, France) and Patricia Probeck (Sanofi Pasteur R&D, Marcy l'Etoile, France) for helpful discussions and Chris Fox (IDRI, Seattle, WA) for reading and commenting on the manuscript.

References

1. Stanberry LR, Simon JK, Johnson C, Robinson PL, Morry J, Flack MR, Gracon S, Myc A, Hamouda T, Baker JR Jr (2012) Safety and immunogenicity of a novel nanoemulsion mucosal adjuvant W805EC combined with approved seasonal influenza antigens. Vaccine 30:307–316
2. Ott G, Van Nest G (2007) Development of vaccine adjuvants: a historical perspective. In: Singh M (ed) Vaccine adjuvants and delivery systems. Wiley, Hoboken, NJ, pp 1–31
3. Allison AC (1999) Squalene and squalane emulsions as adjuvants. Methods 19:87–93
4. Vogel FR, Caillet C, Kusters IC, Haensler J (2009) Emulsion-based adjuvants for influenza vaccines. Expert Rev Vaccines 8:483–492
5. O'Hagan DT, Ott GS, Van Nest G, Rappuoli R, Giudice GD (2013) The history of MF59® adjuvant: a phoenix that arose from the ashes. Expert Rev Vaccines 12:13–30
6. Fox CB, Haensler J (2013) An update on safety and immunogenicity of vaccines containing emulsion-based adjuvants. Expert Rev Vaccines 12:747–758
7. http://www.novartis.ca. Accessed 30 Mar 2016

8. http://www.seqirus-us.com. Accessed 30 Mar 2016
9. O'Hagan DT, Ott GS, De Gregorio E, Seubert A (2012) The mechanism of action of MF59—an innately attractive adjuvant formulation. Vaccine 30:4341–4348
10. Brito LA, O'Hagan DT (2014) Designing and building the next generation of improved vaccine adjuvants. J Control Release 190:563–579
11. Ott G, Barchfeld GL, Chernoff D, Radhakrishnan R, van Hoogevest P, Van Nest G (1995) MF59: design and evaluation of a safe and potent adjuvant for human vaccines. In: Powell MF, Newman MJ (eds) Vaccine design: the subunit and adjuvant approach. Plenum Press, New York, pp 277–296
12. Shah RR, Dodd S, Schaefer M, Ugozzoli M, Singh M, Otten GR, Amiji MM, O'Hagan DT, Brito LA (2015) The development of self-emulsifying oil-in-water emulsion adjuvant and evaluation of the impact of droplet size on performance. J Pharm Sci 104:1352–1361
13. Bachmann MF, Jennings GT (2010) Vaccine delivery: a matter of size, geometry, kinetics and molecular patterns. Nat Rev Immunol 10:787–796
14. Garçon N, Vaughn DW, Didierlaurent AM (2012) Development and evaluation of AS03, an Adjuvant System containing α-tocopherol and squalene in an oil-in-water emulsion. Expert Rev Vaccines 11:349–366
15. Morel S, Didierlaurent A, Bourguignon P, Delhaye S, Baras B, Jacob V, Planty C, Elouahabi A, Harvengt P, Carlsen H, Kielland A, Chomez P, Garçon N, Van Mechelen M (2011) Adjuvant System AS03 containing α-tocopherol modulates innate immune response and leads to improved adaptive immunity. Vaccine 29:2461–2473
16. Haensler J, Probeck P, Su J, Piras F, Dalençon F, Cotte J-F, Chambon V, Iqbal SM, Hawkins L, Burdin N (2015) Design and preclinical characterization of a novel vaccine adjuvant formulation consisting of a synthetic TLR4 agonist in a thermoreversible squalene emulsion. Int J Pharm 486:99–111
17. Shinoda K, Saito H (1969) The stability of O/W type emulsions as functions of temperature and the HLB of emulsifiers: the emulsification by PIT-method. J Colloid Interface Sci 30:258–263
18. Förster T, Schambil F, von Rybinski W (1992) Production of fine disperse and long term stable oil-in-water emulsions by the phase inversion temperature method. J Disper Sci Technol 13:183–193
19. Miles AP, McClellan HA, Rausch KM, Zhu D, Whitmore MD, Singh S, Martin LB, Wu Y, Giersing BK, Stowers AW, Long CA, Saul A (2005) Montanide® ISA 720 vaccines: quality control of emulsions, stability of formulated antigens, and comparative immunogenicity of vaccine formulations. Vaccine 23:2530–2539
20. Fox CB, Sivananthan SJ, Mikasa TJ, Lin S, Parker SC (2013) Charged aerosol detection to characterize components of dispersed-phase formulations. Adv Colloid Interface Sci 199–200:59–65
21. Cotte J-F, Sonnery S, Martial F, Dubayle J, Dalençon F, Haensler J, Adam O (2012) Characterization of surfactants in an oil-in-water emulsion-based vaccine adjuvant using MS and HPLC-MS: structural analysis and quantification. Int J Pharm 436:233–239
22. Klang V, Matsko NB, Valenta C, Hofer F (2012) Electron microscopy of nanoemulsions: an essential tool for characterisation and stability assessment. Micron 43:85–103
23. Yeo HC, Shibamato T (1992) Formation of formaldehyde and malonaldehyde by photooxidation of squalene. Lipids 27:50–53
24. Fox CB (2009) Squalene emulsions for parenteral vaccine and drug delivery. Molecules 14:3286–3312
25. Fox CB, Anderson RC, Dutill TS, Goto Y, Reed SG, Vedvick TS (2008) Monitoring the effects of component structure and source on formulation stability and adjuvant activity of oil-in-water emulsions. Colloids Surf B Biointerfaces 65:98–105
26. Brito LA, Chan M, Baudner B, Gallorini S, Santos G, O'Hagan DT, Singh M (2011) An alternative renewable source of squalene for use in emulsion adjuvants. Vaccine 29:6262–6268
27. Fox CB, Carter D, Baldwin SL, Reed SG (2012) Innovations in emulsion technology. In: Reed SG, Fox CB, Carter D (eds) Emulsion-based vaccine adjuvants. Future Medicine, London, UK, pp 38–51
28. Broeker M (2011) Production of squalene from hyper-producing yeasts. Eu Patent 2268823, 5 Jan 2011
29. Haubricht A, Korb G, Trotzier J-F (2014) Production of squalene and/or sterol from cell suspensions of fermented yeast. Patent WO/2014/139989
30. Fox CB, Baldwin SL, Duthie MS, Reed SG, Vedvick TS (2011) Immunomodulatory and physical effects of oil composition in vaccine adjuvant emulsions. Vaccine 29:9563–9572
31. Calabro S, Tritto E, Pezzotti A, Taccone M, Muzzi A, Bertholet S, De Gregorio E,

O'Hagan DT, Baudner B, Seubert A (2013) The adjuvant effect of MF59 is due to the oil-in-water emulsion formulation, none of the individual components induce a comparable adjuvant effect. Vaccine 31:3363–3369

32. Klucker M-F, Dalençon F, Probeck P, Haensler J (2012) AF03, an alternative squalene emulsion-based vaccine adjuvant prepared by a phase inversion temperature method. J Pharm Sci 101:4490–4500
33. Wong PT, Wang SH, Ciotti S, Makidon PE, Smith DM, Fan Y, Schuler CF 4th, Baker JR Jr (2014) Formulation and characterization of nanoemulsion intranasal adjuvants: effects of surfactant composition on mucoadhesion and immunogenicity. Mol Pharm 11:531–544
34. Ott G, Singh M, Kazzaz J, Briones M, Soenawan E, Ugozzoli M, O'Hagan DT (2002) A cationic sub-micron emulsion (MF59/DOTAP) is an effective delivery system for DNA vaccines. J Control Release 79:1–5
35. Brito LA, Chan M, Shaw CA, Hekele A, Carsillo T, Schaefer M, Archer J, Seubert A, Otten GR, Beard CW, Dey AK, Lilja A, Valiante NM, Mason PW, Mandl CW, Barnett SW, Dormitzer PR, Ulmer JB, Singh M, O'Hagan D, Geall AJ (2014) A cationic nanoemulsion for the delivery of next-generation RNA vaccines. Mol Ther 22:2118–2129
36. Ott G, Radhakrishnan R, Fang J-H, Hora M (2000) The adjuvant MF59: a ten year perspective. In: O'Hagan D (ed) Vaccine adjuvants: preparation methods and research protocols. Humana Press, New York, pp 211–228
37. Anderson RC, Fox CB, Dutill TS, Shaverdian N, Evers TL, Poshusta GR, Chesko J, Coler RN, Friede M, Reed SG, Vedvick TS (2010) Physicochemical characterization and biological activity of synthetic TLR4 agonist formulations. Colloids Surf B Biointerfaces 75:123–132
38. Saheki A, Seki J, Nakanishi T, Tamai I (2012) Effect of back pressure on emulsification of lipid nanodispersions in a high-pressure homogenizer. Int J Pharm 422:489–494
39. Rueck H, Scheffczik H (2015) Arranging interaction and back pressure chambers for microfluidization. US Patent 2015/0258191

Chapter 13

Methods to Prepare Aluminum Salt-Adjuvanted Vaccines

Sachin G. Thakkar and Zhengrong Cui

Abstract

Many human vaccines contain certain insoluble aluminum salts such as aluminum oxyhydroxide and aluminum hydroxyphosphate as vaccine adjuvants to boost the immunogenicity of the vaccines. Aluminum salts have been used as vaccine adjuvants for decades and have an established, favorable safety profile. However, preparing aluminum salts and aluminum salt-adjuvanted vaccines in a consistent manner remains challenging. This chapter discusses methods to prepare aluminum salts and aluminum salt-adjuvanted vaccines, factors to consider during preparation, and methods to characterize the vaccines after preparation.

Key words Vaccine adjuvants, Aluminum oxyhydroxide, Aluminum hydroxyphosphate, Antigen adsorption, In situ precipitation, Antigen evaluation

1 Introduction

Mineral salts such as insoluble aluminum salts and calcium phosphate have been used as adjuvants in vaccine formulations. Aluminum salt-based adjuvants have been used in immunization programs for decades to help induce early, high-titer, and long-lasting protective immunity. Aluminum compounds, including aluminum oxyhydroxide, aluminum hydroxyphosphate, amorphous aluminum hydroxyphosphate sulfate, and alum-precipitated vaccines are currently the most commonly used adjuvants in human and veterinary vaccines. According to the World Health Organization (WHO), in 2015, the global vaccine market is valued at more than $41 billion, compared to $24 billion in 2013. More than half of these vaccines contain aluminum salt adjuvants [1–3]. Diphtheria-tetanus-pertussis vaccines, hepatitis A vaccines, hepatitis B vaccines, pneumococcal conjugate vaccines, anthrax vaccine, and rabies vaccines, all contain aluminum salts as adjuvants (Table 1) [4–7]. In fact, 9 out of the top 15 best-selling vaccines of 2012 contain an aluminum salt as an adjuvant [3, 4].

Aluminum salt-containing adjuvants are often referred to as "alum" in the literature. Chemically, alum is potassium aluminum

Christopher B. Fox (ed.), *Vaccine Adjuvants: Methods and Protocols*, Methods in Molecular Biology, vol. 1494,
DOI 10.1007/978-1-4939-6445-1_13, © Springer Science+Business Media New York 2017

Table 1
Examples of licensed vaccines that contain aluminum salt adjuvants

Adjuvant	Vaccine	Brand name	Manufacturer
Aluminum oxyhydroxide	DTaP	Boostrix	GSK biologicals
		Infanrix	
	Hepatitis B	Engerix-B	GSK biologicals
	Hepatitis A	Avaxim	Sanofi Pasteur
		Havrix	GSK biologicals
	Influenza (H5N1)	Panflu	Sinovac Biotech
Aluminum hydroxyphosphate	DTaP	Daptacel	Sanofi Pasteur
	DTaP, Polio	Repevax	
	DTaP, Polio, and Hib	Pediacel	Sanofi Pasteur
		Pentacel	
	DTaP, Hib, and Hepatits B	Quinvaxem	Novartis
	DTaP, Polio, Hib, and Hepatitis B	Infanrix hexa	GSK biologicals
	Influenza (H5N1)	Fluval	Omnivest
	Influenza (H5N1)	Panvax	CSL Biotherapies
	Pneumococcus	Prevnar	Wyeth
		Synflorix	GSK Biologicals
Aluminum hydroxyphosphate sulfate	Hepatitis A	Vaqta	Merck & Co
	Hepatitis B	Recombivax-HB	Merck & Co
	Human papillomavirus (HPV)	Gardasil	Merck & Co
Aluminum phosphate and aluminum hydroxide	DTaP, polio, and hepatitis B	Pediarix	GSK Biologicals
	Influenza (H5N1)	Daronrix	GSK Biologicals
AS04[a]	Hepatitis B	Fendrix	GSK Biologicals
	HPV	Cervarix	

[a]AS04 consists of aluminum hydroxide or aluminum phosphate and monophosphoryl lipid A (MPL)

sulfate ($KAl(SO_4)_2 \cdot 12H_2O$). It has not been widely used as an adjuvant in human vaccines. Aluminum oxyhydroxide and aluminum hydroxyphosphate have different physical characteristics [8] and differ in their adjuvant properties [9]. Historically, potassium alum was used to purify protein antigens, particularly tetanus and diphtheria toxoids, by precipitating them in the presence of anions, which resulted in a mixture of compounds including aluminum phosphate and aluminum hydroxide [10, 11]. While aluminum hydroxide and aluminum phosphate adjuvants are chemically referred to as $Al(OH)_3$ and $AlPO_4$, they are not stoichiometrically true. Aluminum hydroxide is a crystalline aluminum oxyhydroxide, which is positively charged at physiological pH (i.e., isoelectric point (pI) = 11) [9, 12, 13]. Aluminum phosphate is an amorphous aluminum hydroxyphosphate, which is negatively charged at physiological pH (pI = 5–7) [9, 12, 13]. One of the earliest uses of an aluminum salt as an adjuvant was reported by A. T. Glenny and co-workers in 1926, who showed that the suspension of alum-precipitated diphtheria toxoid has a higher immunogenicity than the toxoid alone [14]. Such preparations could be highly heterogeneous depending on the anions present at the time of preparation. Because of the variability in the production, the use of alum-precipitated tetanus and diphtheria toxoids has been remarkably limited [7, 10, 11, 15]. However, aluminum-adjuvanted vaccines have become widely used since then. The immunogenicity of antigens adsorbed onto aluminum salt-based adjuvants depends on several factors, but the most important include the degree of adsorption of the antigens onto the adjuvants and the dose of adjuvants [6, 8, 12, 16].

It is well-known that aluminum salts as adjuvants predominantly help induce antigen-specific humoral immune responses or T helper type 2 (Th2)-biased immune responses [17]. Aluminum salt-containing adjuvants can only weakly boost specific antibody responses, and its inability to help induce cellular immune responses has triggered researchers to search for alternative adjuvants (Table 2) [16, 18]. AS04 contains 3-O-deacylated monophosphoryl lipid A (MPL) derived from the lipopolysaccharide (LPS) of *Salmonella minnesota*, R595 [19] and aluminum hydroxide or aluminum phosphate in a 1 to 10 ratio (w/w) of MPL to aluminum ion [20]. Novartis' MF59 and GlaxoSmithKline's AS03 are both vaccine adjuvants that consist of oil-in-water emulsions; for instance, MF59 comprises 4.3% of squalene oil as the dispersed oil phase, which is stabilized by two non-ionic surfactants (Tween 80 and Span 85), and a low ionic strength citrate buffer as continuous phase [20, 21]. AF03 is a novel squalene-in-water emulsion

Table 2
Examples of licensed adjuvanted vaccines that do not contain aluminum salts

Adjuvant	Vaccine	Brand name	Manufacturer	Comments
AS03	Influenza (H5N1, H1N1)	Prepandrix Pandemrix Arepanrix	GSK Biologicals	• AS03 contains squalene, DL-α-tocopherol, and Tween 80 • Influenza A (H5N1) virus monovalent vaccine, adjuvanted, contains AS03
Virosomes	Hepatitis A Influenza	Epaxal Inflexal V Invivac	Crucell Crucell Solvay	
MF59™	Influenza (H1N1, H5N1)	Focetria Aflunov Fluad	Novartis	Fluad™ was approved in the USA in November 2015
Montanide™ ISA51	Non-small cell lung cancer	CimaVax-EGF	Bioven	Developed in Cuba's Center of Molecular Immunology
AF03	Influenza (H1N1)	Humenza	Sanofi Pasteur	AF03 is squalene-based thermo reversible oil-in-water emulsion

Note: The information in the table is not an exhaustive list. AS03, adjuvant system 03; AS04, adjuvant system 04

manufactured by a phase inversion temperature emulsification process and was recently approved for use in the human influenza vaccine Humenza™ [22, 23]. Montanide™ ISA51 is composed of a light mineral oil and a surfactant designed to make a water-in-oil emulsion [24]. Virosomes are a biodegradable and non-toxic adjuvant system that contains virus envelopes devoid of inner core and genetic materials [25]. Virosomal adjuvant system induces both B- and T-cell responses and is approved in a variety of vaccines [26].

The search for alternative and improved vaccine adjuvants continues today, but aluminum salt-containing adjuvants are likely to remain in vaccine formulations because of their continued safety profile of more than seven decades [6–9, 11, 16, 27]. Due to the popularity of the aluminum compounds as adjuvants in human vaccines, they have become the point of reference for evaluating new adjuvants. Although aluminum salts have been used for decades, their methods of preparation remain traditional, in which antigens are simply adsorbed onto adjuvants. The primary particles of aluminum hydroxide are in the nanometer scale; however, due to their poor water solubility, the primary particles aggregate to form larger microparticles of 1–20 μm when dispersed in water. Therefore, a vaccine that is prepared by binding an antigen with an aluminum salt is physically a suspension of aluminum salt particles with antigens adsorbed on them (*see* **Note 1**). However, adsorption of antigens on aluminum salt-based adjuvants depends on various factors including physical and chemical characteristics of the antigens, the type of aluminum salt used, conditions of adsorption, charges on adjuvants and antigens, the pH of the formulation, the size of the aluminum salt particles, the order of addition of reagents, and the speed of mixing [8, 9, 16, 27–30] (*see* **Notes 1–6**). It is thus critical that optimal formulations of antigens adsorbed onto aluminum salts are prepared.

Vaccines adjuvanted with aluminum salts are generally prepared by following methods: in situ precipitation of aluminum compounds, and adsorption of antigens onto preformed aluminum salt gel [11, 28]. The initial method developed for purifying toxoids, such as tetanus toxoid and diphtheria toxoid, is an in situ precipitation method, which involves growing the toxoid-producing organisms in culture medium supplemented with anions (i.e., phosphate, bicarbonate) and potassium or sodium alum [29, 31]. Vaccines prepared by this method are referred to as "alum-precipitated toxoids" and are a mixture of aluminum compounds, mainly aluminum phosphate and aluminum hydroxide. Although alum-precipitated toxoids show a higher immunogenicity than the soluble preparations of toxoids alone, these kinds of products are inconsistent to prepare [7, 10, 11, 15].

In the method of adsorption of antigen onto preformed aluminum salt gel, an antigen solution is added to a preformed gel of aluminum salts such as aluminum hydroxide, aluminum phosphate or mixed aluminum hydroxide plus phosphate. The resultant preparations are called "aluminum-adsorbed vaccines." Unlike alum-precipitated toxoids, the adsorption of antigens onto aluminum salts is carried out under controlled conditions, resulting in a consistent product. Because it is difficult to manufacture aluminum adjuvants consistently and reproducibly, and a poorly formulated aluminum adjuvant preparation does not have the optimal adjuvant activity [28, 32], Alhydrogel® (aluminum oxyhydroxide) and Adju-Phos® (aluminum hydroxyphosphate) from Superfos Biosector (now Brenntag Biosector, A/S) have been chosen as a scientific standard in an independent scientific workshop in Greece for the evaluation of new adjuvants and to minimize batch-to-batch variability [33, 34].

2 Materials

2.1 Reagents

1. Aluminum sulfate ($Al_2(SO_4)_3 \cdot 16H_2O$) solution (0.145 M).
2. Ammonia solution (13%, w/v).
3. Potassium alum ($KAl(SO_4)_2 \cdot 12H_2O$) solution (10%, w/v).
4. Aluminum chloride ($AlCl_3 \cdot 6H_2O$) solution (0.15–0.4 M), pH 3–4.
5. Sodium hydroxide (NaOH) solution (0.01–5 N), pH 12–14.
6. Physiological salt solution (0.9%, w/v, sodium chloride) (*see* **Notes 5, 6**).
7. Thimerosal ([(o-carboxyphenyl) thio] ethylmercury sodium salt) solution (1%, w/v).
8. Acetic acid (CH_3COOH) solution (5 N).
9. Aluminum hydroxide gel (0.01 M).
10. Alhydrogel® (2% w/v) [equivalent to 9–11 mg/mL aluminum].
11. Trisodium phosphate ($Na_3PO_4 \cdot 12H_2O$) solution (15.75%, w/v).
12. Sodium chloride (NaCl) solution (0.36%, w/v).
13. Aluminum phosphate gel.
14. Adju-Phos® (2%, w/v).
15. Sodium alum ($Na_2SO_4 \cdot Al_2(SO_4)_3 \cdot 24H_2O$) solution (10%, w/v).
16. Disodium phosphate (0.01 M) ($Na_2HPO_4 \cdot 12H_2O$) solution (0.5%, w/v), pH 8.5–9.5.
17. Sodium citrate (10%, w/v).
18. Sterile water for injection or sterile distilled water (*see* **Note 7**).

2.2 Equipment

1. Mixing vessels and tubes.
2. Centrifuge.

3. Water bath sonicator.
4. Kl filter sheets (e.g., BECO® filter sheets from Eaton Co) (*see* **Note 8**).
5. Autoclave.
6. Incubator.
7. Cold room (2–8 °C).
8. PD10 desalting columns.
9. Inductively coupled plasma optical emission spectrometer (ICP-OES, to measure aluminum content).
10. Instrument to characterize micro- and nanoparticles.
11. pH meter.
12. Protein BCA kit.
13. SDS-PAGE kit.

3 Methods

Details of the commercial production of aluminum adjuvants are subject to confidentiality. The methods below are adapted from various research articles, laboratory protocols, and book chapters [11, 12, 14, 31, 35–41]. The WHO has also published a method for preparing aluminum phosphate adjuvant [42]. The solutions listed in Subheading 2.1 should be prepared at the desired volume using distilled water (*see* **Note 7**). The solution is then sterilized by autoclaving or filtration through 0.22 μm filter (*see* **Note 9**). If using sterilization by filtration, it is recommended to test the compatibility of the solute with the filter material. The sterile solutions should be stored at room temperature. Sterile solutions of 5 N acetic acid and/or 5 N NaOH are used to adjust the pH. When using either in situ precipitation or adsorption of antigens to preformed aluminum salt gels, it is recommended to stir the contents continuously during the procedure at 40–60 rpm. The pH of the final preparation could change depending on the particular antigen. When performing the in situ precipitation, sterility should be strictly maintained throughout all operations. Vaccines adjuvanted with aluminum salts should remain stored as a liquid suspension at 2–8 °C from manufacturing to being administered to patients (*see* **Note 10**).

3.1 Preparation of Aluminum Hydroxide-Adjuvanted Vaccines: In Situ Adsorption of Antigens on Aluminum Hydroxide [37, 43]

Generally, aluminum hydroxide adjuvant is prepared by exposing aqueous solutions of aluminum ions in a well-defined and controlled chemical environment to alkaline conditions. Aluminum salts used for preparing aluminum hydroxide include aluminum chloride, aluminum sulfate, and potassium alum. These aluminum ions are then exposed to alkaline environment with the use of sodium hydroxide or ammonia. However, the resultant product is highly dependent on the experimental conditions including concentration, temperature, and rate of mixing. Even slightly different processing conditions can yield aluminum hydroxide with different size and adjuvant properties (*see* **Note 2**). Anions present in the reaction may precipitate and affect the characteristics of the adjuvant. One milligram of the aluminum hydroxide is expected to bind to ~50–200 μg of protein antigens. It is recommended to determine the optimum binding efficiency of an antigen to aluminum hydroxide by mixing the antigen and adjuvant at different ratios (*see* **Note 3**). It is recommended to test various lots of adjuvants to verify consistency in the process.

1. Add 0.29 M aluminum chloride ($AlCl_3 \cdot 6H_2O$), 0.08–0.2 M aluminum sulfate ($Al_2(SO_4)_3 \cdot 16H_2O$), or 10 % potassium alum in a mixing vessel.
2. While stirring, add 0.25–1.25 N sodium hydroxide (NaOH) solution or 5–13 % strong ammonia solution drop wise, and stir continuously until pH reaches 7.0. This forms precipitates of aluminum hydroxide [37, 40].
3. Centrifuge at 1000 × *g* for about 10 min.
4. Remove and discard the supernatant. Wash and resuspend aluminum hydroxide precipitate in physiological saline (*see* **Notes 5, 6**).
5. Add antigen to the aluminum hydroxide gel. One milligram of aluminum hydroxide can bind with ~50–200 μg of protein antigens. It is recommended to prepare the antigen in a saline solution.
6. Incubate the antigen-adjuvant mixture for 20 min to overnight.
7. Add 1 % thimerosal solution to reach a 0.01 % final concentration, if needed.
8. Check the pH and adjust it to optimal pH, depending on the antigen, with 5 N acetic acid or 5 N NaOH.

3.2 Preparation of Aluminum Hydroxide-Adjuvanted Vaccines: Adsorption of Antigens on Preformed Aluminum Hydroxide Gels

As mentioned earlier, processing conditions can introduce significant variability in aluminum hydroxide adjuvant prepared. To reduce the variability, gels of the clinical grade aluminum hydroxide is available. Based on our experience, it is preferred to purchase these preformed gels from a commercial source and design an optimal process for optimal adsorption of antigens. For example, our laboratory purchases Dried Aluminum Hydroxide Gel, Powder, United State Pharmacopeia grade (USP) from Spectrum® Chemical MFG Corp. (Gardena, CA). It is recommended to determine the optimal pH of adsorption as well as optimal binding of antigens to be adsorbed in preliminary studies before adsorption [8, 31, 41, 42]. Aluminum hydroxide gel should be sterilized after preparation (*see* **Note 9**). When dispersed in aqueous solutions, these gels may form reversible flocculates. Therefore, it is recommended to vortex or sonicate the gels briefly before mixing with an antigen solution.

1. Prepare aluminum hydroxide gel in a calculated volume of physiological saline (*see* **Notes 5, 6**).
2. Sonicate aluminum hydroxide gel for 5–10 min to break up flocculates.
3. Adjust the pH to the optimal pH for antigen binding with 5 N acetic acid or 5 N NaOH.
4. Prepare the antigen in saline solution (see **Notes 5, 6**) solution and add it to the aluminum hydroxide gel while stirring.
5. Incubate the antigen-adjuvant mixture for 20 min to overnight while stirring at 4 °C (*see* **Note 4**).
6. Add 1 % thimerosal solution to reach a 0.01 % final concentration, if needed.
7. Check pH of the final formulation again and adjust if desired.

3.3 Preparation of Aluminum Hydroxide-Adjuvanted Vaccines: Adsorption of Antigens onto Commercial Alhydrogel®

Alhydrogel® is a sterilized aluminum hydroxide wet gel/suspension. It is a commercial preparation. Alhydrogel® is generally regarded as safe (GRAS) to use in human vaccines and has been tested free from pyrogenicity. Currently, the most commonly used method for preparation of aluminum-adsorbed vaccines is the adsorption of antigens onto commercially available Alhydrogel®. As with aluminum hydroxide gels prepared with commercial aluminum hydroxide dry gel, determining the optimal binding of antigen to adjuvant using different ratios of antigen to adjuvant is recommended. Before mixing with the antigen solution, the Alhydrogel® suspension should be vortexed or sonicated briefly. If needed, dilute Alhydrogel® with saline solution (*see* **Notes 5, 6**).

1. Vortex or sonicate Alhydrogel® suspension for 5–10 min to break up flocculates (*see* **Note 11**).
2. Adjust the pH, if desired, to the optimal pH for antigen-binding with 5 N acetic acid or 5 N NaOH.
3. Prepare the antigen solution in saline solution (*see* **Note 5**) and add to the Alhydrogel® while stirring.
4. Incubate the antigen-adjuvant mixture for 20 min to overnight while stirring.
5. Add 1 % thimerosal solution to reach a 0.01 % final concentration, if needed.
6. Check pH of the final formulation again to adjust to optimal pH.

3.4 Titration of Antigen with Alhydrogel®

For best results, antigen solution should be titrated against Alhydrogel® to identify the amount of antigen and Alhydrogel® and the optimal ratio of antigen to adjuvant. Below is a procedure for antigen titration to Alhydrogel® [43–45].

1. Place 1 mL of antigen solution into 12 tubes.
2. Add 1.1 mL of water to the first tube, 1.0 mL to the second, and so on. The last tube receives no water.

3. Make a 1 in 9 (tenfold) dilution of Alhydrogel® in distilled water. Add 0.1 mL to the first tube, 0.2 mL to the second, and so on. The last tube receives 1.2 mL.
4. Rapidly mix the contents of each tube by a single inversion, and then allow to stand undisturbed.
5. The first tube to show flocculation contains the correct proportions. If the flocculation is first seen in either first or last tube, then another test must be run with more suitable dilutions of the antigen or the Alhydrogel®. Qualitative immunoelectrophoresis is suggested as a method for determining the adsorption capacity of the gel [44].

3.5 Preparation of Aluminum Hydroxide-Adjuvanted Vaccines: Adsorption of Antigens on Aluminum Hydroxide Nanoparticles [18]

The primary particles of aluminum hydroxide and aluminum phosphate are in the nano meter scale, as mentioned above. For example, the dimensions of aluminum hydroxide particles are of $4.5 \times 2.2 \times 10$ nm [46]. However, the particles aggregate to form larger microparticles when dispersed in water [47]. Despite the favorable safety profile of aluminum hydroxide, it only weakly potentiates antigen-specific antibody responses and is not able to help induce cellular immune responses [16]. Recently, our group showed that that the size of the aluminum hydroxide particles plays an important role in their adjuvant activity. Small-size aluminum hydroxide nanoparticles (~110 nm) have more potent adjuvant activity than larger aluminum hydroxide microparticles (9 μm) [18]. Here is a brief description of the adsorption of antigens on aluminum hydroxide nanoparticles. We have also prepared aluminum phosphate nanoparticles and showed that the nanoparticles have a more potent adjuvant activity than the traditional aluminum phosphate microparticles (*see* **Note 12**) [48].

1. Add of 3.6 mg/mL $AlCl_3{\cdot}6H_2O$ solution (0.15 M) into a mixing vessel.
2. Add equal volume of 0.04 M NaOH solution to the above solution.
3. Add a small volume of 0.01 M NaOH until the pH is adjusted to 7.0.
4. After 20 min of stirring at room temperature, sonicate the suspension for 15 min to decrease the particle size.
5. Pass the suspension through a PD10 desalting column to remove sodium chloride.
6. Determine the particle size and the aluminum content in the final nanoparticle preparation.
7. Prepare the antigen solution and add to the nanoparticle preparation while stirring.
8. Incubate the antigen-adjuvant mixture for 20 min to overnight while stirring.

3.6 Preparation of Aluminum Phosphate-Adjuvanted Vaccines: In Situ Adsorption of Antigens on Aluminum Phosphate

As with aluminum hydroxide, aluminum phosphate adjuvant can be prepared by in situ precipitation in a similar way as described above for the in situ precipitation of aluminum hydroxide gels, except that the adjuvant is precipitated with phosphate ions (e.g., trisodium phosphate). Recently, in situ precipitation is not performed because of the same reasons of variability in the product with different processing conditions.

In general, aluminum phosphate adjuvant is prepared by exposing solutions of aluminum ions in a well-defined chemical environment with phosphate ions. Commonly used aluminum ions include aluminum chloride and aluminum sulfate. These aluminum ions are then exposed to phosphate ions such as trisodium phosphate. Below is the common procedure for preparing aluminum phosphate [42, 49]. WHO also provides methods for producing aluminum phosphate adjuvant on a large scale. There are two different ways of producing suitable suspensions of aluminum phosphate, starting either from alum or from aluminum chloride [50].

3.6.1 Method Starting from Aluminum Chloride (WHO Method)

1. Filter 150 L of distilled water through Kl filter sheets (*see* **Note 8**) into a container of 300 L capacity.
2. Slowly add 30 L of $AlCl_3$ solution (0.4 M) while mixing.
3. Add Na_3PO_4 with vigorous stirring until a pH of 5.0 is reached.
4. Add 30 L of distilled water and mix the suspension well.
5. Leave the suspension standing for 7 days.
6. Siphon off supernatant after 7 days and add same volume of distilled water.
7. Mix the suspension well and leave standing for 7 days.
8. Siphon off the clear supernatant after 7 days, and add distilled water to bring the volume to 150 L.
9. Add 100 L of 0.36% NaCl to a total volume of 250 L.
10. Distribute the suspension of $AlPO_4$ with continuous mixing into 6 L volumes in 10 L bottles.
11. Autoclave the suspension at 121 °C.
12. Check the sterility of the phosphate suspension after 2 or 3 days.
13. This procedure yields bottles each containing 6 L of $AlPO_4$ suspension with 6 mg of $AlPO_4$/mL or 1.32 mg of Al/mL.
14. Add the antigen to aluminum phosphate based on the binding efficiency of the protein antigen. It is recommended to prepare antigen in a saline solution.
15. Check the pH and adjust it to optimal pH, depending on the antigen, with 5 N acetic acid or 5 N NaOH.

3.6.2 Method Starting from Alum (WHO Method)

1. Prepare potassium alum ($KAl(SO_4)_2 \cdot 12H_2O$) in 6 L of water (0.194 M).

2. Filter and keep at 37 °C, as it is slightly over saturated at room temperature.
3. Prepare trisodium phosphate ($Na_3PO_4 \cdot 12H_2O$) in 6 L of water (0.3 M).
4. Pour both solutions at the same time with mixing into 21 L of water.
5. Centrifuge the precipitate and resuspend the sediment in 13 L of water.
6. Centrifuge the suspension again, and resuspend with saline to a total volume of 8.1 L.
7. Homogenize the suspension and adjust the pH with 5 N NaOH to 6.0.
8. Autoclave for 1 h at 120 °C.
9. This quantity is sufficient for preparing 66 L of a vaccine with 3 mg $AlPO_4$/mL or 0.66 mg Al/mL.
10. Add the antigen to aluminum phosphate based on the binding efficiency of the protein antigen. It is recommended to prepare antigen in a saline solution.
11. Check the pH and adjust it to optimal pH, depending on the antigen, with 5 N acetic acid or 5 N NaOH.

3.7 Preparation of Aluminum Phosphate-Adjuvanted Vaccines: Adsorption of Antigens on Preformed Aluminum Phosphate Gel

Similar to aluminum hydroxide, aluminum phosphate prepared by in situ adsorption in the lab is known to have some variability due to processing conditions, and commercial preparation of aluminum phosphate of clinical grade is available for optimal adsorption and to reduce the variability. As with aluminum hydroxide, it is advisable to design optimal process for adsorption with aluminum phosphate gel. Aluminum phosphate is negatively charged at physiological pH [9, 12, 13], and hence antigens should be chosen that could have optimum adsorption at this pH. Aluminum phosphate gel should be vortexed or sonicated briefly to remove any aggregates.

1. Prepare aluminum phosphate gel in calculated volume of physiological saline.
2. Sonicate aluminum phosphate gel for 5–10 min to break up flocculates.
3. Adjust the pH to the optimal pH of the antigen with 5 N acetic acid or 5 N NaOH.
4. Prepare the antigen solution and add it to the aluminum phosphate gel while stirring.
5. Incubate the antigen-adjuvant mixture for 20 min to overnight while stirring at 4 °C.
6. Add 1 % thimerosal solution to reach a 0.01 % final concentration, if needed.
7. Check pH of the final formulation again and adjust if desired.

3.8 Preparation of Aluminum Phosphate-Adjuvanted Vaccines: Adsorption of Antigens onto Commercially Available Adju-Phos®

As mentioned above, to address the issue of variability in the production of aluminum phosphate, Adju-Phos® was chosen as a scientific standard for preparing aluminum phosphate adjuvanted vaccines. Adju-Phos® is a commercial sterilized aluminum phosphate wet gel suspension. Adju-Phos® has been tested to be free of pyrogenicity. At physiological pH, Adju-Phos® has a net negative charge and is well suited for adsorption of net positively charged antigens. Adju-Phos® should be vortexed or sonicated briefly before mixing with antigen solution.

1. Sonicate Adju-Phos® suspension for 5–10 min to break up flocculates.
2. Adjust the pH, if desired, to the optimal pH of the antigen with 5 N acetic acid or 5 N NaOH.
3. Prepare the antigen solution and add to the Adju-Phos® while stirring.
4. Incubate the antigen-adjuvant mixture for 20 min to overnight while stirring.
5. Add 1 % thimerosal solution to reach a 0.01 % final concentration, if needed.
6. Check pH of the final formulation again to adjust to optimal pH.

3.9 Method to Prepare Aluminum-Precipitated Toxoid Vaccines by In Situ Precipitation

As mentioned above, alum-precipitated toxoids are known to produce inconsistent product and are not very common in current lab practice. Here, we provide a brief overall procedure for preparing alum-precipitated toxoids [31, 41]. In situ precipitation is carried out by adding aluminum salts to the toxoid-containing anions. Source of aluminum can come from aluminum chloride ($AlCl_3{\cdot}6H_2O$), aluminum sulfate $Al_2(SO_4)_3{\cdot}16H_2O$, potassium alum ($KAl(SO_4)_2{\cdot}12H_2O$), or sodium alum ($Na_2SO_4{\cdot}Al_2(SO_4)_3{\cdot}24H_2O$).

1. Stir the contents continuously during the procedure at 40–60 rpm.
2. Maintain sterility throughout all operations.
3. Add the purified toxoid (~9 L) to a mixing vessel and allow to stand in the incubator at 37 °C for one-half hour to one hour.
4. Add 1 L aluminum chloride solution ($AlCl_3{\cdot}6H_2O$) or 10% sodium alum ($Na_2SO_4{\cdot}Al_2(SO_4)_3{\cdot}24H_2O$) to the purified toxoid.
5. This makes the pH of the solution to around 4.5 and a precipitate of aluminum phosphate is formed.
6. Transfer the mixing vessel to cold room (2–8 °C) and keep overnight.
7. Spin down the precipitates and wash twice with physiological salt solution.
8. Resuspend the precipitates in the same solution or 0.5% sodium phosphate solution ($Na_2HPO_4{\cdot}12H_2O$) solution equal to the original volume of the toxoid.

9. Add 1% thimerosal solution to reach a final concentration of 0.01%.
10. Adjust final pH (depending on the antigen, *see* **Note 2**) with 5 N NaOH or 5 N acetic acid.

3.10 Evaluation of Antigens Adsorbed onto Aluminum Salt-Based Adjuvants

It is very important to characterize the vaccines prepared with aluminum adjuvants in terms of physicochemical and adjuvant properties.

3.10.1 Adsorption Ratio of Protein Antigen Aluminum Salts

There has been mixed opinions regarding the effect of the degree of antigen adsorption on the adjuvant activity of aluminum salts [51]. In some cases adsorption of antigens onto aluminum adjuvants at 50% or even lower has proved efficacious. Nonetheless, it is known that the degree of antigen adsorption drives the immunogenicity of aluminum salt-adjuvanted vaccines [6, 8, 16] (*see* **Note 13**). The degree of adsorption is a parameter that could be controlled during the preparation. For example, the WHO recommends at least 80% of tetanus and diphtheria toxoids should be adsorbed onto aluminum salts [50]. Various tests can be employed to assess the degree of adsorption depending on the nature of the antigen [16]. Generally, the suspension of the adsorbed vaccines is centrifuged at 1000 × *g* for 10 min. The amount of antigen left in the supernatant is assessed. If the amount of antigen is assessed by optical density, the adsorption ratio of the antigen to the precipitate is expresses by the following equation [40]:

$$\text{Adsorption ratio} = \frac{[\text{Ag}]_{\text{added}} - [\text{Ag}]_{\text{in supernatant}}}{[\text{Ag}]_{\text{added}}} \times 100$$

Besides the commonly used centrifugation method, gel electrophoresis may also be used to determine the adsorption efficiency of the antigen to the aluminum adjuvant [52]. This is particularly useful when determining the extent to which protein antigens are adsorbed onto aluminum hydroxide nanoparticles as a much higher centrifugation speed is needed to precipitate nanoparticles. Aluminum adsorbed vaccine is applied to SDS-PAGE gel and subjected to electrophoresis. The intensity of the protein antigen bands are quantified after staining. Adsorption efficiency is then calculated by subtracting the percentage of unbound proteins from the total proteins. The rationale behind calculating adsorption efficiency is that protein antigens strongly adsorbed onto aluminum salts will not migrate out of the loading well of the SDS-PAGE gel [52].

3.10.2 Desorption of Antigens [12, 50]

If the aluminum-adsorbed vaccines are exposed to high concentrations of salts (e.g., sodium citrate) or phosphate ions, antigens are desorbed from the aluminum salts (*see* **Note 5**). It is a common procedure to desorb antigens from aluminum salts for direct measurement of antigens. Desorption is also performed to determine the identity of the product as per the requirement of regulatory agencies. The most commonly used solutions for desorption are sodium citrate and sodium phosphate solutions [50]. Sodium citrate or sodium phosphate solution is directly added to aluminum-adsorbed vaccines at a final concentration of 10%. The solution is mixed until all the granules are dissolved. This mixture is then incubated at 37 °C overnight or longer. All the samples are then centrifuged to determine the antigen content in the supernatant. Theoretically after desorption, all the protein antigens should be in the supernatant.

3.10.3 Quantitation of Aluminum Adjuvants

Chapter 21 of the US Code of Federal Regulations [610.15(a)] governs the amount of aluminum permitted in the recommended single human dose of a product between 0.85 and 1.25 mg. Therefore, quantitation of aluminum in the final bulk product is one of the quality-control parameters. Different methods available for the quantitation purposes [50, 53] include inductively coupled plasma optical emission spectroscopy (ICP-OES) [54], direct current plasma (DCP) [55, 56], and wet chemistry methods in which aluminum is dissolved (in either concentrated sulfuric or nitric acid) and titrated against zinc sulfate [57–59]. There is a wet chemistry method available from the WHO manual for quantitation of aluminum [50]. The readers are suggested to refer to the manual or the prior literature for more detailed procedure on quantitation of aluminum [12].

4 Notes

1. Although the adsorption of antigens onto aluminum adjuvants is heavily dependent on electrostatic attraction, ligand exchange occurs with phosphorylated antigens and is the strongest adsorption force. Phosphate binds more strongly to aluminum than hydroxyl and displaces surface hydroxyl groups from aluminum hydroxide and aluminum phosphate adjuvant [60]. Ovalbumin (OVA) contains up to two phosphate groups thus it can adsorb to positively charged aluminum hydroxide by both electrostatic interaction and ligand exchange. The adsorption of OVA with phosphate-treated aluminum hydroxide showed that ligand exchange may occur even when an electrostatic repulsive force is present [60].
2. Various factors affect the adsorption of antigens onto aluminum adjuvants. The major mechanisms by which antigens adsorb to aluminum adjuvants include electrostatic attraction, hydrophobic forces, van der Waals forces, and ligand exchange. Antigen adsorption heavily depends on electrostatic attraction [8, 9, 16, 61]. Other interactions, including hydrogen bonding and van der Waals forces, may not be effective if electro-

static repulsive forces are present. Electrostatic forces are driven by isoelectric point (pI) of aluminum adjuvants and the pI value of the antigens. Aluminum hydroxide and aluminum phosphate have different pI values [9, 13]. The pI of aluminum hydroxide is 11, and 5–7 for aluminum phosphate. Vaccine formulations are formulated with a pH close to physiological pH, in the range of 6–8, to reduce any discomfort. At neutral pH, these gels have different net charges; aluminum phosphate is negatively charged, and aluminum hydroxide is positively charged. The adjuvant that has the opposite charge of the antigen is chosen for optimum adsorption [62].

3. The adsorption capacity of each antigen to aluminum salt adjuvants should be determined. This is usually done by adding increasing concentrations of the antigen to a series of samples of the adjuvant at a controlled pH. Each sample should have the same concentration of adjuvant but different concentrations of the antigen. The samples are allowed to equilibrate, and after centrifugation, the concentration of the antigen in the supernatant is determined.
4. In general, incubation of the aluminum salt and antigen mixture at room temperature for 1–2 h or overnight at 4 °C is recommended to allow better and complete adsorption.
5. Ionic strength and pH can alter the charge on the aluminum salt gel and antigens. Ionic strength should be kept as low as possible. Polyols may be used in place of salts to adjust the tonicity. Pretreatment with phosphate anion could change the pI of aluminum hydroxide from 11.4 to 4.6 [60]. It is thus recommended to avoid phosphate buffers (i.e., absence of phosphate ions and low ionic strength) in the mixture for the optimal adsorption of antigens onto aluminum adjuvants [29, 30].
6. Alhydrogel® could be diluted if needed in physiological saline (to avoid phosphate ions) before it is adsorbed to the antigen. However, diluting the final vaccine preparation any further could affect the reactivity of the aluminum hydroxide gel [63].
7. Sterile water for injection or sterile distilled water free from endotoxin is recommended for preparing any of the adjuvant formulations. All chemicals should be of USP or NF grades.
8. BECO® standard range filter products from Eaton Company are available for filtration of liquids. K1 filter sheets from BECO® are designed for clarifying filtration and coarse filtration [64].
9. Limulus amoebocyte lysate (LAL) testing to determine endotoxin content is recommended for aluminum adjuvants.
10. Vaccines adjuvanted with aluminum salts must remain stored as a liquid suspension at 2–8 °C from manufacturing to being administered to patients. The reason for this is that aluminum

adjuvants are sensitive to freezing and freezing-induced irreversible coagulation or aggregation of the gel particles [65]. Aluminum salts are suspensions of hydrated colloid particles with slow sedimentation in water. The reasons for the slow sedimentation include the oriented water molecules that give buoyancy and the charges on the salts that give electrical repulsion among the particles in the suspension. Freezing irreversibly damages the hydrated colloid structures [66]. During slow freezing, free water, as well as the oriented water molecules, will freeze, and upon thawing will not take up their original positions, leading to irreversible damages [67, 68]. However, it is worth pointing out that there are technologies to make aluminum salt-adjuvanted vaccines not sensitive to freezing conditions [52, 65, 69, 70].

11. Aluminum oxyhydroxide particles are known to flocculate in suspension, and the flocculants can be easily broken up upon quick vortexing or sonication. Figure 1 shows how the particle size distribution changes from an X_{90} value of ~30 to ~3 µm upon quick vortexing (*see* Fig. 1). For this reason, it is advisable to vortex Alhydrogel® suspension quickly before use.

12. Our laboratory has also prepared aluminum phosphate nanoparticles. Here an aqueous solution of aluminum chloride ($AlCl_3$, 180 mM) was added to an aqueous solution of dibasic hydrogen phosphate (108 mM). The resultant suspension is then probe sonicated and centrifuged at a low speed.

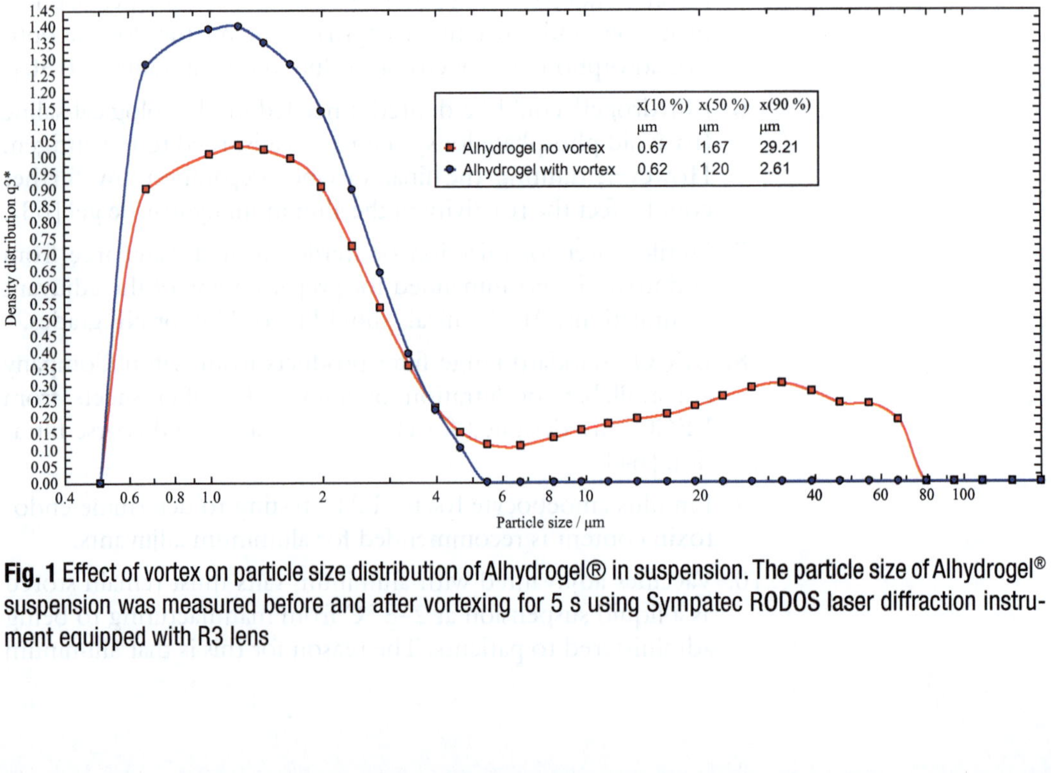

Fig. 1 Effect of vortex on particle size distribution of Alhydrogel® in suspension. The particle size of Alhydrogel® suspension was measured before and after vortexing for 5 s using Sympatec RODOS laser diffraction instrument equipped with R3 lens

The supernatant gives aluminum phosphate nanoparticles [48]. The aluminum phosphate nanoparticles have more potent adjuvant activity than aluminum phosphate microparticles [48].

13. The degree of antigen adsorption or binding efficiency appears to drive the immunogenicity of the antigens adsorbed onto aluminum adjuvants [6, 8, 16], and is considered a critical parameter for formulating aluminum-adjuvanted vaccines [8]. In general, an adsorbed vaccine is centrifuged, and the supernatant is assayed for total proteins (by protein assay such as Lowry assay, BCA assay) or antigenicity, depending on the antigen. In some cases, the proteins in the supernatant are assayed by enzyme-linked immunosorbent assay (ELSIA) [49]. SDS-PAGE gel electrophoresis may also be used to determine the binding efficiency of the antigen to an adjuvant.

References

1. Global vaccine market in 2015. http://www.statista.com/statistics/265102/revenues-in-the-global-vaccine-market/
2. Global vaccine market. http://www.who.int/immunization/programmes_systems/procurement/market/world_vaccine_market_trends.pdf
3. Top 15 Vaccines of 2012. http://www.genengnews.com/insight-and-intelligence/top-15-vaccines-of-2012/77899844/?page=2
4. FDA complete list of vaccines [updated 12/03/2015].http://www.fda.gov/BiologicsBloodVaccines/Vaccines/ApprovedProducts/ucm093833.htm
5. Cox JC, Coulter AR (1992) Advances in adjuvant technology and application. In: Yong W (ed) Animal parasite control utilizing biotechnology. CRC Press, Boca Raton, FL, pp 49–112
6. Gupta RK, Siber GR (1995) Adjuvants for human vaccines—current status, problems and future prospects. Vaccine 13(14):1263–1276
7. Gupta RK, Relyveld EH, Lindblad EB, Bizzini B, Ben-Efraim S, Gupta CK (1993) Adjuvants—a balance between toxicity and adjuvanticity. Vaccine 11(3):293–306
8. Gupta RK, Rost BE, Relyveld E, Siber GR (1995) Adjuvant properties of aluminum and calcium compounds. In: Powell MF, Newman MJ (eds) Vaccine design. Springer, New York, pp 229–248
9. Hem SL, White JL (1995) Structure and properties of aluminum-containing adjuvants. In: Powell MF, Newman MJ (eds) Vaccine design. Springer, New York, pp 249–276
10. Holt LB (1950) Developments in diphtheria prophylaxis. William Heinemann Medical Books, London, pp 1–181
11. Aprile MA, Wardlaw A (1966) Aluminium compounds as adjuvants for vaccines and toxoids in man: a review. Can J Public Health 57:343–354
12. Gupta RK, Rost BE (2000) Aluminum compounds as vaccine adjuvants. In: Vaccine adjuvants. Springer, New York, pp 65–89
13. Al-Shakhshir R, Regnier F, White JL, Hem SL (1994) Effect of protein adsorption on the surface charge characteristics of aluminium-containing adjuvants. Vaccine 12(5):472–474
14. Glenny AT, Pope CG, Waddington H, Wallace U (1986) XXIII- The antigenic value of toxoid precipitated by potassium alum. J Pathol Bacteriol 29:38–39
15. van Ramshorst J (1949) The adsorption of diphtheria toxoid on aluminium phosphate. Recl Trav Chim Pays-Bas 68(2):169–180
16. Gupta RK (1998) Aluminum compounds as vaccine adjuvants. Adv Drug Deliv Rev 32(3):155–172
17. Coffman RL, Sher A, Seder RA (2010) Vaccine adjuvants: putting innate immunity to work. Immunity 33(4):492–503
18. Li X, Aldayel AM, Cui Z (2014) Aluminum hydroxide nanoparticles show a stronger vaccine adjuvant activity than traditional aluminum hydroxide microparticles. J Control Release 173:148–157
19. Qureshi N, Mascagni P, Ribi E, Takayama K (1985) Monophosphoryl lipid A obtained from

lipopolysaccharides of Salmonella minnesota R595. Purification of the dimethyl derivative by high performance liquid chromatography and complete structural determination. J Biol Chem 260(9):5271–5278
20. Mbow ML, De Gregorio E, Valiante NM, Rappuoli R (2010) New adjuvants for human vaccines. Curr Opin Immunol 22(3):411–416
21. O'hagan D, Wack A, Podda A (2007) MF59 is a safe and potent vaccine adjuvant for flu vaccines in humans: what did we learn during its development? Clin Pharmacol Ther 82(6):740–744
22. Klucker MF, Dalençon F, Probeck P, Haensler J (2012) AF03, an alternative squalene emulsion-based vaccine adjuvant prepared by a phase inversion temperature method. J Pharm Sci 101(12):4490–4500
23. Shinoda K, Arai H (1964) The correlation between phase inversion temperature in emulsion and cloud point in solution of nonionic emulsifier. J Phys Chem 68(12):3485–3490
24. Aucouturier J, Dupuis L, Deville S, Ascarateil S, Ganne V (2002) Montanide ISA 720 and 51: a new generation of water in oil emulsions as adjuvants for human vaccines. Expert Rev Vaccines 1(1):111–118
25. Cryz SJ, Que JU, Glück R (1996) A virosome vaccine antigen delivery system does not stimulate an antiphospholipid antibody response in humans. Vaccine 14(14):1381–1383
26. Herzog C, Hartmann K, Künzi V, Kürsteiner O, Mischler R, Lazar H et al (2009) Eleven years of Inflexal® V—a virosomal adjuvanted influenza vaccine. Vaccine 27(33):4381–4387
27. Nicklas W (1992) Aluminum salts. Res Immunol 143(5):489–494
28. Edelman R (1980) Vaccine adjuvants. Rev Infect Dis 2(3):370–383
29. Bomford R (1989) Aluminium salts: perspectives in their use as adjuvants. In: Immunological adjuvants and vaccines. Springer, New York
30. Lindblad E, Sparck J (1987) Basic concepts in the application of immunological adjuvants. Scand J Lab Anim Sci 14(1):1–13
31. Seal S, Johnson SJ (1941) Studies on the purification of alum-precipitated diphtheria toxoid. J Infect Dis 69:102–107
32. Alving CR, Detrick B, Richards RL, Lewis MG, Shafferman A, Eddy GA (1993) Novel adjuvant strategies for experimental malaria and AIDS vaccines. Ann N Y Acad Sci 690:265–275
33. Stewart-Tull D (1989) Recommendations for the assessment of adjuvants (immunopotentiators). In: Greogoriadis G, Allsion A, Poste G (eds) Immunological adjuvants and vaccines. Springer, New York, pp 213–226
34. Stewart-Tull D (1991) The assessment and use of adjuvants. In: Vaccines. Springer, New York, pp 85–92
35. Dresser DW (1967) Immunization of experimental animals. In: Weir DM (ed) Handbook of experimental immunology. Blackwell, Oxford, p 8.10.1
36. Williams CA, Chase MW (1967) Production of antiserum. In: Methods in immunology and immunochemistry, vol 1. Academic, London, pp 197–209
37. Nail SL, White JL, Hem SL (1976) Structure of aluminum hydroxide gel I: initial precipitate. J Pharm Sci 65(8):1188–1191
38. Hem SL, HogenEsch H (2007) Aluminum-containing adjuvants: properties, formulation, and use. In: Vaccine adjuvants and delivery systems. Wiley, Hoboken, NJ, pp 81–114
39. Glenny AT, Buttle AH, Stevens MF (1931) Rate of disappearance of diphtheria toxoid injected into rabbits and guinea pigs:toxoid precipitated with alum. J Pathol Bacteriol 34:267–275
40. Hu J-G, Kitagawa T (1990) Studies on the optimal immunization schedule of experimental animals. VI. Antigen dose-response of aluminum hydroxide-aided immunization and booster effect under low antigen dose. Chem Pharm Bull 38(10):2775–2779
41. Ericsson H (1946) Purification and adsorption of diphtheria toxoid. Nature 158(350):1
42. WHO (1977) World Health Organization Manual for the production and control of vaccines: diptheria toxoid; Appendix D.21: Preparation of aluminum phosphate suspension.: BLG/UNDP/77.1.Rev.1
43. Herbert WJ (1973) Mineral-oil adjuvants and the immunization of laboratory animals. In: Weir D (ed) Handbook of experimental immunology, vol 3. Blackwell Scientific Publications, Oxford, pp A 3.1–A 3.15
44. Weeke B, Weeke E, Løwenstein H (1975) The adsorption of serum proteins to aluminium hydroxide gel examined by means of quantitative immunoelectrophoresis. Scand J Immunol 4(s2):149–154
45. Technical data sheet 'Alhydrogel®'. http://www.invivogen.com/PDF/Alhydrogel_TDS.pdf
46. Romero Mendez IZ, Shi Y, HogenEsch H, Hem SL (2007) Potentiation of the immune response to non-adsorbed antigens by aluminum-containing adjuvants. Vaccine 25(5):825–833
47. Hem SL, Hogenesch H (2007) Relationship between physical and chemical properties of alu-

minum-containing adjuvants and immunopotentiation. Expert Rev Vaccines 6(5):685–698
48. Ruwona TB, Xu H, Taylor A, Cui Z (2016) Towards understanding the mechanism underlying the strong adjuvant activity of aluminum salt nanoparticles. Vaccine 34(27):3059–3067
49. Gupta RK, Siber GR (1994) Comparison of adjuvant activities of aluminium phosphate, calcium phosphate and stearyl tyrosine for tetanus toxoid. Biologicals 22(1):53–63
50. WHO (1977) Manual for the production and control of vaccines-Tetanus toxoid: BLG/UNDP/77.2 Rev 1
51. Corbel M, Griffiths E, Winsnes R (1997) Workshop on standardisation of aluminium adsorbed vaccines. Biologicals 25(3):351–353
52. Li X, Thakkar SG, Ruwona TB, Williams RO, Cui Z (2015) A method of lyophilizing vaccines containing aluminum salts into a dry powder without causing particle aggregation or decreasing the immunogenicity following reconstitution. J Controlled Release 204:38–50
53. May JC, Progar J, Chin R (1984) The aluminum content of biological products containing aluminum adjuvants: determination by atomic absorption spectrometry. J Biol Stand 12(2):175–183
54. Olesik JW (1991) Elemental analysis using ICP-OES and ICP/MS. Anal Chem 63(1): 12A–21A
55. Urasa IT (1984) Determination of arsenic, boron, carbon, phosphorus, selenium, and silicon in natural waters by direct current plasma atomic emission spectrometry. Anal Chem 56(6):904–908
56. Urasa I, Ferede F (1987) Use of direct current plasma as an element selective detector for simultaneous ion chromatographic determination of arsenic (III) and arsenic (V) in the presence of other common anions. Anal Chem 59(11):1563–1568
57. Kenkel J (2010) Analytical chemistry for technicians. CRC Press, Boca Raton, FL
58. United States Pharmacopeia and National Formulary (USP 38-NF 33). 2015:2130.
59. European Pharmacopoeia 2.5.11.
60. Chang M-F, White JL, Nail SL, Hem SL (1997) Role of the electrostatic attractive force in the adsorption of proteins by aluminum hydroxide adjuvant. PDA J Pharm Sci Technol 51(1):25–29
61. Al-Shakhshir RH, Regnier FE, White JL, Hem SL (1995) Contribution of electrostatic and hydrophobic interactions to the adsorption of proteins by aluminium-containing adjuvants. Vaccine 13(1):41–44
62. Seeber SJ, White JL, Hem SL (1991) Predicting the adsorption of proteins by aluminium-containing adjuvants. Vaccine 9(3):201–203
63. Kerkhof NJ, White JL, Hem SL (1975) Effect of dilution on reactivity and structure of aluminum hydroxide gel. J Pharm Sci 64(6):940–942
64. BECO standard range filters. http://www.eaton.com/Eaton/ProductsServices/Filtration/DepthFiltration/DepthFilterSheets/FilterSheets/BECOStandardRange/index.htm
65. Kristensen D, Chen D, Cummings R (2011) Vaccine stabilization: research, commercialization, and potential impact. Vaccine 29(41): 7122–7124
66. Rowe RC, Sheskey PJ, Quinn ME, Association AP, Press P (2009) Handbook of pharmaceutical excipients. Pharmaceutical press, London
67. Organization WH (1998) Safe vaccine handling, cold chain and immunizations. World Health Organization, Geneva
68. Galazka A, Milstien J, Zaffran M (1998) Thermostability of vaccines. World Health Organization, Global Programme for Vaccines and Immunization, Geneva
69. Maa YF, Zhao L, Payne LG, Chen D (2003) Stabilization of alum-adjuvanted vaccine dry powder formulations: mechanism and application. J Pharm Sci 92(2):319–332
70. Randolph TW, Clausi A, Carpenter JF, Schwartz DK (2008) Method of preparing an immunologically-active adjuvant-bound dried vaccine composition. USA

Chapter 14

Production of Adjuvant-Loaded Biodegradable Particles for Use in Cancer Vaccines

Cristina Maria de Barros*, Emad Ibrahim Wafa*, Khanidtha Chitphet*, Kawther Ahmed*, Sean M. Geary, and Aliasger K. Salem

Abstract

Immune adjuvants, such as ligands for pathogen-associated molecular patterns (PAMPs), have been showing promise in boosting immune responses to tumor associated antigens, and delivering these adjuvants as discrete packages is considered advantageous over delivery in soluble form. Here we describe in detail, methods for independently loading a range of adjuvants into polymer-based biodegradable particles. We also describe the means by which to characterize these particles with respect to adjuvant loading and release kinetics as well as in terms of particle size, shape, and zeta-potential. These adjuvant-loaded particles have the potential to be used in dendritic cell-based uptake experiments performed in vitro or to be used in preclinical cancer vaccine research applications where they can be co-delivered with antigen-loaded particles or some other vaccine component comprising antigenic material.

Key words Adjuvant delivery systems, Cancer vaccine, Dendritic cells, Antitumor immune response, Toll-like receptors, Poly(D,L-lactide-*co*-glycolide)

1 Introduction

The purpose of most cancer vaccines is to not only generate strong immune responses but to do so in a therapeutic setting where the individual already has the disease (cancer) prior to vaccination. There is a wide range of variously formulated antitumor vaccines that are at different stages of preclinical and clinical investigation [1, 2]. A promising approach to enhancing cancer vaccines is the use of biodegradable polymeric particles, primarily designed to deliver antigens with or without adjuvants, to dendritic cells (DCs), the quintessential antigen-presenting cells [3, 4]. Such particle-based vaccines offer versatility in their ability to carry a range of antigenic and immune potentiating agents, potentially improving

*Authors contributed equally to this work

Christopher B. Fox (ed.), *Vaccine Adjuvants: Methods and Protocols*, Methods in Molecular Biology, vol. 1494,
DOI 10.1007/978-1-4939-6445-1_14, © Springer Science+Business Media New York 2017

vaccine delivery of tumor antigens (TAs) in the form of purified proteins/peptides, tumor lysates and plasmid DNA-based vaccines. Biodegradable particles loaded with antigenic material and/or adjuvants possess many advantages over soluble vaccine systems which include [5]: (1) the ability to co-deliver antigens and adjuvants to the same DC, (2) the potential to stimulate robust Th1-type responses, (3) the ability to mimic microbial pathogens thereby facilitating DC-mediated uptake and antigen presentation, and (4) the capacity to enhance antigen stability and allow for sustained release of antigens/adjuvants from particles.

Unlike microbial proteins, TAs are considerably less immunogenic and require delivery with strong adjuvants in order to generate effective antitumor immune responses. Aluminum-based adjuvants possess a poor capacity to promote cellular immune responses that are essential in controlling cancer [6, 7]. A diverse group of adjuvants receiving a great deal of attention for more than a decade now are pathogen-associated molecular patterns, or PAMPs, which have shown promising beneficial effects in increasing the immunogenicity of cancer vaccines [7]. PAMPs are highly conserved microbial molecular motifs that are recognized by the host's innate immune cells as "danger signals" through pattern recognition receptors (PRRs), of which the most intensely studied to date have been the family of Toll-like receptors (TLRs) [8–10]. Interaction with PAMPs and PRRs on host innate immune cells, such as DCs, results in the induction of a cocktail of inflammatory cytokines (Th1 type response), including type I interferons, designed to have immediate antimicrobial effects as well as long term influences on antigen-specific adaptive immunity. Salient examples of TLR agonists include: polyriboinosinic-polyribocytidylic acid (Poly I:C), monophosphoryl Lipid A (MPLA), CpG oligonucleotides (CpG ODNs), and imiquimod. These TLR agonists are included in the National Cancer Institute's ranking of immunotherapeutic agents with the highest potential to boost cancer immunotherapy [11]. More recently, most of the PAMPs used in clinical and preclinical studies have been synthesized, rather than purified from microbial sources, to avoid contamination; however, these synthetic agents are still capable of potent stimulation of their respective PRRs.

Of all the PAMPs studied thus far, the only one to be approved for use by the US Food and Drug Administration (FDA) is MPLA, a nontoxic derivative of lipopolysaccharide (LPS) that targets the TLR-4 receptor [12]. MPLA is a component of Cervarix® (GSK Biologicals) human papillomavirus (HPV) vaccine [13, 14]. Poly I:C and its derivative, poly I:C stabilized with poly-L-lysine and carboxymethylcellulose (poly-ICLC) are synthetic analogs of viral double stranded RNA that interact with endosomal TLR-3, causing increased production of type I IFN and inflammatory cytokines [12, 14]. Poly I:C and poly-ICLC are also being studied as cancer vaccine adjuvants in particulate systems aiming to improve its safety and efficacy [15]. Imiquimod (a TLR-7 agonist) and resiquimod (a TLR-7/8 agonist) are synthetic imidazoquinoline compounds. These molecules exert their stimulatory effects via TLR-7 or TLR-8, inducing the production of TNF-α and other inflammatory cytokines by DCs. Imiquimod is currently FDA licensed as a topical drug for genital warts and basal cell skin cancer [12, 16, 17]. CpG ODNs are synthetic single stranded oligonucleotide motifs based on unmethylated sequences found in bacterial DNA. They interact with TLR-9, stimulating innate immunity and the production of cytokines that promote Th1 immunity. In contrast to bacteria, most mammalian DNA is methylated, therefore the presence of unmethylated DNA containing CpG motifs in a mammalian host flags the possibility of a bacterial infection and thereby triggers the innate immune system. CpG ODNs are one of the most potent adjuvants and have shown great promise as cancer vaccine adjuvants [18].

When manufacturing antigen and adjuvant-loaded biodegradable particles for use as cancer vaccines one needs to take into account a number of factors in determining the desired final formulation. In particular, the particle size will be dictated by (1) optimal size for uptake by DCs and (2) loading efficiency and release kinetics of loaded antigen/adjuvant [19–21]. Particles much greater than 500 nm in size are less likely to be taken up by DCs and are therefore more likely to behave as depots, whilst particle sizes of <200 nm will often have inefficient loading, undesired burst release kinetics and be taken up more readily by non-phagocytic cells, thereby diminishing the potential for the formulation to promote Th1-type immune responses. Here we focus on the manufacture of particles loaded solely with adjuvant; however, co-loading with antigen is often feasible. It should be noted that co-loading of adjuvant and antigen can result in dramatically reduced loading efficiencies for both components compared to when either component is loaded alone.

Finally, different types of biodegradable polymers have the potential to be used as carriers in cancer vaccine formulations [1, 22, 23]. The use of particles based on the well-established polymer, poly(lactic-co-glycolic) acid (PLGA), is an attractive approach for controlled release of antigens and adjuvants [24, 25]. Here we highlight the use of PLGA because it is widely used, easy to obtain and work with, FDA approved and versatile due to being highly tunable and readily chemically modified at its termini. We specifically focus on describing how to generate PLGA particles (~500 nm diameter) loaded with CpG, Poly I:C, resiquimod, or MPLA, followed by instructions on how to characterize these particles in terms of size, charge, loading, loading efficiencies, and release kinetics. These particles can be subsequently used in cancer vaccine formulations by combining with tumor antigens (e.g., purified tumor antigens or in the form of tumor derived lysates) loaded independently into particles.

2 Materials

2.1 Preparation of adjuvant-loaded particles

1. Resomer® PLGA polymers (PLGA RG 503) (Boehringer Ingelheim KG) (*see* **Note 1**).
2. Polyvinyl alcohol (PVA) (Mowiol®8-88, Mw 67000, 88% hydrolysis) (Sigma-Aldrich) (*see* **Note 2**).
3. Dichloromethane (DCM).
4. 0.1 M 2-(*N-morpholino*)ethanesulfonic acid (MES) buffer, pH 5.
5. Phosphate buffered saline (PBS; 1×): 0.01 M phosphate buffer, 0.0027 M potassium chloride, and 0.137 M sodium chloride, pH 7.4
6. Ultrapure water (NANOpure Diamond™, Barnstead International) or any other source of sterile water.
7. Chloroform.
8. Methanol.
9. 150-mL glass Pyrex® beaker and 100-ml glass Pyrex® round bottom flask.
10. Stir bar and magnetic stirrer.
11. Sonic dismembrator Model 100 equipped with an ultrasonic converter probe.
12. 50-mL conical tube.
13. 7-mL and 20-mL glass scintillation vials.
14. Rotary Evaporator (e.g., Laborota 4000-efficient, Heidolph).
15. Centrifuge.
16. FreeZone 4.5 Freeze Dry System (Labconco Corporation).
17. Cytosine-phosphate-guanosine-oligodeoxynucleotide: CpG ODN class B 1826 (Integrated DNA Technologies) prepare stock in PBS at highest concentration possible (*see* **Note 3**).
18. Polyinosinic-polycytidylic acid sodium salt: Poly I:C (Sigma-Aldrich): Prepare stock solution at 12.5 mg per mL in PBS.
19. Resiquimod (R848, InvivoGen): Prepare resiquimod stock in chloroform at 8 mg/ml, dispense into 250-μl aliquots and store at −20 °C.
20. Monophosphoryl lipid A (MPLA, Avanti Polar Lipids, Inc.): Prepare MPLA stock in chloroform–methanol (4:1) at 10 mg/mL, dispense into 100-μL aliquots and store at −20 °C.

2.2 Characterization of PLGA Nanoparticles

2.2.1 Size and Zeta-Potential Measurement

1. Adjuvant-loaded particles (prepared as described below).
2. Blank particles (*see* **Note 4**).
3. NANOpure Diamond™ ultrapure water or equivalent.
4. Zetasizer Nano ZS (Malvern Instrument Ltd).

2.2.2 Particle Shape and Surface Morphology

1. Adjuvant-loaded particles (prepared as described below).
2. Blank particles (*see* **Note 4**).
3. NANOpure Diamond™ ultrapure water or equivalent (Barnstead International).
4. Argon beam K550 sputter coater (Emitech Ltd.).
5. Hitachi S-4800 Scanning Electron Microscopy (SEM) (Hitachi High-Technologies).
6. Silicon wafer and aluminum stubs.

2.2.3 Adjuvant Loading and Release Profile

1. Adjuvant-loaded particles (prepared as described below).
2. Blank particles (*see* **Note 4**).
3. 0.3 N NaOH and 1 N HCl solutions.
4. Dimethylsulfoxide (DMSO).
5. 0.01 M PBS, pH 7.4
6. OliGreen® kit (Molecular Probes).
7. Endotoxin assay (Kinetic-QCL™ LAL Assay, Lonza).
8. 96-well plate (Celltreat Scientific Products).
9. 96-well quartz plate (Corning-Costar).
10. SpectraMax M5 Microplate reader (Sunnyvale).

3 Methods

CpG-loaded particles and Poly I:C-loaded particles are most commonly prepared by the double emulsion-solvent evaporation method while resiquimod-loaded particles and MPLA-loaded particles are most commonly prepared by the single emulsion-solvent evaporation method (*see* **Note 5**).

3.1 Preparation of CpG-Loaded PLGA Particles (With Average Particle Size of ~500 nm in Diameter)

1. Dissolve 100 mg of PLGA RG503 in 1.25 mL DCM in a 7-mL glass scintillation vial (oil phase).
2. Dilute CpG stock in PVA solution to make a solution of 2 mg CpG in 50 μL of 1 % PVA (water1 phase) in a 0.5-mL microfuge tube.
3. Prepare 4 mL of 2.5 % PVA in 0.1 M MES buffer or PBS in a 20-mL glass scintillation vial (water2 phase) (*see* **Note 6**).
4. Prepare 22 mL of 1 % PVA in 0.1 M MES buffer or PBS in a 150-mL glass beaker (external aqueous phase).
5. Prepare primary emulsion (water1-in-oil) by sonicating the water1 phase into the oil phase for 30 s at 40 % amplitude (*see* **Note 7**). Specifically, pipette 50 μL of water1 phase into the 1.25 mL oil phase whilst simultaneously sonicating as described.

6. Prepare secondary emulsion (water1-in-oil-in-water2) by sonicating the primary emulsion into water2 phase for 30 s at 40% amplitude. Specifically, transfer the entire volume of the primary emulsion using a glass Pasteur pipette into the water2 phase whilst simultaneously sonicating as described.
7. Pour secondary emulsion into external aqueous phase already stirring on magnetic stirrer at 380 rpm and maintain stirring in a fume hood for 90 min to allow complete evaporation of DCM.
8. Transfer the emulsion to a 50-mL conical tube and centrifuge at 800 × *g* for 5 min and discard oversized particles (pellet) (*see* **Note 8**).
9. Transfer supernatant to a 50-mL conical tube and centrifuge at 10,000 × *g* for 10 min.
10. Wash the particle pellet three times with sterile water (top up volume to 30 mL each time). The pellet should be resuspended after each wash using a 1-mL pipette (do not vortex!).
11. Resuspend the pellet in 3–5 mL sterile water and freeze at −80 °C for at least 3 h (*see* **Note 9**).
12. Lyophilize the particles overnight using a Freezone 4.5 Freeze Dry System (*see* **Note 10**).
13. Store dried particles protected from moisture at −20 °C until ready to use (*see* **Note 11**).

3.2 Preparation of Poly I:C-Loaded PLGA Particles (With Average Particle Size of ~500 nm in Diameter)

1. Dissolve 200 mg of PLGA RG503 in 2.5 mL DCM in a 7-mL glass scintillation vial (oil phase).
2. Mix 150 μL of Poly I:C stock solution with 30 μL 5% PVA (water1 phase).
3. Prepare 8 mL of 2.5% PVA in PBS in a 20-mL glass scintillation vial (water2 phase) (*see* **Note 6**).
4. Prepare 22 mL of 2.5% PVA in PBS in a 150-mL beaker (external aqueous phase).
5. Prepare primary emulsion (water1-in-oil) by sonicating water1 phase into the oil phase for 45 s at 40% amplitude. Specifically, pipette 180 μL of water1 phase into the 2.5 mL oil phase whilst simultaneously sonicating as described.
6. Prepare secondary emulsion (water1-in-oil-in-water2) by sonicating the primary emulsion into water2 phase for 2 min at 60% amplitude (*see* **Note 7**). Specifically, transfer the entire volume of the primary emulsion using a glass Pasteur pipette into the water2 phase whilst simultaneously sonicating as described.
7. Pour the secondary emulsion into external aqueous phase and maintain stirring on a magnetic stirrer in a fume hood for 2 h to allow complete evaporation of DCM.

8. Transfer the emulsion to a 50-mL conical tube and centrifuge at 800×*g* for 5 min and discard oversized particles (pellet) (*see* **Note 8**).
9. Transfer supernatant to a 50-mL conical tube and centrifuge at 10,000×*g* for 20 min.
10. Please follow **steps 10–13** described in Subheading 3.1.

3.3 Preparation of Resiquimod-Loaded PLGA Particles (With Average Particle Size of ~500 nm in Diameter)

1. Mix together 100 mg PLGA (in 550 μL chloroform) and 2 mg resiquimod (in 250 μL chloroform)—giving a final volume of 800 μL in a 2-mL microcentrifuge tube (oil phase).
2. Prepare 4 mL of 9% PVA in PBS in a 20-mL glass scintillation vial (water phase).
3. Prepare 10 mL of 5% PVA in PBS in a 150-mL beaker (external water phase).
4. Prepare emulsion (oil in water) by sonicating the oil phase into the water phase for 2 min at 60% amplitude (*see* **Notes 7** and **12**). Specifically, pipette 800 μL of the oil phase into the 4 mL water phase whilst simultaneously sonicating as described.
5. Pour the emulsion into the external water phase and maintain stirring on a magnetic stirrer at 380 rpm in a fume hood for 1 h.
6. Transfer to a 100-mL round bottom flask and place on a rotary evaporator for 3 h and set pressure at 46 mbar to evaporate organic solvent (*see* **Note 13**).
7. Transfer particle suspension to a 50-ml conical tube and top up volume to 30 mL with sterile water. Centrifuge at 800×*g* for 3 min and discard oversized particles (pellet) (*see* **Note 8**).
8. Transfer supernatant to a 50-mL conical tube and centrifuge at 10,000×*g* at 4 °C for 10 min.
9. Wash the particle pellet three times with 30 mL sterile water. The pellet should be resuspended after each wash using a 1-mL pipette (do not vortex!).
10. Resuspend the pellet in 3–5 mL of sterile water and freeze at -80 °C for at least 3 h (*see* **Note 9**).
11. Lyophilize the particles overnight in a Freezone 4.5 Freeze Dry System (*see* **Note 10**).
12. Store dried particles protected from moisture at -20 °C until ready to use (*see* **Note 11**).

3.4 Preparation of MPLA-Loaded PLGA Particles (Average Particle Size of ~500 nm in Diameter)

1. Mix together 100 mg PLGA (in 700 μL chloroform) and 1 mg MPLA (in 100 μL 4:1 chloroform–methanol)—giving a final volume of 800 μL in a 2-mL microcentrifuge tube (oil phase).
2. Please follow **steps 2–12** described in Subheading 3.3.

3.5 Characterization of Prepared Particles

1. *Size*:

   Resuspend 1 mg particles in 1 mL nanopure water. Determine the size using a Zetasizer (Nano-ZS).

2. *Particle shape and surface morphology:*

   Particle morphology can be examined using scanning electron microscopy (SEM). Resuspend 1 mg of lyophilized particles in 1 mL of nanopure water and place a drop (30–50 μL) of this suspension on a silicon wafer attached to an aluminum stub. Allow the liquid to evaporate to obtain a dry film of particles. Coat the particles with gold-palladium for 3 min using an Argon beam K550 sputter coater prior to imaging via SEM at 2 kV accelerating voltage.

3. *Particle zeta-potential:*

   Resuspend 1 mg lyophilized particles in 1 ml nanopure water. Determine the zeta-potential by using Zetasizer (Nano-ZS). It may be necessary to dilute further in water until the solution is almost clear. If the particles are too concentrated this may yield inaccurate data.

4. *Adjuvant loading:*

   Degrade 5–10 mg of particles loaded with CpG, MLPA, or Poly I:C by adding 0.3 N NaOH (use 100 μl per 1 mg particles) and incubating at room temperature until a clear solution is obtained (approximately 1 h). Neutralize this solution with 1 N HCl (one can use pH paper to test solution), and record all volumes added.

   1. *CpG and Poly I:C:*

      Loading of CpG and Poly I:C can be measured using an OliGreen® ssDNA kit according to kit instructions. Briefly, prepare a working solution of the Oligreen reagent by making 200-fold dilution. Add 100 μL of working reagent to 100 μL of different known concentrations of CpG (or Poly I:C) solutions, so as to create a standard curve, as well as to test samples with unknown CpG (or Poly I:C) concentrations in a 96-well plate. Incubate the plate at room temperature, in the dark, for 5 min. Using a SpectraMax® M5 multi-mode microplate reader, measure the fluorescence intensity of the solutions at λex 480 and λem 520 nm. Construct and use the standard curve to determine the concentrations of CpG (or Poly I:C) in the test samples. Calculate loading and percentage encapsulation efficiency (%EE) by using Eqs. (1) and (2), respectively.

   2. *MPLA:*

      Loading of MPLA can be measured indirectly using a Limulus amebocyte lysate (LAL) endotoxin assay kit according to kit instructions (*see* **Note 14**).

3. *Resiquimod:*

   Dissolve 5–10 mg particles in 500 μL DMSO. Make serial dilutions in DMSO and distribute 100 μL of samples into the wells of a 96-well quartz plate. Make a serial dilution of 1 mg/mL resiquimod solution in DMSO to generate a standard curve. Measure samples using fluorescence λex 280 and λem 365 nm. The standard curve should be linear over a range of 1–15 μg/mL. Calculate loading and percentage encapsulation efficiency (%EE) by using Eqs. (1) and (2), respectively.

$$\text{loading}\left(\mu\text{g adjuvants per mg PLGA particles}\right)=\frac{\text{conc.}\left(\mu\text{g / mL}\right)\times\text{volume}\left(\text{mL}\right)}{\text{weight of particles used}\left(\text{mg}\right)} \quad (1)$$

conc. = concentration of adjuvant in the solution of degraded particles as calculated from standard curve (μg/mL); volume = volume of neutralized solution of degraded particles (mL).

$$\%\text{EE}\left(\text{encapsulation efficiency}\right)=\frac{\text{total weight of particles collected}\left(\text{mg}\right)\times\text{loading}\left(\mu\text{g / mg}\right)}{\text{initial weight of adjuvants used}\left(\mu\text{g}\right)}\times 100 \quad (2)$$

5. *Release profile:*

   To determine release profiles of loaded adjuvants, suspend 25–30 mg particles in 5 mL PBS in capped glass vials and incubate in a shaker (300 rpm/min) at 37 °C. At specified time points: 0, 1, 3, 6, 12, 24, 48, 72, 120 h, and every 2–3 days afterward (*see* **Note 15**), centrifuge the samples at 10,000 × *g* for 10 min and take 0.5 mL of the supernatant. Replenish samples with 0.5 ml of fresh PBS (*see* **Note 16**). Calculate the amount released in each sample using the assays described for loading estimation. Construct a release profile curve by plotting % adjuvant release versus time.

4 Notes

1. PLGA is available in different lactic acid–glycolic acid ratios. As the lactide content increases, the hydrophobicity of the polymer and consequently of the prepared particles increases. This affects the loadings and release rates of the loaded cargo and overall degradation times of the prepared particles. However, PLGA 50:50 is an exception to the rule being the polymer with the fastest degradation [26]. In addition, the inherent viscosity of PLGA is directly proportional to the chain length and can consequently affect degradation rates of PLGA particles.

2. Polyvinyl alcohol (PVA) is a commonly used surfactant/emulsifier which dissolves in the aqueous phase. PVA is available in different molecular weights and varying degrees of hydrolysis. These parameters can affect the size and structure of the particles. The fully hydrolyzed PVA is less surface active than partially hydrolyzed PVA. Moreover, residual PVA will also affect the zeta-potential of the particles [27, 28].
3. CpG stock should be prepared in a buffer such as 1× (Tris–EDTA) TE buffer (pH 8) or 1× PBS (pH 7.4) at a high concentration (for example 100 mg/ml) and then diluted with higher concentrations of PVA to achieve a final 1 % PVA solution containing CpG to prepare the particles.
4. Blank particles are prepared using the same methods used for preparing adjuvant-loaded particles without adding the adjuvants in the water1 phase for water soluble adjuvants or oil phase for lipid soluble adjuvants.
5. The choice of the method depends mainly on the particle size required. In general, for vaccine purposes, particles need to be within the size range suitable for uptake by DCs (preferably <500 nm) [27]. However, the smaller the particles, the lower the loading efficiency and the higher the percent burst release. The emulsion solvent evaporation method can be tailored to formulate particles of different sizes by changing formulation parameters. For water soluble cargo, one should use the double emulsion method where the cargo will be incorporated in the internal aqueous phase while for water insoluble cargo, one should use the single emulsion method where the cargo will be incorporated in the oil phase.
6. One can use PVA in water but the incorporation of buffers or any salts results in higher loading due to the effect of buffer in reducing the difference in osmotic pressure between water1 phase and water2 phase and thereby decreasing drug outward diffusion during the fabrication process [29]. MES buffer is useful if the free carboxylic end groups on the polymer are to be activated for consequent protein and/or peptide binding while PBS can be used merely for improved loading purposes. The pH of the buffer can be varied according to need. Other additives like NaCl or glucose have also been used.
7. Changing the sonication conditions will affect particle size such that higher amplitudes and longer times will yield smaller particles. However, one should be aware that the sonication process generates heat that might affect the stability of loaded cargo. To avoid such an effect, one can perform the sonication in an ice bath.
8. The double emulsion method generally yields particles with a broad size distribution. For vaccine purposes and to ensure that particles used are within the desired range for uptake by

DCs, step-wise centrifugation is advisable [30]. The particles pelleted in the first step of the methods described here should have a size of approximately 1–3 μm in diameter.

9. The volume of the particle suspension per sc is not important. The idea is to use the smallest volume possible such that the freezing and the lyophilization process does not take extended times. If one is preparing multiple batches simultaneously, it is advisable to pool particle suspensions before freezing to minimize the amount of particles lost to the walls of multiple tubes.
10. The time required for drying the particles can vary depending on the initial volume of the particle suspension. Excessive lyophilization can make the particles difficult to handle due to the particles acquiring static electrical charge.
11. Particles can be stably stored for up to 4 months at −20 °C unless the loaded cargo is particularly labile when stored for extended durations. In general, if the particles can be freely redispersed in liquid with no signs of aggregation, they are suitable for downstream use.
12. The emulsion will be very thick due to the high concentration of PVA used. One will need to move the vial around during the sonication process to ensure homogenous emulsion formation.
13. One can leave particle suspensions stirring in the hood for extended times if no rotary evaporation is available. However, one should be aware that extended times will have a negative impact on loading.
14. The endotoxin assay is very sensitive to any contamination (e.g., bacterial or LPS contaminants) and therefore requires the use of clean and endotoxin-free reagents and glassware to obtain reproducible results. Additionally, since this is an indirect assay and it will report the result in endotoxin units rather than amount MPLA, one should run two standards: one using an endotoxin standard and the other using an MPLA standard. Thus one can convert the endotoxin unit obtained directly from the kit to amount MPLA. More laborious HPLC methods have been described for MPLA-like molecules.
15. PLGA particles generally exhibit multiple phases in the release profile: an initial burst release phase during the first 24 h followed by a sustained release phase and then another burst release due to particle break down. The later phase can be seen at different time points depending on the specific formulation of PLGA used (*see* **Note 1**). One needs to collect samples at early time points to be able to characterize the burst release; however, one can choose when to end the study depending on the desired application of the particles [31]. In general, release studies are carried out for a minimum of 1 month when particles are to be used in an in vivo study.

16. It is important to maintain sink conditions throughout the release study to drive adjuvant release. The total volume of the release media used is dictated by the solubility of the adjuvant in the release media and the total amount of adjuvant (loaded into particles) used in the release study.

References

1. Palucka K, Banchereau J (2013) Dendritic-cell-based therapeutic cancer vaccines. Immunity 39(1):38–48
2. Finn OJ (2003) Cancer vaccines: between the idea and the reality. Nat Rev Immunol 3(8):630–641
3. Ahmed KK, Geary SM, Salem AK (2014) Applying biodegradable particles to enhance cancer vaccine efficacy. Immunol Res 59(1-3):220–228
4. Eldridge JH et al (1991) Biodegradable microspheres as a vaccine delivery system. Mol Immunol 28(3):287–294
5. Hamdy S et al (2011) Targeting dendritic cells with nano-particulate PLGA cancer vaccine formulations. Adv Drug Deliv Rev 63(10-11):943–955
6. Schijns VE, Lavelle EC (2011) Trends in vaccine adjuvants. Expert Rev Vaccines 10(4): 539–550
7. Tefit JN, Serra V (2011) Outlining novel cellular adjuvant products for therapeutic vaccines against cancer. Expert Rev Vaccines 10(8):1207–1220
8. Janeway CA Jr, Medzhitov R (2002) Innate immune recognition. Annu Rev Immunol 20:197–216
9. Medzhitov R (2007) Recognition of microorganisms and activation of the immune response. Nature 449(7164):819–826
10. Kumar H, Kawai T, Akira S (2011) Pathogen recognition by the innate immune system. Int Rev Immunol 30(1):16–34
11. Cheever MA (2008) Twelve immunotherapy drugs that could cure cancers. Immunol Rev 222(1):357–368
12. Steinhagen F et al (2011) TLR-based immune adjuvants. Vaccine 29(17):3341–3355
13. Giannini SL et al (2006) Enhanced humoral and memory B cellular immunity using HPV16/18 L1 VLP vaccine formulated with the MPL/aluminium salt combination (AS04) compared to aluminium salt only. Vaccine 24(33-34):5937–5949
14. Ammi R et al (2015) Poly(I:C) as cancer vaccine adjuvant: knocking on the door of medical breakthroughs. Pharmacol Ther 146: 120–131
15. Hafner AM, Corthesy B, Merkle H (2013) Particulate formulations for the delivery of poly(I:C) as vaccine adjuvant. Adv Drug Deliv Rev 65(10):1386–1399
16. Hemmi H et al (2002) Small anti-viral compounds activate immune cells via the TLR7 MyD88-dependent signaling pathway. Nat Immunol 3(2):196–200
17. Kobold S et al (2014) Modes of action of TLR7 agonists in cancer therapy. Immunotherapy 6(10):1085–1095
18. Bode C et al (2011) CpG DNA as a vaccine adjuvant. Expert Rev Vaccines 10(4):499–511
19. Yan S, Gu W, Xu Z (2013) Re-considering how particle size and other properties of antigen-adjuvant complexes impact on the immune responses. J Colloid Interface Sci 395:1–10
20. Gutierro I et al (2002) Size dependent immune response after subcutaneous, oral and intranasal administration of BSA loaded nanospheres. Vaccine 21(1-2):67–77
21. Katare YK, Muthukumaran T, Panda AK (2005) Influence of particle size, antigen load, dose and additional adjuvant on the immune response from antigen loaded PLA microparticles. Int J Pharm 301(1-2):149–160
22. Rueckert C, Guzman CA (2012) Vaccines: from empirical development to rational design. PLoS Pathog 8(11):e1003001
23. Mellman I, Coukos G, Dranoff G (2011) Cancer immunotherapy comes of age. Nature 480(7378):480–489
24. Colditz GA et al (1994) Efficacy of BCG vaccine in the prevention of tuberculosis. Meta-analysis of the published literature. JAMA 271(9):698–702
25. Nabel GJ (2013) Designing tomorrow's vaccines. N Engl J Med 368(6):551–560
26. Makadia HK, Siegel SJ (2011) Poly lactic-co-glycolic acid (PLGA) as biodegradable controlled drug delivery carrier. Polymers (Basel) 3(3):1377–1397
27. Shaffie KA et al (2010) Effect of polyvinyl alcohol of different molecular weights as protective colloids on the kinetics of the emulsion polymerization of vinyl acetate. J Am Sci 6(10):1202–1212

28. Foged C et al (2005) Particle size and surface charge affect particle uptake by human dendritic cells in an in vitro model. Int J Pharm 298(2):315–322
29. Sah E, Sah H (2015) Recent trends in preparation of poly(lactide-co-glycolide) nanoparticles by mixing polymeric organic solution with antisolvent. J Nanomater 2015:1–22
30. Joshi VB, Geary SM, Salem AK (2013) Biodegradable particles as vaccine delivery systems: size matters. AAPS J 15(1):85–94
31. Hines DJ, Kaplan DL (2013) Poly(lactic-co-glycolic) acid-controlled release systems: experimental and modeling insights. Crit Rev Ther Drug Carrier Syst 30(3):257–276

Chapter 15

Lyophilization of Adjuvanted Vaccines: Methods for Formulation of a Thermostable Freeze-Dried Product

Michelle Y. Chan, Timothy S. Dutill, and Ryan M. Kramer

Abstract

Lyophilization of vaccines is advantageous for the distribution and storage of thermally labile products, particularly in regions where cold chain management is difficult. To date, current lyophilized vaccines do not contain an adjuvant. Instead, adjuvanted vaccines may be presented as a two vial system, that require bedside-mixing prior to immunization. Here we present an example of a lyophilization cycle that we have used to successfully freeze-dry an adjuvanted protein formulation in a single vial.

Key words Lyophilization, Freeze-drying, Thermostable, Formulation, Adjuvant, Nanoemulsion

1 Introduction

The lyophilization of vaccines is of great interest. Many vaccines are thermally labile, which can challenge distribution and storage of vaccines in countries where cold-chain management is difficult [1]. The development of thermostable products can help with the distribution of vaccines in these areas, and can also help reduce waste of product that has inadvertently been stored at temperatures that exceed or fall below specified storage temperatures. In addition, lyophilized formats have potential to provide for longer product shelf lives.

Current available lyophilized vaccines do not contain adjuvant and are presented as a two vial system. A vial containing the lyophilized protein is reconstituted using a diluent prior to immunization. Adjuvants are rarely used with lyophilized vaccines but in some cases are administered with the diluent [2, 3]. We recently reported that lyophilization of a multicomponent antigen–adjuvant system is possible with thermostability of at least 1 month at 50 °C without impaired immunological activity [4]. Here we present an example of a lyophilization cycle that we have used to successfully freeze-dry protein formulated with an oil-in-water emulsion adjuvant in a single vial.

Christopher B. Fox (ed.), *Vaccine Adjuvants: Methods and Protocols*, Methods in Molecular Biology, vol. 1494, DOI 10.1007/978-1-4939-6445-1_15, © Springer Science+Business Media New York 2017

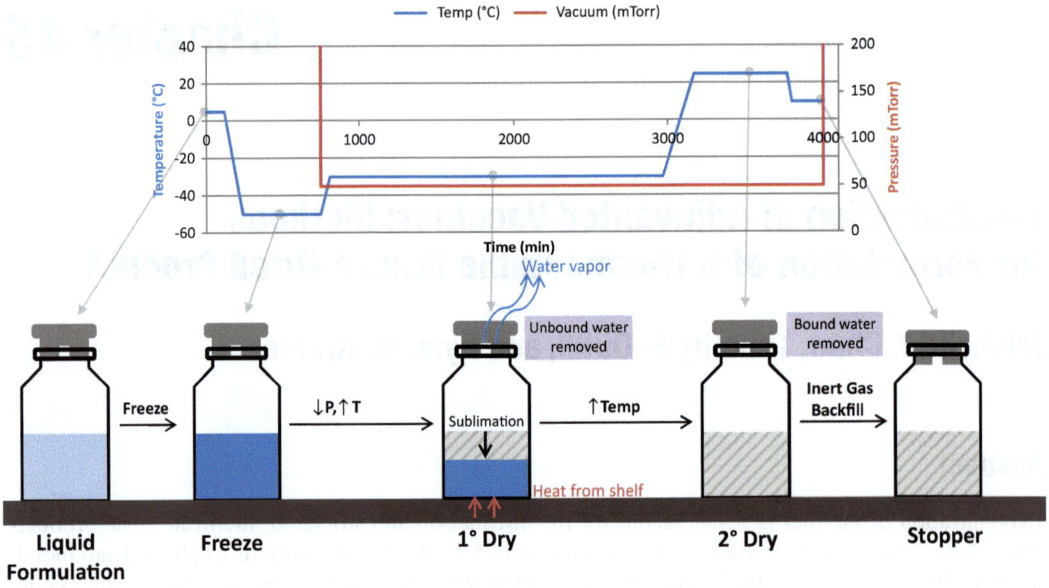

Fig. 1 The five main stages of lyophilization include formulation, freezing, primary (1°) drying, secondary (2°) drying, and stoppering. In liquid formulation, excipients are added to the active ingredient and then vialed and half stoppered. Samples are then frozen. During primary drying, a vacuum is pulled to lower pressure and heat is applied by increasing the shelf temperature. This allows sublimation to occur, removing unbound water from the samples. During secondary drying, temperature is increased and bound water is removed from the samples. Samples are then brought back to atmospheric pressure, blanketed with an inert gas, and stoppered

Lyophilization is a complex process which can be divided into several steps, and each step has several parameters that can be varied. Freeze drying consists of five main stages: formulation, freezing, primary drying, secondary drying, and stoppering (*see* Fig. 1). The science and theory on how these steps collectively produce a lyophilized product are widely published [3, 5–7]. In a simplified explanation, a vaccine is prepared with excipients (e.g., sucrose, trehalose, mannitol) that act as lyoprotectants and bulking agents to protect the active ingredients during the freeze-dry process and in the dried state post-lyophilization. The samples are frozen and then pressure in the chamber is reduced, allowing water in the samples to sublimate and collect as ice on a condenser. In primary drying, the sublimation is driven by a pressure differential between the vapor pressure of ice at the sublimation front and the partial pressure of water vapor in the chamber. Temperature may then be increased during secondary drying to drive off additional water that remains. Once sufficiently dry, atmospheric pressure is restored and an inert gas may be used to blanket the samples. The samples are then stoppered and ready for use (*see* Fig. 2).

While many different types of freeze dryers exist, the protocol presented here is for the use of a single shelf Virtis AdVantage 2.0 EL benchtop freeze dryer from SP Scientific (Gardiner, NY). The protocol is an example of a conservative lyophilization cycle that has been employed for successful freeze drying of adjuvanted

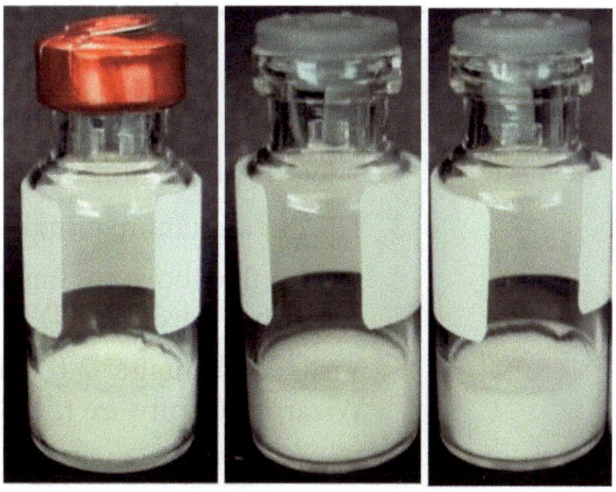

Fig. 2 Images of a protein and GLA-SE (an oil in water nanoemulsion adjuvant) lyophilized with 10 % sucrose (*left*), 0.5 % glycine (*middle*), and 1 % mannitol (*right*) in 10 mM sodium citrate

protein formulations, including protein formulated with oil-in-water emulsion adjuvants. Other similar cycles have been used for liposome-containing formulations. This particular cycle is designed to be suitable for a range of amorphous formulations such as disaccharide, glycine, and mannitol based formulations. Additives such as detergents or anionic salts may be included. Formulations containing 5–10% (w/v) sucrose or trehalose with up to 1% (w/v) mannitol have been particularly successful for maintaining physicochemical properties after reconstitution and conveying thermostability. The formulations are prepared in bulk and then filled into 3-mL 13-mm glass vials with a 1-mL fill volume. Vials are packed onto a removable bottom tray and transferred to the shelf of the freeze dryer. Samples are first cooled to −50 °C at atmospheric pressure, and then subjected to a primary drying step at −30 °C and a secondary drying step at 25 °C with vacuum applied at 50 mTorr. In this case, the cycle is performed by a microprocessor-based Wizard 2.0 controller (*see* **Note 1**). At the completion of the cycle, samples are brought back to atmospheric pressure, blanketed with high purity nitrogen, and stoppered prior to being removed from the freeze-dryer chamber. To monitor the lyophilization of these samples, four product temperature probes are placed in vials containing samples. The resulting temperature probe plot, along with recorded shelf temperatures and vacuum pressures, are reviewed to verify that the lyophilization run was executed as intended.

It is important to note that vial type, stopper type, fill volumes, cycle parameters, blanketing gas type, and the freeze dryer itself can and should be adjusted for specific applications. Lyophilization cycle temperatures and times for a particular formulation can be systematically investigated and should be refined to produce an acceptable final product using the fastest and most economical cycle that is safe, effective, and robust. Some tips on modifications, such as the inclusion of an annealing step or the use of excipients, are included in section 4 (*see* **Notes 2** and **3**).

2 Materials

1. 3-mL 13-mm glass vials (Afton Scientific, Charlottesville, VA).
2. 2-leg lyophilization stoppers (Wheaton, Millville, NJ).
3. 13-mm aluminum crimps (Wheaton, Millville, NJ).
4. Removable bottom stainless steel tray, 10″×14″×1.5″ (SP Scientific, Gardiner, NY).
5. Virtis AdVantage 2.0 EL-85 benchtop freeze dryer with Wizard 2.0 software (SP Scientific, Gardiner, NY).
6. Vacuum Pump.
7. High purity nitrogen gas.
8. Product temperature probes and 13-mm stoppers equipped with 1” guide tubes (SP Scientific, Gardiner, NY).
9. Sucrose solution (5 % w/v).
10. Sample of interest (e.g., protein antigen in oil-in-water emulsion) and lyophilization excipients (e.g., sucrose, trehalose, mannitol).

3 Methods

1. Assemble the removable bottom tray by placing the rectangular rack into the tray bottom. The front of the tray is the short edge of the tray with the rim. The back of the tray is rimless.
2. Carefully add 1 mL of sample, compounded with the excipients of interest, to the vials, avoiding splashing on the vial walls (*see* **Note 4**).
3. Insert stoppers halfway, making sure there is an opening for exchange between the inside and the outside of the vials (*see* **Note 5**).
4. Place filled vials in the center of the assembled removable bottom tray.
5. Add four vials containing temperature probes to the tray in the four quadrants as shown in Fig. 3. To prepare these vials follow **steps 6–9** below.
6. Add 1 mL of sample to four separate vials (*see* **Note 6**).
7. Fully cap using the stoppers equipped with 1” guide tubes (*see* **Note** 7).
8. Feed probes through the guide tube, to the bottom center of the vial so that thermocouples are as close to the bottom of the vial as possible without touching it.
9. Secure the position of the probe by taping the external wire to the vial with a piece of lab tape.

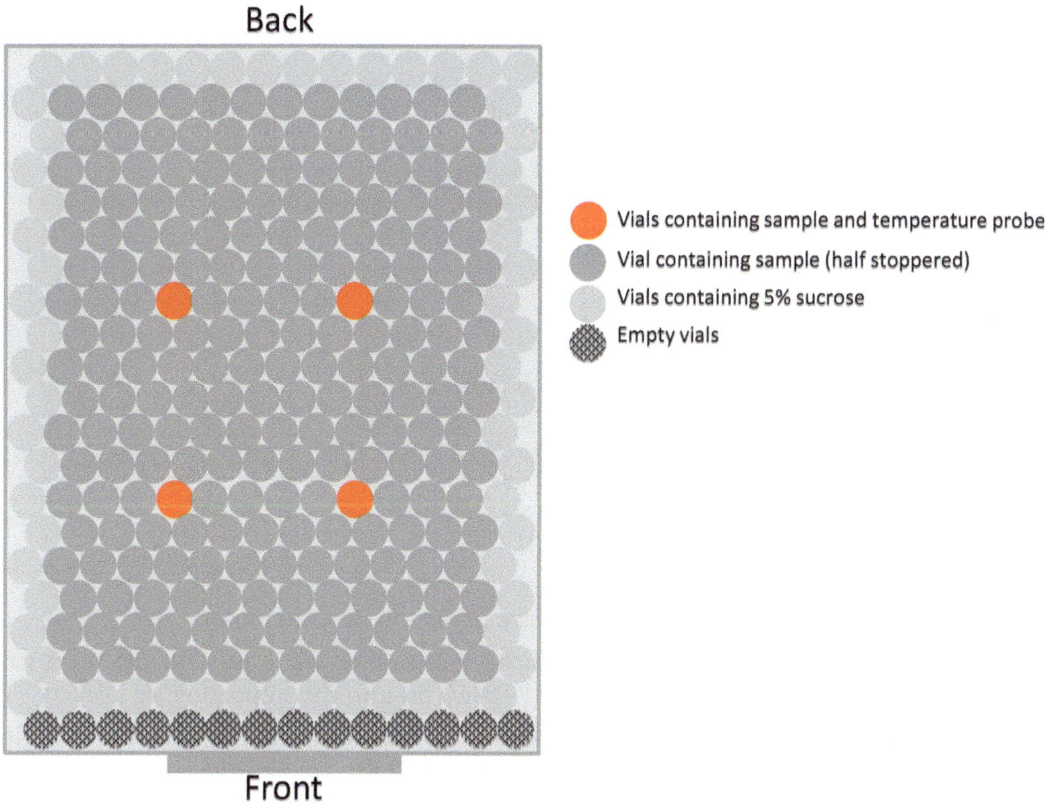

Fig. 3 An example schematic of a removable bottom tray fully packed with vials containing samples (*dark grey*), vials containing 5 % sucrose (*light grey*), and empty vials (*hatched*), as well as four vials containing sample and product temperature probes (*orange*)

10. Tightly pack the remaining space in the tray with empty vials so that vials containing sample are clustered together in the center of the tray (*see* **Note 8**).
11. Fill the surrounding ring of empty vials that have immediate contact with sample vials with 1 mL of 5 % sucrose solution (*see* **Notes 9** and **10**).
12. Load samples onto the freeze dryer shelf as described in **steps 13** and **14** below.
13. Place the tray assembly containing samples onto the shelf, carefully centering it. Make sure that the front side of the tray is in the front.
14. Hold the rack in place and carefully remove the tray bottom by sliding it out from underneath the vials. The rack stays in the chamber and the vials now sit directly on the shelf for more optimal heat transfer.
15. Arrange the wires of the product temperature probes so that they do not interfere with the samples, fan, or condenser by tucking them into the space underneath the shelf.
16. Close the chamber door and cover with aluminum foil to minimize heat radiation from the room (*see* **Note 11**).

Table 1
Lyophilization cycle

Procedure	Step	Temp (°C)	Time (min)	Vacuum (mTorr)	Ramp/hold
Freeze	1	5	120	N/A	H
	2	-50	120	N/A	R
	3	-50	480	N/A	H
	4	-50	30	50	H
Primary drying	1	-30	60	50	R
	2	-30	2160	50	H
Secondary drying	1	25	200	50	R
	2	25	600	50	H
Post-run	1	10	Until manual shutoff	50	H

17. Turn on the freeze dryer and vacuum pump.
18. Turn on the nitrogen gas, allowing 1 psi into the inert gas backfill inlet and 40–60 psi into the stoppering air inlet.
19. In the lyophilization control software, program the cycle in Table 1 (*see* **Notes 12** and **13**):
20. Start the run.
21. Upon completion of the cycle, the freeze dryer will maintain the post-run conditions until the user manually stops the run. Stop the run.
22. Wait for the chamber to come to atmospheric pressure (760 Torr). In this time, vials are being backfilled with nitrogen gas.
23. Stopper vials by activating the stoppering lever on the freeze dryer. This triggers the pneumatic stoppering platen to drop, fully inserting the stoppers into the vials. Return the stoppering lever to its original position to lift the platen.
24. Open the chamber door and remove lyophilized samples. To remove the samples, hold the tray bottom against the edge of the lyophilizer shelf. Slowly and carefully pull out the rack and allow the samples to transfer onto the tray bottom one row at a time, until the full tray assembly is in one piece (all vials should be on the tray bottom in the tray assembly).
25. Turn off the nitrogen supply.
26. Review temperatures and pressures achieved in the cycle as collected by the product temperature probes (*see* Fig. 4).
27. Crimp the vials using aluminum seals to secure the stoppers.

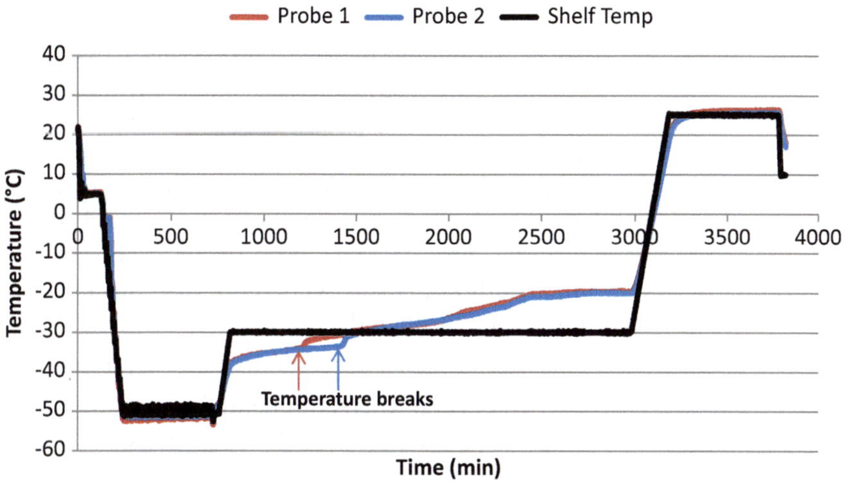

Fig. 4 An example of a product temperature probe plot. The shelf temperature is shown in *black*. Two product temperature probes were placed in two separate vials containing 2 % GLA-SE and either 5 % sucrose or 5 % trehalose, shown in *red* and *blue*. The temperature of the samples closely follows the shelf temperature during the freezing step at −50 °C, but diverge at the start of primary drying. Samples remain cooler than the shelf until the inflection point (temperature break) when samples rise above the shelf temperature. The temperature break is the point at which the sublimation front reaches and surpasses the location in the vial where the temperature probe is placed (ideally in the bottom center of the vial). A cycle should be designed so that the sample temperatures remain below critical temperatures until after the temperature break when sublimation is complete. Shelf and sample temperatures are then increased during secondary drying. At the completion of the cycle, samples are held at 10 °C

4 Notes

1. Cycle shelf temperatures are set so that sample temperatures, as measured by the product temperature probes, remain approximately 3 °C below critical temperatures during the sublimation phase of primary drying. Critical temperatures are determined by thermal analysis of samples that contain excipients of interest such as 5–10 % (w/v) sucrose or trehalose (*see* **Note 3**). It is beneficial to understand the thermal capabilities of the specific lyophilizer in use. Set shelf temperatures can be different from the actual temperature experienced by the sample since heat transfer between the shelf and sample is imperfect and temperatures of the chamber can be raised by external factors such as heat radiation through an acrylic glass chamber door. Additionally, depending on the construction of the shelf, it is common to have warm and cool spots (e.g., the corners) where temperatures deviate from the rest of the shelf. Temperature mapping can be performed [8] to locate these areas and to help assess the calibration of the unit. This information can be referred to when setting shelf temperatures and determining sample vial placement to maintain the target sample temperatures.

2. Excipient selection: Excipients provide the active ingredient with a surrounding matrix to protect its active properties and to produce a visually satisfactory final product. A good place to begin is to use excipients that have been used successfully in approved lyophilized products [6] and are reported in the literature. Excipients can be combined to synergistically provide the active ingredient protection during and after the harsh freeze-dry process. The purpose of each can be generally binned, although many serve more than one purpose. Some of these excipients include:
   - Disaccharide lyoprotectants: Sucrose, trehalose, lactose

     In general, we recommend formulating below 10 % solids so as not to impede mass transfer of water during sublimation.
   - Bulking agents: Mannitol

     The inclusion of mannitol generally yields a more pharmaceutically elegant cake. Crystallization of mannitol can be controlled by adding an annealing step during the freezing phase of lyophilization (*see* **Note 3**).
   - Buffers: Tris, sodium phosphate, amino acids (glycine, histidine)

     Sodium phosphate is known to drop in pH (as low as pH 4) upon freezing due to salt precipitation. This loss of buffering capacity may or may not be harmful to the active ingredient. These pH shifts can be minimized when formulating with less concentrated sodium phosphate [9].
   - Surfactants/Detergents: Tween 80, Poloxamer 188
   - Other: Chelators (EDTA), isotonicity agents (sodium chloride, glycerol), antioxidants (ascorbic acid)

     Minor collapse of cakes in our samples was evident with the inclusion of glycerol at <0.5 %.
3. Cycle should be optimized for formulation.
   - Freeze: The shelf temperature is first equilibrated at 5 °C to evenly cool all samples. Samples are then frozen at −50 °C. The freezing rate of the sample determines the size of the ice crystals formed and the porosity of the matrix. Generally, a slow freezing rate induces large crystal growth while a fast freezing rate induces small crystal growth. Large ice crystal growth has more potential to disrupt protein complexes but create larger channels for sublimation, thereby yielding faster drying. The freeze step causes freeze concentration of solutes which can be detrimental to formulations. It may be of interest to add an annealing step after freezing, when working with crystalline excipients such as mannitol. This forces a controlled crystallization of mannitol and can increase ice crystal size

by Oswald Ripening. To anneal, after freezing the samples, samples are then warmed to and held at a temperature above the glass transition temperature (T_g') and then returned to the original freezing temperature. The annealing temperature is the temperature at which crystallization occurs and can be determined using differential scanning calorimetry (DSC) [10, 11]. For example, for a mannitol containing sample which has a crystallization temperature of −15 °C, samples are frozen at −50 °C for 8 h, then warmed to −12 °C for 2 h, and then returned back to −50 °C for 2 h prior to continuing on to primary drying.

- Primary Drying: The condenser is activated, the pressure is reduced, and the temperature is increased. The condenser maintains a temperature of −80 °C throughout the rest of the lyophilization cycle and acts to condense the water vapor being sublimated off the sample. Pressure is reduced to 50 mTorr and the sample shelf is brought to −30 °C. The shelf temperature should be set so that samples remain below critical temperatures during this phase. Critical temperatures T_g' and collapse temperature can be determined by DSC and freeze dry microscopy (FDM) respectively. While remaining below critical temperatures, the warmer the shelf temperature (increased heat transfer), the faster sublimation can occur. This is due to achieving a greater pressure differential between the vapor pressure of ice at the sublimation front and the partial pressure of water vapor in the chamber. Refer to a vapor pressure of ice chart. The primary drying phase will be the longest phase in the cycle and should last at least until sublimation is complete. This time can be estimated using product temperature probes.
- Secondary Drying: The shelf temperatures are increased to 25 °C to facilitate desorption of bound water. The final moisture level achieved is dependent upon target shelf temperature and time. Care must be taken not to exceed glass transition of the dried layer during warming or sample may collapse.

4. As a general guideline, fill volume should not exceed ½ of the maximum vial volume. An appropriate vial should be selected to maximize sample-air interface to facilitate sublimation while still allowing for good cake formation. For example, a 1 mL fill in a 50 mL vial gives high sample-air interface but would result in a dried film instead of a cake.
5. Consider the pretreatment of stoppers since they have direct contact with the inside of sample vials. Autoclave sterilization can introduce moisture into the stopper matrix, which if not sufficiently dried, can slowly leach into the sample vial. Autoclaving can be followed with an additional drying step by

placing stoppers in a 50 °C oven for 4–8 h. Stoppers are also available with coatings that reduce the risk of interaction between the sample and the stopper (e.g., FluroTec® coating from West Pharmaceutical Services).

6. If conservation of sample is desired, the vials containing the temperature product probes may be filled with mock sample to estimate the product temperature profile. This mock sample may be made to contain excipients only. For example, to conserve protein, a mock sample of a formulation containing protein, adjuvant, and 5 % (w/v) sucrose in buffer may contain 5 % (w/v) sucrose in buffer or 5 % (w/v) sucrose and adjuvant in buffer. The mock sample is a good substitute only if the component removed is at very low concentrations. Removing components at high concentrations would likely change the temperature profile of the sample.
7. The top of the guide tubes should line up flush with the top of the stopper. The purpose of the guide tube is to allow a path for the temperature probe into the sample vial. Alternatively, a more ideal set up would be to use the actual stoppers used for the samples, placed in the same half-stoppered position. The stopper can be pierced and a hole can be made to allow for the temperature probe to enter the sample vial.
8. By fully packing the tray, vials are physically held in place. Avoid placing actual samples around the perimeter of the tray (*see* **Note 9**). This means the total number of samples will be less than the maximum number of vials that can fit in the tray.
9. The vials around the perimeter of the tray provide the outer ring of samples with neighboring vials that contain solution. This allows all samples to experience a more uniform heat transfer and vapor pressure environment, minimizing differences seen by samples in the center versus samples in the outermost ring of the cluster. These vials can be half stoppered to mimic actual samples. This is important particularly for small scale lyophilizers which have higher heat radiation effects than pilot or commercial scale units.
10. The fill volume should be matched with the fill volume used for samples. The excipient solution should be matched with the excipients used in formulation to mimic the freeze-drying profile of samples.
11. Aluminum foil is used to cover up an acrylic chamber door to minimize heat radiation from sunlight or light sources in the laboratory.
12. If using the Wizard 2.0 lyophilization control software (synwiz.exe), open the Recipe Manager and program the cycle as follows in Tables 2, 3, 4, 5, and 6. The terminology of each phase is specific to this software. The thermal treatment fields include steps for the starting temperature and freezing steps,

Table 2
Thermal treatment

	Temp (°C)	Time (min)	Ramp/Hold
Step 1	5	120	H
Step 2	-50	120	R
Step 3	-50	480	H

Table 3
Freeze, condenser, vacuum phases

Freeze (°C)	-50
Extra freeze (min)	0
Condenser (°C)	-40*
Vacuum (mTorr)	500

*The -40 °C set point is the condenser temperature that will start the vacuum phase. The condenser is either on or off and automatically cools to -80 °C.

Table 4
Primary drying

	Temp (°C)	Time (min)	Vacuum (mTorr)	Ramp/Hold
Step 1	-50	30	50	H
Step 2	-30	60	50	R
Step 3	-30	1000	50	H
Step 4	-30	1160	50	H
Step 5	25	200	50	R
Step 6	25	600	50	H

Table 5
Post heat

Temp (°C)	Time (min)	Vacuum (mTorr)
10	30	50

Table 6
Secondary set point

Temp (°C)
35**

**The secondary set point is an emergency temperature threshold. If the temperature exceeds this set point, the lyophilizer will automatically enter safe mode.

and the primary drying fields include steps for both primary and secondary drying.

From the Recipe Manager, write the recipe to the Wizard by selecting "Write to Wizard F7" under the recipe tab.

13. All temperatures listed in this protocol are shelf target temperatures. Product temperatures typically do not match shelf temperature and are dependent on many factors including heat radiation, shelf calibration and accuracy, and hold time at each temperature. Product temperature probes can be used in sample vials to estimate the temperatures that samples experience.

Acknowledgements

This project has been funded with Federal funds from the National Institute of Allergy and Infectious Diseases, National Institutes of Health, Department of Health and Human Services, under Contract No. HHSN272201400041C. We thank Edward H. Trappler of Lyophilization Technologies, Inc for advice while developing this method.

References

1. Brandau DT, Jones LS, Wiethoff CM, Rexroad J, Middaugh CR (2003) Thermal stability of vaccines. J Pharm Sci 92(2):218–231
2. Summary of stability data for licensed vaccines. Working in Tandem, Ltd., PATH Vaccine and Pharmaceutical Technologies Group. https://www.path.org/publications/files/TS_vaccine_stability_table.pdf. Accessed 18 July 2016
3. Adams GJ (2003) Lyophilization of vaccines. In: Robinson A, Hudson M, Cranage M (eds) Vaccine protocols. Humana, New York, pp 223–243
4. Orr MT, Kramer RM, Barnes VL, Dowling QM, Desbien AL, Beebe EA, Laurance JD, Fox CB, Reed SG, Coler RN, Vedvick TS (2014) Elimination of the cold-chain dependence of a nanoemulsion adjuvanted vaccine against tuberculosis by lyophilization. J Control Release 177:20–26
5. Costantino HR, Pikal MJ (2004) Lyophilization of biopharmaceuticals. AAPS Press, Arlington, VA
6. Schwegman JJ, Hardwick LM, Akers MJ (2005) Practical formulation and process development of freeze-dried products. Pharm Dev Technol 10(2):151–173
7. Kennedy J, Turan N (2000) Freeze-drying/lyophilization of pharmaceutical and biological products. Bioseparation 9(2):118–118, Louis Rey and Joan C May (editors)
8. Dutill T, Sunderland W (2014) Methods for measuring shelf temperature uniformity in a lyophilizer. Lyophilization Technology Inc.
9. Gomez G, Pikal MJ, Rodriguez-Hornedo N (2001) Effect of initial buffer composition on pH changes during far-from-equilibrium freezing of sodium phosphate buffer solutions. Pharm Res 18(1):90–97
10. taPrime Consulting. The Use of Mannitol. http://www.ta-prime.co.uk/assets/file/Mannitol.pdf. Accessed 22 Oct 2015
11. Searles JA, Carpenter JF, Randolph TW (2001) Annealing to optimize the primary drying rate, reduce freezing-induced drying rate heterogeneity, and determine T(g)′ in pharmaceutical lyophilization. J Pharm Sci 90(7):872–887

Chapter 16

Stressed Stability Techniques for Adjuvant Formulations

Manvi Hasija, Anthony Sheung, Nausheen Rahman, and Salvador F. Ausar

Abstract

Stressed stability testing is crucial to the understanding of mechanisms of degradation and the effects of external stress factors on adjuvant stability. These studies vastly help the development of stability indicating tests and the selection of stabilizing conditions for long term storage. In this chapter, we provide detailed protocols for the execution of forced degradation experiments that evaluate the robustness of adjuvant formulations against thermal, mechanical, freeze-thawing, and photo stresses.

Key words Forced degradation, Thermostability, Mechanical stress, Freeze-thawing, Photostability

1 Introduction

Adjuvants are key components of modern vaccines that are formulated with antigens to enhance and promote adequate antigen-specific immune responses. They comprise a variety of molecules ranging from simple mineral salts, to more complex chemical entities or biological macromolecules. Adjuvants can be divided into three groups: (1) immunopotentiators; (2) delivery systems; and (3) combination systems [1]. Immunopotentiators are generally specific components of whole pathogens that elicit their effects by direct activation of immune cells to increase the immune response. Delivery systems, such as emulsions, aluminum salts, liposomes and other particulates, largely work by promoting the uptake of co-administered antigens into the immune cells and may also have immunostimulatory effects on their own. Combination systems comprise the majority of adjuvant formulations; in this group a delivery system such as an aluminum salt is used as a carrier for both the immunopotentiator and the antigen of interest [2].

During the formulation development of adjuvants, there are a number of critical attributes that should be controlled to ensure quality, consistency, and effectiveness of the formulation [1, 3], as antigens and adjuvants are exposed to a variety of stress conditions

Christopher B. Fox (ed.), *Vaccine Adjuvants: Methods and Protocols*, Methods in Molecular Biology, vol. 1494,
DOI 10.1007/978-1-4939-6445-1_16, © Springer Science+Business Media New York 2017

that may induce losses in vaccine effectiveness. Many physicochemical characteristics of the adjuvant, such as particle size, surface charge, chemical integrity, and crystallinity, can be affected by external factors which may significantly impact the antigen–adjuvant interaction and affect the vaccine's immunogenicity [4, 5]. One of the main objectives of the formulation development of adjuvants is to develop a formulation that can withstand external stress factors during manufacturing stages and storage. Conducting stability stress testing on adjuvant formulations is essential in early stage development as it provides preliminary information on degradation pathways of adjuvant components, aid in the identification of stabilizing conditions, and supports the development of stability indicating assays and analytical tools [3, 4].

One of the most common stress conditions used in forced degradation studies in the industry is thermal stress. In such studies, the formulation is exposed to extreme temperatures to assess changes in the physicochemical properties of the adjuvant, and to investigate potential stabilizing conditions. Thermal stress can be conducted alone or in conjunction with other types of stresses such as extreme pH and oxidizing conditions. Thermal stress experiments provide insight into the degradation kinetics of the adjuvant. A key parameter of kinetic studies is the rate constant, which provides a measure of the rate of degradation under a given set of conditions. This information, with the use of modeling software, can be analyzed to predict the behavior of the physiochemical properties of the adjuvant when the vaccine is exposed to adverse conditions during manufacturing, storage, distribution, and administration [6]. Appropriate temperature conditions for testing should be selected on a case-by-case basis. For example, mineral salts such as aluminum are relatively resistant to thermal degradation and would require higher temperature stress conditions than emulsion, peptide or liposome containing adjuvants to manifest detectable changes.

Mechanical stress testing is another key component of forced degradation studies, as this type of stress can result in undesirable damage in adjuvants, particularly for shear sensitive formulations. Experimental design and setup of mechanical stress experiments can include agitation, stirring, and pumping, depending on the stage of development and the condition being studied. A typical mechanical stress study used in early stage development of adjuvants involves shaking samples at 250–350 rpm on a laboratory shaker for several hours at room temperature. This simple and rapid test can unveil potential physical instability issues of the adjuvant and help in the selection of appropriate stabilizing conditions [4].

Freeze–thaw testing is useful to assess the robustness and stability of the adjuvant against intended or accidental freezing, and to identify excipients that stabilize the adjuvant during freezing or frozen storage. Freezing and thawing of vaccines containing aluminum adjuvants is well known to induce gross aggregation and precipitation, leading to losses in vaccine potency [7]. For other adjuvants, it has been observed that freeze-thawing may significantly affect colloidal stability, particularly in emulsion and liposome containing formulations [8, 9].

Photo-induced damage of the adjuvant can occur at different points of a vaccine's life cycle, from production to delivery. The evaluation of photodegradation is of particular importance for those molecules known to be sensitive to photochemical reactions, which usually lead to oxidation and hydrolysis [10]. Regulatory agencies have acknowledged the importance of photo-stress testing, and as such, drafted a detailed International Conference on Harmonization (ICH Q1B) guideline [11]. The guideline recommend that photostability testing is to be performed using either a light source that is designed to produce an output similar to artificial daylight (i.e., a fluorescent lamp combining visible and ultraviolet (UV) light), or with both cool white light and UVA light. Samples should be exposed to a minimum of 1.2 million lux hours and 200 W·h/m^2 of light, as per ICH Q1B requirements. However, to fully characterize the adjuvant robustness against photodegradation, it is important to conduct photo-testing beyond the recommended ICH Q1B exposure conditions [4].

In this chapter, we provide detailed protocols for the examination of stress stability testing of adjuvant formulations with respect to temperature, mechanical, freeze-thawing, and photo stresses. Representative results obtained during stress stability testing of adjuvants are illustrated with appropriate examples.

2 Materials

1. Adjuvant candidate.
2. Sterile glass vials with rubber stoppers and aluminum caps—West Pharmaceuticals (Exton, USA), or equivalent.
3. Laboratory incubators capable of sustaining stable temperatures up to 70 °C (*see* **Note 1**).
4. Stability and kinetics analysis software—AKTS software version 4.05 (Siders, Switzerland), or equivalent.
5. RP-HPLC System—Agilent 1100 series (Santa Clara, USA) or equivalent.
6. Orbital shaker with built-in adjustable clamps capable of speeds up to 500 rpm—VWR standard 5000 orbital shaker (Radnor, USA), or equivalent.
7. Particle size analyzer—Malvern Mastersizer 2000 with 2000S accessory (Malvern, UK), or equivalent.
8. Laboratory freezer capable of maintaining temperatures as low as −80 °C (*see* **Note 1**).

9. Photostability Chamber—Caron 6540 Series (Caron, Marietta, OH), or equivalent.
10. Aluminum foil.

3 Methods

3.1 Thermal Stress

Thermal incubation is commonly executed to elucidate the degradation kinetics of biological products. Similarly, adjuvant stability can be assessed by subjection to selected stress temperatures for determined periods of time and evaluated by stability indicating tests. The method below describes a forced degradation experiment by thermal stress for an adjuvant.

1. Aliquot the candidate adjuvant into clear glass vials, then stopper and cap the vials. Fill volumes should be consistent for all test groups.
2. Label all vials clearly, stating the incubation temperature and incubation duration.
3. Place vials in appropriate incubators.
4. Incubate test samples at the temperatures of 4, 37, 45, 55 or 65 °C for up to 12 weeks (*see* **Note 2**).
5. Collect sample vials at the end of the incubation periods following the experimental outline.
6. Store the pulled vials at 4 °C or −80 °C (*see* **Note 3**) until ready for further testing.
7. In the example of Fig. 1, an RP-HPLC method was used as a stability indicating assay to investigate TLR9 degradation imparted by thermal and pH stresses (*see* **Notes 4** and **5**). A short term pH screening study under stress temperature of 55 °C suggested improved stability under neutral and slightly acidic pH when compared to alkaline conditions (Fig. 1a). A long term accelerated stability study was then performed to compare the stability of the product formulated at pH 6.5 and pH 7.5 (Fig. 1b, c). The results were analyzed using AKTS software version 4.05 [6] (an advanced kinetic modeling software, *see* **Note 6**) to obtain a complex two step (no autocatalysis) kinetic model with a combination of first and second order kinetics, which predicted a shelf life of greater than 5 years for both pH conditions.

3.2 Mechanical Stress

Adjuvants can be susceptible to various mechanical stresses during any stage of the product life cycle. To assess whether these mechanical and shear stresses affect adjuvant stability, horizontal/vertical shakers, stirring reactors and pumps are commonly utilized as stress testing methods. The method below describes a forced degradation experiment by mechanical stress for an adjuvant using a horizontal shaker.

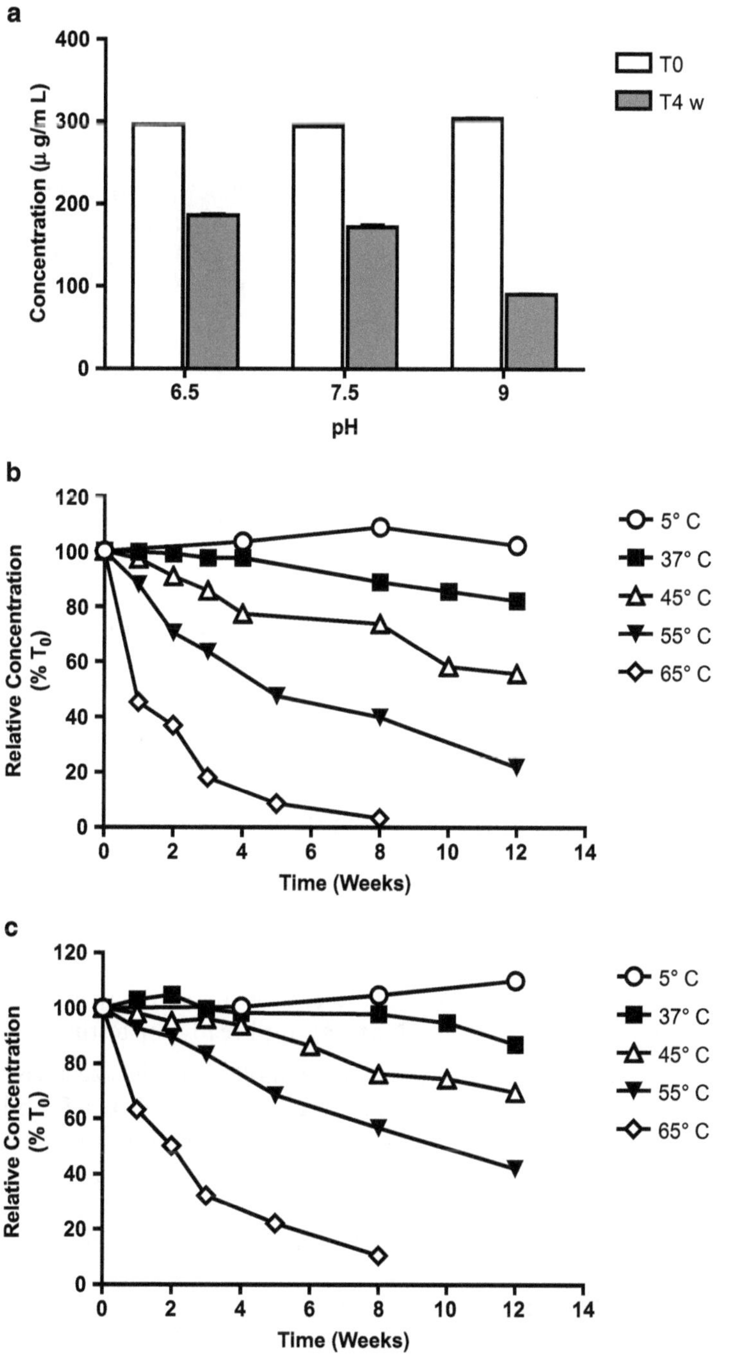

Fig. 1 Effect of temperature and pH on the stability of a TLR9-containing adjuvant. (**a**) Short term pH screening under stress temperature 55 °C. The results for a long term accelerated stability study for pH 7.5 and pH 6.5 are shown in (**b**) and (**c**) respectively

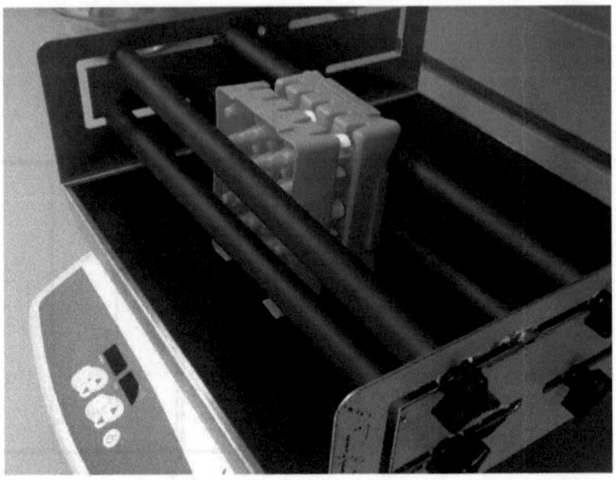

Fig. 2 Example of glass vials placed between vial racks secured with built-in clamps on an orbital shaker

1. Aliquot the candidate adjuvant into clear glass vials, then stopper and cap the vials. Fill volumes should be consistent for all test groups.
2. Label all vials clearly, stating the agitation duration. Set aside control vials (non-agitated) at room temperature (same temperature conditions as the shaker).
3. Secure vials tightly in vial racks and place on the orbital shaker in a horizontal position (*see* Fig. 2).
4. Set shaker speed at 250 rpm and start agitation for up to 96 h (*see* **Note 7**).
5. Collect samples from the shaker according to the designated agitation durations. Place vials under quiescent condition until the last time point is completed.
6. At the end of the study, store all vials at 4 °C or −80 °C (*see* **Note 3**) until ready for testing.
7. In this example, particle size assessment was used as a stability indicating assay (*see* **Notes 5** and **8**) to determine changes imparted by mechanical stress (*see* Fig. 3). An exponential decrease in particle size was observed after 96 h of continuous agitation. This result can be explained by the disruption of adjuvant particles due to mechanical stress.

3.3 Freeze-Thawing

Frozen storage is commonly used as a method of preserving biological products; however the formation of an ice-water interface, in addition to low temperatures, can lead to destabilization of the product. Temperature excursions while in storage and distribution can also occur for products that are stored using refrigeration only, potentially leading to freeze–thaw cycles. To examine whether a candidate adjuvant can withstand frozen storage, freeze–thaw studies are highly recommended. The method below describes a forced degradation experiment by repeated freeze-thawing for an adjuvant.

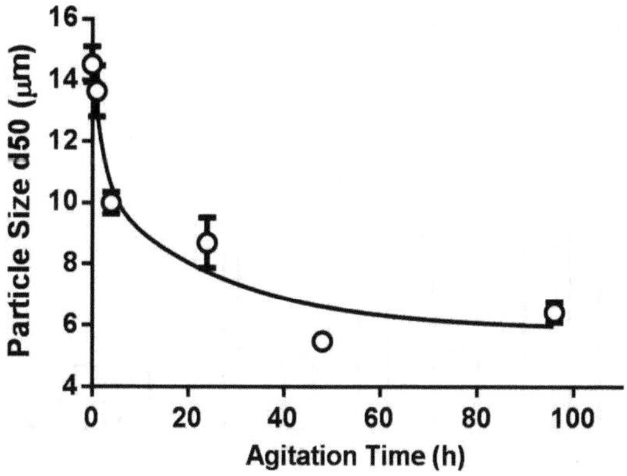

Fig. 3 Effect of agitation stress on particle size of a TLR9-containing adjuvant formulation measured by laser diffraction

1. Aliquot the candidate adjuvant into clear glass vials, then stopper and cap the vials. Fill volumes should be consistent for all test groups.
2. Label all groups and indicate the target number of freeze–thaw cycles to be performed.
3. Place non-frozen control samples at 4 °C.
4. Place test samples in the −80 °C freezer for up to 24 h to ensure samples are adequately frozen (*see* **Note 9**).
5. Thaw all test samples at room temperature (*see* **Note 10**).
6. Repeat **steps 4** and **5** for up to six cycles (*see* **Note 11**).
7. Store samples that have completed the target amount of freeze–thaw cycles at 4 °C or −80 °C until ready for further testing (*see* **Notes 3** and **12**).
8. In the example depicted in Fig. 4, the candidate adjuvant formulation was subjected to six freeze–thaw cycles and characterized by particle size measurements (*see* **Notes 5** and **8**) on cycle 0, 3, and 6 in the presence of potential cryoprotectants and compared to the control formulation. In this example, the particle size assessment showed a significant increase on cycle 3 and 6 for the control formulation, suggesting high sensitivity to freeze–thaw induced aggregation. Formulation 3 and 4 were found to inhibit the freeze–thaw induced aggregation (*see* **Note 8**).

3.4 Photodegradation

To determine whether an adjuvant is photosensitive and to elucidate degradation pathways, light exposure experiments using a photostability chamber with both visible and UVA radiation, is recommended by the ICH Q1B Guideline. The method below

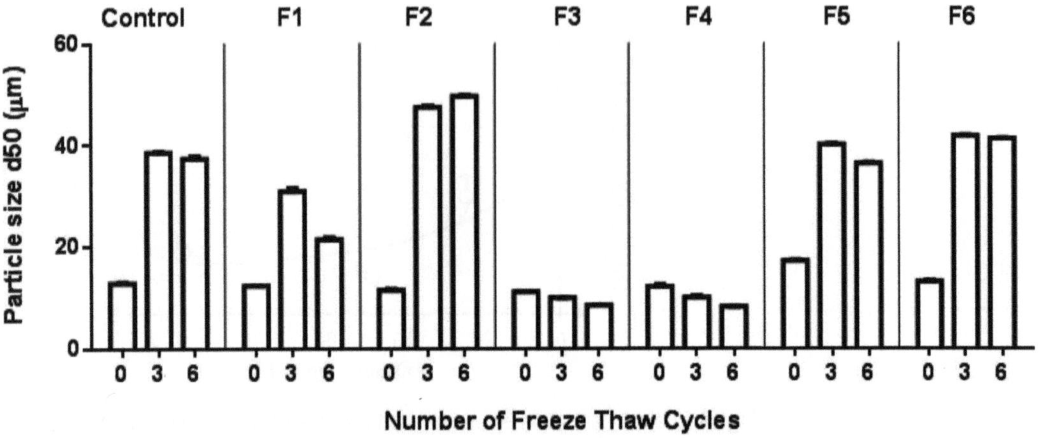

Fig. 4 Freeze-thawing stress on particle size of a TLR9-containing adjuvant formulation. Adjuvant control sample and adjuvant in the presence of potential cryoprotectants (*F1–F6*) were subjected to six freeze–thaw cycles and the particle size was measured by laser diffraction at T_0 and cycles 3 and 6

describes a forced degradation experiment by photo-exposure for an adjuvant.

1. Aliquot candidate adjuvant into clear glass vials, then stopper and cap the vials. Fill volumes should be consistent for all test groups.
2. In this example, vials will be exposed at 0% (non-exposed control), 50%, 100%, or 200% of the ICH Q1B recommended conditions (*see* **Note 13**). For non-exposed control vials, vials are wrapped in aluminum foil to block light.
3. To distinguish between test groups, glass vials should be labeled with a water and alcohol resistant marker on the aluminum caps only. Avoid labeling with a sticker or marker on the glass vials which may block light.
4. Turn on the photostability chamber and allow the chamber to acclimatize to the set temperature. A temperature of 25 °C was used in this example (*see* **Note 14**).
5. Place all sample vials horizontally on a flat, stable tray (*see* Fig. 5). If UVA exposure is performed first, place tray in the center of the UVA chamber to maximize exposure (*see* **Note 15**).
6. Set exposure to 100 W·h/m^2 (50% ICH Q1B guideline for UVA) (*see* **Note 13**) and start exposure.
7. When UVA exposure is complete, transfer all vials to the center of VIS exposure chamber.
8. Set exposure to 600k lux (50% ICH guideline for VIS) (*see* **Note 13**) and start exposure.
9. When VIS exposure is complete, wrap sample vials designated for 50% ICH Q1B exposure (now completed) in aluminum foil.
10. Repeat **steps 5–9** for groups designated for higher exposures.

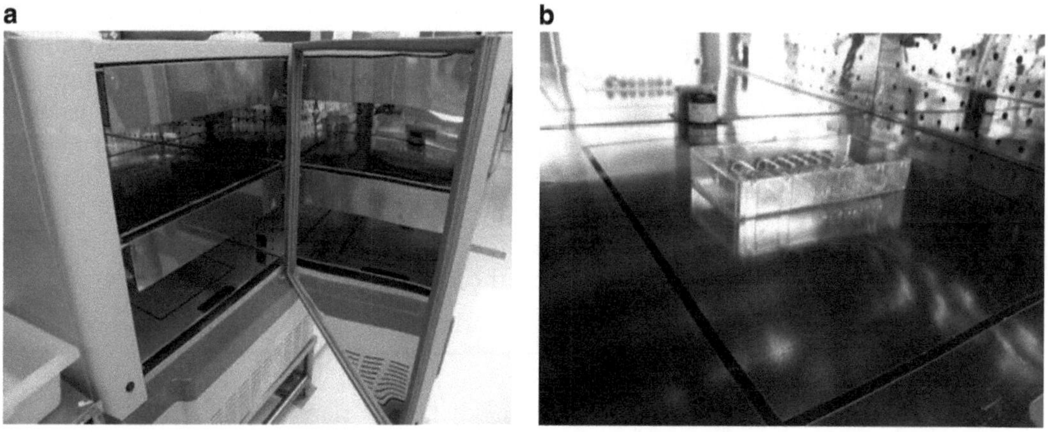

Fig. 5 (**a**) An example of a photostability unit; (**b**) example of glass vials placed in the center of a photo-exposure chamber

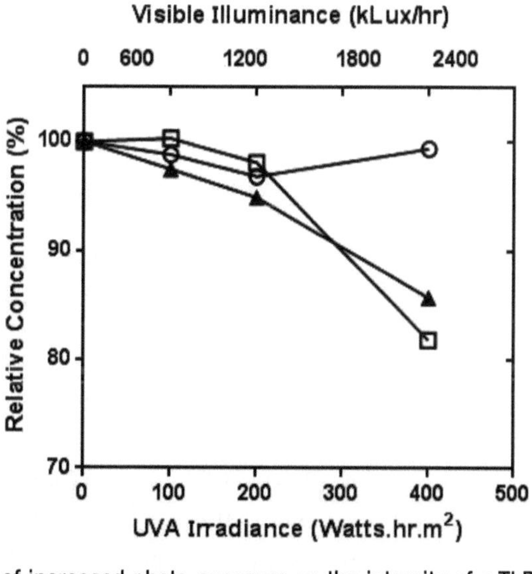

Fig. 6 Effect of increased photo-exposure on the integrity of a TLR9-containing adjuvant as measured by RP-HPLC. The potential protective effects of nitrogen blanketing (*filled triangle*) and secondary packaging (*open circle*) compared to the control (*open square*) are illustrated

11. To avoid imparting any differences due to temperature variation, sample vials (including the non-exposed control) which have completed their designated exposure setting should remain in the photostability chamber with other test groups until the completion of all photo-exposure runs (*see* **Note 16**).
12. Store the pulled vials at 4 °C or −80 °C (*see* **Note 3**) until ready for further testing.
13. In this example, RP-HPLC was used as a stability indicating assay to determine changes imparted by photo-exposure (*see*

Notes 4 and **5**). Figure 6 shows a TLR9-Containing adjuvant exposed to increasing irradiance (UV and VIS), and the effects of nitrogen blanketing or secondary packaging on photodegradation. As studied by RP-HPLC, the concentration of intact adjuvant decreased by nearly 20% after maximum photo-exposure. The secondary packaging, but not nitrogen blanketing, was shown to fully protect the TLR9 against photo-exposure for up to two times the irradiance recommended by the ICH Q1B guideline.

4 Notes

1. It is recommended that all temperature regulated units (incubators or freezers) are connected to a monitored Building Automation System (BAS) to detect temperature excursion events.
2. There are two types of stress temperature experiments:
   (a) Short term experiment—Screening experiments in which one stress temperature is used to compare changes with a control sample to identify top formulation candidates.
   (b) Long term experiment—Temperature conditions and time points selected based on prediction software recommendations.
3. The stable storage temperature for the candidate adjuvant tested is dependent on the properties of each specific adjuvant. Generally, temperatures of 4 °C or −80 °C are used. If freezing temperatures are used, preliminary studies are recommended to assess the product's sensitivity to freeze–thaw cycles.
4. RP-HPLC was performed using the Agilent Model 8453 HPLC unit (Agilent Technologies, Santa Clara, USA).
5. Examples of potential stability indicating assays that could be used to assess the effects of stress conditions on candidate adjuvants are listed in Table 1. Alternative assay methods may also be used and should be product-dependent.
6. Typical approaches to analyze data and predict long term stability from accelerated stability studies is based on a simple kinetic model (zero- or first-order kinetic models) to obtain the rate constant for two or more temperatures. However, stability predictions based on the above are very often too simplified for biological products, which frequently undergo complex and multistep degradation pathways. More sophisticated degradation kinetic models may be useful to describe degradation of biological products. Using AKTS (AKTS software version 4.05) ex situ data analysis, a more complicated approach in which a one-step, two-step kinetic model, including an *n*th order and an autocatalytic component can be identified.

Table 1
A list of potential stability indicating assay methods used for characterization of adjuvant formulations and application examples

Method	Principle	Application example
Chromatography (liquid or gas)	Separation, identification, and quantification of components in a mixture	TLR agonists; peptides; lipids (i.e., squalene)
X-Ray diffraction	Crystallite characterization by reflection of X-ray diffraction pattern analysis	Aluminum based adjuvants
Dynamic light scattering	Size distribution profiling of small particle suspension by light scattering	Liposome based adjuvants; Emulsions
Laser diffraction	The size of particles is measured by the intensity of light scattered as a laser beam passes through a dispersed particulate sample. The scattering pattern is analyzed to calculate the size of the particles in a sample	Aluminum based adjuvants, aluminum salts–TLR agonist combinations
Zeta potential	Electrophoretic mobility determination for estimation of colloidal stability	Aluminum based adjuvants, Aluminum salts-TLR agonist combinations, Liposome based adjuvants, Emulsions

7. 250 rpm was used in this example but higher or lower speeds may be used depending on the product.
8. Particle size measurement was performed by laser diffraction using the Mastersizer 2000 instrument fitted with the 2000S accessory (Malvern Instruments, UK). Other methods for particle characterization are described in Table 1.
9. In this protocol, a conventional freezer is used whereby the product is placed until frozen. Freezing by using a controlled-rate freezer or flash-freezing by liquid nitrogen may also be used.
10. Thawing was performed by leaving the frozen adjuvant on a benchtop at room temperature. Different methods of thawing may also be used, such as placing the product in an incubator at 25 °C or thawing with a temperature controlled water-bath.
11. A range of 3–6 cycles of freeze-thawing is generally recommended.
12. If testing cannot be completed immediately and the candidate adjuvant requires freezing temperatures as a storage temperature, thawing for testing is considered one extra freeze–thaw cycle.
13. The ICH Q1B photostability guideline recommends that confirmatory studies are to be illuminated with not less than 1.2 million lux hours of visible light (400 800 nm) and an integrated near ultraviolet energy (320–400 nm) of not less than

200 W·h/m^2—this is denoted as the "100% ICH" condition. In experiments where underexposure or overexposure are compared to the recommended exposure limit in ICH Q1B, the "50% ICH" condition consists of 600,000 lx hours of visible light and 100 W·h/m^2 of near UV; and the "200% ICH" condition consists of 2.4 million lux hours of visible light and 400 W·h/m^2 of near UV.

14. If the adjuvant being tested is temperature sensitive, photoexposure can alternatively be conducted at 4 °C provided that the photostability chamber supports cooling functionality.
15. UVA exposure requires a shorter duration. It is recommended to perform UVA exposure first to minimize waiting time and proceed to VIS exposure to be performed overnight.
16. If the candidate adjuvant is temperature sensitive, each photoexposure condition tested can be accompanied by its own foil-wrapped non-exposed control, with both groups pulled and stored at a stabilizing temperature prior to testing.

References

1. Reed SG, Orr MT, Fox CB (2013) Key roles of adjuvants in modern vaccines. Nat Med 19(12):1597–1608
2. Fox CB, Kramer RM, Barnes VL, Dowling QM, Vedvick TS (2013) Working together: interactions between vaccine antigens and adjuvants. Ther Adv Vaccines 1(1):7–20
3. Dey AK, Malyala P, Singh M (2014) Physicochemical and functional characterization of vaccine antigens and adjuvants. Expert Rev Vaccines 13(5):671–685
4. Hasija M, Li L, Rahman N, Ausar SF (2013) Forced degradation studies: an essential tool for the formulation development of vaccines. Vaccine (Auckl) 3:11–33
5. Hem SL, HogenEsch H, Middaugh CR, Volkin DB (2010) Preformulation studies—The next advance in aluminum adjuvant-containing vaccines. Vaccine 28(31):4868–4870
6. Clénet D, Imbert F, Probeck P, Rahman N, Ausar SF (2014) Advanced kinetic analysis as a tool for formulation development and prediction of vaccine stability. J Pharm Sci 103(10):3055–3064
7. Gupta RK (1998) Aluminum compounds as vaccine adjuvants. Adv Drug Deliv Rev 32(3):155–172
8. Ghosh S, Coupland JN (2008) Factors affecting the freeze–thaw stability of emulsions. Food Hydrocoll 22(1):105–111
9. Crommelin DJA, van Bommel EMG (1984) Stability of liposomes on storage: freeze dried, frozen or as an aqueous dispersion. Pharm Res 1(4):159–163
10. Kerwin BA, Remmele RL Jr (2007) Protect from light: photodegradation and protein biologics. J Pharm Sci 96(6):1468–1479
11. ICH Q1B (1997) Guidelines for photostability testing of new drug substances and products. Fed Regis 62: 27115–27122

Chapter 17

Particle Sizing of Nanoparticle Adjuvant Formulations by Dynamic Light Scattering (DLS) and Nanoparticle Tracking Analysis (NTA)

Michelle Y. Chan, Quinton M. Dowling, Sandra J. Sivananthan, and Ryan M. Kramer

Abstract

Dynamic light scattering (DLS) and nanoparticle tracking analysis (NTA) are two orthogonal and complementary methods of measuring size of particles in a sample. These technologies use the theory of Brownian motion by analyzing the random changes of light intensity scattered by particles in solution. Both techniques can be used to characterize particle size distribution of proteins and formulations in the nanometer to low micron range.

Each method has benefits over the other. DLS is a quick and simple measurement that is ideal for monodisperse particles and can also analyze a distribution of particles over a wide range of sizes. NTA provides a size distribution that is less susceptible to the influence of a few large particles, and has the added benefit of being able to measure particle concentration. Here we describe methods for measuring the particle size and concentration of an oil-in-water nanoemulsion.

Key words Particle size, Dynamic light scattering, DLS, Nanoparticle tracking analysis, NTA

1 Introduction

Particle size is an important characteristic of a sample. In the fields of vaccines and therapeutics where the use of adjuvants or delivery vehicles such as nanoemulsions and liposomes are utilized, particle size is one of many physicochemical characteristics that can be used to design and engineer effective drug products. It has been shown that particle size can affect organ (such as draining lymph nodes) or tumor targeting and can impact intracellular uptake of the antigen or drug [1]. Manufacturing particles smaller than 200 nm is necessary for sterilization by 0.2-μm filtration. Particle size measurements can also be used to determine protein size distributions and aggregate formation, characterize and monitor the stability of a formulation, and provide a measure of quality control in a manufacturing process [2–5].

Christopher B. Fox (ed.), *Vaccine Adjuvants: Methods and Protocols*, Methods in Molecular Biology, vol. 1494, DOI 10.1007/978-1-4939-6445-1_17, © Springer Science+Business Media New York 2017

Two complementary particle sizing methods will be described in this chapter: dynamic light scattering (DLS) technology, also known as photon correlation spectroscopy (PCS) or quasi-elastic light scattering (QELS), and nanoparticle tracking analysis (NTA). Both methods are commonly used to measure the size distribution of samples in the nanometer to micron range, including nanoparticles (emulsions, liposomes) and macromolecules (protein) [6–9]. Size determination is based on Brownian motion, the theory that particles in solution undergo constant random movement. The movement of individual particles depends on their size, where small particles will move faster than large particles. The velocity due to Brownian motion of a spherical particle suspended in a liquid with a known viscosity at a constant temperature is proportional to the particle's diameter according to the Stokes-Einstein equation. By solving the equation from collected particle velocity data, algorithms can be used to determine the particle size distribution of a sample.

Stokes–Einstein equation:

$$D_{\mathrm{h}} = \frac{kT}{3\pi\eta D_t}$$

where D_{h} = hydrodynamic diameter, k = Boltzmann's constant, T = temperature, η = solution viscosity, and D_{t} = translational diffusion coefficient (velocity of Brownian motion). k, T, and η are known and D_{t} is measured, solving for D_{h}.

DLS is a non-destructive and simple measurement effective in measuring particles in the range of approximately 1 nm to 10 μm. A laser illuminates the sample in a cuvette and light that is scattered by particles in solution is collected by a detector. Common detector positions are back angle (173°) and right angle (90°) relative to the incident laser. By inputting the refractive index and the viscosity of the diluent or sample medium, particle size can be determined. To determine D_t, the light that is scattered by the sample over a period of time (in microseconds) is digitally processed in a correlator to derive an autocorrelation function, where the exponential decay can be analyzed. The decay constant, representing the movement of particles, is directly proportional to D_t. Particle diffusion rate can be affected by factors including the ionic strength of the solution and surface structure [10]. From this information, the intensity weighted mean size, Z-average (Z_{avg}), and the polydispersity index (PDI) describing the broadness of size distribution of the sample can be obtained. When a sample has more than one particle size population (multimodal distribution), a multi-exponential fit is used to describe the autocorrelation function and the result is a distribution of relative light intensities scattered by particles of different size populations. Using light scattering theories and algorithms, these size distributions can be represented as number, volume, or intensity-weighted. A comprehensive review of theory and data interpretation can be found in the literature [11–14].

Nanoparticle tracking analysis (NTA) is a relatively new method in the field of nanoparticle characterization. Advances in digital camera and video processing technologies have led to a significant increase in object tracking capabilities. NTA uses those capabilities to track the movement of individual particles in solution. Particles are illuminated with a laser and scattered light is imaged using a high-speed camera and microscope. Compared to DLS, NTA size measurements are not as susceptible to the influence of polydispersity. Furthermore, the particle size distribution measured by NTA is a more direct measurement because the measurement is based on the tracking of individual particles and does not rely on curve fitting as used for DLS. Also, because the volume visible to the camera is known, the particle concentration can be determined by counting the number of particles within the volume. NTA is effective for particles between 10 and 1000 nm in diameter. The lower size limit depends on sensitivity of the camera and refractive index of the particle while above 1000 nm the error associated with finding the center of particles by the software approaches the same magnitude as the Brownian motion of the particle. Using a syringe pump to flow sample through the laser beam at a constant rate increases the number of particles measured and thereby improves the size and concentration statistics.

A common limitation between DLS and NTA methods is the assumption that is made that the particles being measured are solid and spherical, which is often not the case, particularly for macromolecules or rod-shaped particles. By modeling the diffusional properties of these particles, the calculated size reflects a hydrated and dynamic particle, deriving the term "hydrodynamic diameter" [15, 16]. The calculated hydrodynamic diameter describes the diameter of a spherical particle that diffuses in solution in the manner detected.

2 Materials

2.1 DLS

1. Nano-ZS (Malvern) or equivalent. The Nano-ZS is a commonly used DLS instrument that employs a 173° angle backscatter detector and has other capabilities this chapter does not include such as the measurement of zeta potential and protein molecular weight.
2. Disposable polystyrene micro cuvettes for size measurement at 173° back-scattering angle (ZEN0040, Malvern Instruments Limited) (*see* **Note 1**).
3. 200 nm and/or 60 nm polystyrene size standards (3000 Series Nanosphere™, Thermo Scientific). Dilute by adding three drops of standard into 1 mL of 10 mM sodium chloride (*see* **Note 2**). Invert several times to mix well.

2.2 NTA

1. NanoSight 405 nm laser LM10 (Malvern) with an Orca Flash 2.8 sCMOS camera (Hamamatsu), a syringe pump (Harvard Apparatus) and a HH804U thermometer (OMEGA Engineering).
2. Milli-Q® or equivalent ultrapure water.
3. 25 mm Anotop® Syringe Filter (Whatman), 0.02-μm pore size.
4. Water for cleaning: Prepare a 1-mL slip-tip syringe filled with water. Attach a filter. Push the water through the filter to eliminate air, then refill the syringe and reattach the filter. Fill a 50-mL conical vial with water. Use this to refill the syringe as needed (*see* **Note 3**).
5. Water for sample dilutions: Prepare 10 mL of water through a filter into a 15 mL conical vial (*see* **Notes 3** and **4**).
6. Bacteriostatic 10% v/v ethanol in water storage solution: Aliquot 5 mL 200-proof ethanol into a 50 mL conical vial. QS to 50 mL. Filter the resulting 10% ethanol solution through a filter into a new conical vial. (*see* **Note 3**).

3 Methods

3.1 DLS [17]

1. Turn on instrument and open Malvern Zetasizer software (version 7.11) (*see* **Note 5**). Wait 30 min for the laser to stabilize before use (*see* **Note 6**).
2. Dilute sample to the appropriate concentration using water or buffer if required (*see* **Notes** 7 and **8**).
3. Using a pipette, slowly add 40 μL of the sample to the bottom of the cuvette, avoiding the introduction of bubbles (*see* **Notes 9** and **10**).
4. Open lid and insert the cuvette into the cell holder with a polished side facing forward (towards the user). Many cuvettes have a triangle that indicates the front of the cuvette. Close the lid.
5. Open a new measurement (.dts) file. All subsequent measurements will automatically be saved to this file until it is closed or another .dts file is opened.
6. In the Measure menu, select Manual.
7. In the Manual Measurement editor, input sample information (*see* **Note 11**) as described below in **steps 8–11.**
8. Measurement type: Size.
9. Sample: Input sample name, Material: Polystyrene latex, Dispersant: Water, General options: Use default Mark-Houwink parameters, Temperature: 25.0 °C; Equilibration time: 25 s, Cell: Disposable cuvettes (ZEN0040).

10. Measurement: 173° back-scatter (NIBS default); Automatic measurement duration; Three measurements with a 3 s delay between measurements. Advanced: Extend duration for large particles: No; Positioning method: Seek for optimum position; Automatic attenuation selection: Yes.
11. Data Processing: General purpose (normal resolution), Reports: N/A (deselect print report), Export: N/A (do not export results).
12. Save settings if the method will be used in the future. Press "OK" to go to the Manual Measurement window.
13. To start the measurement, press the "start" button in the Manual Measurement window. The instrument will equilibrate to temperature according to the user-defined settings prior to beginning measurements. A status bar will appear in the lower left hand corner of the window, indicating the progress of the measurement. The intensity particle size distribution (PSD) results, as well as Z-average size and PDI, can be viewed as they are collected (*see* **Note 12**). The screen will display the average of all collected acceptable data.
14. Once the measurement has completed, the quality of the measurement can be checked in the Expert Advice Tab in the Manual Measurement window. This will indicate if the measurement meets quality criteria or if unwanted attributes exist (e.g., the presence of aggregates).
15. Retrieve cuvette and discard.
16. To measure additional samples, repeat steps. In the Manual Measurement window, select the "Settings" button to change the sample name and any settings if needed.
17. View data in the Measurement (.dts) file. Each measured sample will appear in measured order in the records view tab. Z-average and PDI will be displayed along with other data such as peak means and mean count rate. This tab can be customized to show additional collected mean data under Tools menu > Settings > Configure Workspace > Add Workspace > Record View Parameters. The remaining tabs will show reports generated for size measurements (e.g., Intensity PSD, Volume PSD, Number PSD) or data quality (Expert Advice). The correlation data (Correlogram) and data fits (Cumulants Fit and Distribution Fit) can also be seen, among many other results. These tabs can also be customized to display the desired result types under Tools menu > Settings > Configure Workspace > Add Workspace > Report Pages.

3.2 NTA

1. Prepare instrument as described in **steps 2–8** below:
2. Consult NanoSight Operating Manual for instrument schematic [18].

3. Plug the power supply into the camera and turn on laser module.
4. Ensure that the temperature probe is plugged into the brass temperature port on the LM10 top plate and turn on the thermometer.
5. Check that the outlet line from the sample chamber is placed in a waste container.
6. Start the NTA software (NTA 3.1).
7. In the "Capture" tab in the top left panel of the NTA software click "Start Camera" to connect to the sCMOS camera.
8. Center the viewfinder over the laser beam as described in **steps 9–12** below:
9. Increase camera sensitivity to more easily locate the laser beam: Select the "Hardware" tab from the right side of the lower main panel. Select the "Adv Camera" tab from the top of the main panel. Slide the "Shutter" control to its maximum value. Using the right mouse button narrow the Camera Histogram range to maximize sensitivity.
10. In small increments move the microscope stage up and down in the Y-direction until the laser beam is centered in the display. If the laser beam cannot be found, move the microscope stage incrementally in the X-direction and repeat Y movements until the laser beam appears in the display.
11. Locate the "thumbprint" where the laser beam leaves the optical flat by moving the stage in the X-direction along the laser beam. Move the stage so that the "thumbprint" is just out of the display to the right. This position ensures the best possible measurement.
12. Approximately focus the camera on the laser beam.
13. Clean sample cell as described in **steps 14–18** below:
14. Always ensure a liquid-to-liquid contact when connecting a syringe to the fill line. This will prevent air from entering the sample chamber (*see* **Note 13**).
15. Hold the Luer-Lok end of the fill line below the level of the outlet line so that liquid flows into the Luer-Lok fitting.
16. Push a small droplet of liquid out of the end of the cleaning syringe filter.
17. Touch the droplet to the liquid in the Luer-Lok fitting, then seat the syringe filter. This will ensure that no air is introduced into the sample chamber.
18. Rinse the cell with at least 2 mL filtered water. Check the display for particles. When there are no visible particles the sample chamber is clean (*see* **Note 14**).
19. Prepare sample as described in **steps 20–23** below.

20. To account for dilution errors make three independent 10^5 dilutions as follows: Fill three sets of three 1.7 mL microcentrifuge tubes with 990, 990, and 900 μL filtered water.
21. Aliquot 10 μL sample into the first set of three microcentrifuge tubes containing 990 μL filtered water. Cap and finger-flick or vortex the vial briefly to mix (100-fold dilution).
22. Transfer 10 μL of the 100-fold dilution sample into the second set of three Eppendorf tube containing 990 μL filtered water. Cap and finger-flick or vortex the vial briefly to mix (10^4-fold dilution).
23. Transfer 100 μL of the 10^4-fold dilution sample into the third set of three microcentrifuge tubes containing 900 μL filtered water. Cap and finger-flick or vortex the vial briefly to mix (10^5-fold dilution) (*see* **Note 15**).
24. Measure sample as described in **steps 25–31** below.
25. Fill a 1-mL slip-tip syringe with sample. Carefully connect the syringe to the fill line without introducing air as described in **step 17** of Subheading 3.2.
26. Advance 0.5 mL sample into the fill line. This should be a sufficient volume to displace the water in the sample chamber.
27. Adjust the focus so that particles on the left side of the display are slightly blurry and particles on the right side of the display have small diffraction rings around them (i.e., center the focal plane in the camera window) (*see* **Note 16**).
28. Adjust the camera settings to their maximum value to check for dim particles, then starting with the camera gain, turn

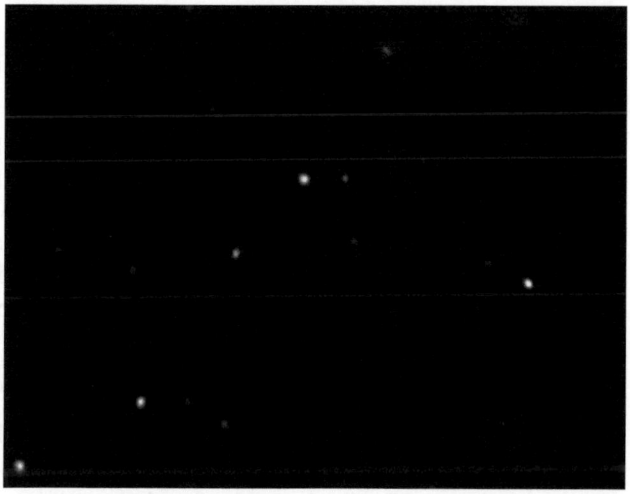

Fig. 1 An example of good camera settings. This sample is somewhat dilute and will require longer collection times

down settings until an optimum image is reached (Fig. 1, *see* **Note 17**) as described in **steps 29–31** below.

29. Shutter setting: 1000.
30. Camera Gain: 300.
31. Intensity Histogram: High and low bounds adjusted to narrowly encompass the intensity of the sample scattering.
32. Start the syringe pump. Select the "Syringe Pump" tab at the top of the lower main panel. Turn the infusion rate up to 200 (arbitrary units) until particle flow stabilizes, then turn flow back down to 20 (*see* **Note 18**).
33. Load the measurement script and set the base filename by clicking on the "SOP" tab on the right side of the lower main panel (*see* **Note 19**).
34. Select the "SOP Standard Measurement script" and click "Load Script."

    Script

    SYRINGELOAD 15

    TEMPERATURE 22.4

    CAPTURE 60

    DELAY 1

    CAPTURE 60

    DELAY 1

    CAPTURE 60

    DELAY 1

    CAPTURE 60

    DELAY 1

    SYRINGESTOP
35. To set the base filename for each sample and data export location click the "..." button.
36. Click "Run" and enter appropriate information when prompted. The script will prompt the user for sample information first, then request that the user set appropriate camera settings (which can be skipped since this was done earlier). At the end of each run the user will be prompted for the sample temperature. This value must be entered before the next run starts.
37. Clean and shutdown as described in **steps 38–41** below.
38. After each sample rinse the sample chamber with 2 mL filtered water.
39. At the end of each experiment thoroughly rinse the cell out with water and fill the cell with 1 mL 10% v/v ethanol (*see*

Note 20). Leave the instrument with the syringe used to fill the chamber with ethanol connected to the fill line.

40. In the "Capture" tab of the top left panel click "Stop Camera." Unplug the camera and gently drape the power cord over the back of the microscope.
41. Turn off the laser.
42. Analyze data as described in **steps 43–47** below.
43. Open an experiment by selecting the "Analysis" tab in the main lower panel. Click the "Open Experiment" button and select the desired experiment file. In the panel below the buttons double click on the first run to load the run.
44. Evaluate the run by sliding the time slider in the main display. If the slider is not found, make sure to select the top-most plot in the upper right hand corner of the main display. The screen gain can be temporarily set high to help decipher between particles and noise. While moving the time slider, look for over-sensitivity as characterized by multi-centered particles and the detection of noise as particles. Also look for under-sensitivity where particles are not being detected. Choose a "Detection Threshold" that will be used in the next step.
45. Select all of the runs and click "Process Selected Files." The user will be prompted to adjust the "Detection Threshold" in the top left panel. Set the detection threshold to 5 or the value determined in the previous step (*see* **Note 21**).
46. Click "Ok" in the prompt window to start the analysis.
47. Export the analysis at the end of processing by clicking the "Export Results" button in the lower main panel. Click "Ok" when prompted, or adjust export settings as desired.

4 Notes

1. Many cuvettes, including generic brands, are available that can be used in the Malvern Nano-ZS. Cuvettes should have an outside dimension (O.D.) of 12 × 12 × 45 mm with a 10 mm pathlength and should be acceptable for assays in 340–750 nm spectral range. When selecting cuvettes, consider available sample volume, solvent and temperature compatibility, and price. Polystyrene cuvettes should not be used with organic solvents and for measurements performed above 70 °C. Disposable cuvettes can easily be scratched so they are not recommended for multiple uses [19].
2. 10 mM sodium chloride is used for the dilution of the standards as described in the international standard for DLS (ISO22412:2008) [20]. Measuring the size of standards

diluted in demineralized water (low conductivity) can increase the thickness of the electric double layer of the particles (Debye length), slowing particle movement and resulting in a size 15 % higher than the reported size [16].

3. Maintaining a particle free environment is critical for accurate particle concentration measurements. Prior to sample measurements, check to make sure none of the containers used to hold diluent or sample are shedding particles. Fill representative containers with particle free water and shake or vortex, then load an aliquot into the LM10 sample compartment and check for the presence of particles. If there are more than one or two particles, consider a particle free water wash, use newer containers, or find a different container supplier.
4. Some nanoparticles or proteins are not stable in ultrapure water and will need an appropriate dilution buffer. Most common buffers are compatible with the LM10 and with Anotop® filters. If a dilution buffer is used, filter it through a 0.02-μm Anotop® filter to ensure the diluent is particle free.
5. It is recommended to keep the Zetasizer software updated with the latest revision. Additionally, it is important that all computers accessing the same pool of data files have the exact Zetasizer software revision. Once an existing data file has been accessed using a newer version, it will automatically overwrite the file and be unable to revert back to the outdated version, thus rendering the file permanently inaccessible via the older software version.
6. Generally, Zetasizers are always left powered on and are only turned off if not used for an extended period of time (e.g., a week).
7. The appropriate dilution can be empirically determined by performing a dilution series and measuring the particle size of each dilution. The ideal dilution range will give reproducible sizes with good data quality results as determined by the software. The concentration of the analyte must be in the range where scattering intensity of the particles achieve acceptable signal-to-noise ratio but does not exceed a critical concentration where multiple scattering interferes with data collection. Multiple scattering is a phenomenon where a scattered photon is rescattered by neighboring particles. Note that more recent backscatter (173°) DLS technology has largely overcome these issues since measurements are being made at a shallow penetration into the cell, limiting the reach of multiple scattering signals into the detector. With these advances, turbid solutions can be measured. Because larger particles scatter more light, a sample containing large particles will need to be diluted more than a sample containing small particles [16, 17]. A 1:100 dilution in water is commonly used for nanoemulsions and liposomes. Protein solutions can often be measured without dilution.

8. Use the same buffer as is used to prepare the sample for dilution. Ultrapure water is often substituted for the dilution of robust particles, such as emulsions and liposomes, and the assumption is often made that the change in ionic strength of the medium does not change particle size. This should first be empirically determined.
9. The fill volume of a cuvette should be at a height above the measurement line but should not be excessive. In the Nano-ZS, measurements are made 8 mm from the bottom of the cuvette. Therefore, the minimum fill volume is 10 mm from the bottom of the cuvette to avoid interference from the meniscus. It is recommended that the fill height should not exceed 15 mm from the bottom of the cuvette to avoid thermal gradients within the sample that can affect temperature control [19].
10. Bubbles can be removed using a pipette or by tapping the cuvette gently against the lab bench. Sonication can also be used if it is not destructive to the sample.
11. Input appropriate sample parameters according to sample type. The parameters shown are used for a nanoemulsion.
12. The type of data displayed in the results page can be customized by right-clicking on the graph and selecting the desired result type, including Count Rate, Correlation Function, Intensity PSD, Volume PSD, and Number PSD.
13. If the LM10 sample cell is dry or has large air bubbles present, remove the cell from the microscope stage and hold it so that the exit port is facing up. Push filtered water into the cell slowly so that the meniscus moves smoothly across the cell. If air bubbles are visible use a series of short, harder bursts to dislodge the bubbles.
14. If a buffer other than water is going to be used, rinse the cell with 2 mL of filtered buffer before adding sample.
15. It is important to find the proper dilution for each sample type. Completely opaque samples like nanoemulsions at 10 % v/v oil will likely need to be diluted 10^6-fold. Liposomes and aqueous formulations will likely require diluting 10^4-fold. Proteins typically will be measured without dilution. Use a 0.02-μm filter to prepare buffer. It is important that buffers for dilution be particle free. Create a dilution series going one or two dilutions more than the expected appropriate dilution. Load the dilution series starting with the most dilute samples. A proper dilution should have approximately 50–100 particles in view at a time. Fewer particles will require longer measurement times to attain acceptable statistics. Too many particles will interfere with the accuracy of concentration and size values. The optimum particle concentration is approximately 10^8–10^9 particles per mL depending on size and the width of

the size distribution. Turn the shutter and gain up all the way to check for any dim particles that might otherwise be missed.

16. The laser beam travels through the sample at a slight inclination, thus particles illuminated on the left side of the sample are a little higher than particles illuminated on the right. As a result, the focal plane transects the visible particles, only those particles that are illuminated in the focal plane will be in perfect focus, and this region will move left and right as the focal plane is moved up and down. If the section of particles in perfect focus is centered in the camera view the software will compensate for those particles that are out of the focal plane.
17. For most protein and liposome samples maximize the sensitivity of the camera settings so that the faintest particles can be detected while still minimizing the noise. Emulsions usually do not require maximizing sensitivity. NTA measurements are dominated by the brightest particles regardless of their size. Thus, bright particles tend to wash out small particles. Also, bright particles that are not perfectly spherical have large moving interference patterns, which the NTA software has a difficult time tracking and accurately measuring. When a sample contains bright particles and the shutter, gain, and histogram (CMOS Camera) are not set appropriately, bright particles are systematically undersized. This can be corrected by increasing the minimum expected particle size, except that doing so may exclude legitimate small, weakly scattering particles. To ensure the most accurate measurement of particles choose gain, shutter, and histogram settings that result in accurate sizing of the brightest particles with the knowledge that all of the particles sized are sized correctly but that a portion of the true particle distribution was not sized at all. Thus, though the distribution is accurate, it is not complete. On the other hand, if inappropriate settings were chosen, the distribution would be complete (all particles sized), but not accurate (particles assigned the wrong size). The former option, accurate and incomplete, is likely a better option because it allows for the user to subsequently select sampling conditions to measure the weakly scattering particles, for example by dilution to the point where there are so few bright particles that they do not contribute significantly to the total population measured.
18. The syringe pump speed should be adjusted so that the flow rate allows for particles to travel across the field of view in 5–10 s. The speed is in arbitrary units and pump calibration is not required. The NanoSight syringe pump operating manual states that for LM10 models, syringe pump speed should typically be between 20 and 50 units. As long as the flow is in the appropriate range, the speed does not affect measured size as it is compensated for by the NTA software [21].

19. On the correct length of time to collect data: as the population distribution widens, the number and length of each measurement should subsequently increase. This is a simple statistics problem. Assuming two populations of particles, it will take twice as long at the same total particle concentration to collect data for two populations as it will to collect data for one population. Thus, as the heterogeneity of the sample increases, so should the number of samples collected and the length of the collection measurement. Remember though, that as measurement time increases concentration tends to decrease because of particle adsorption to the sample chamber.
20. If a dilution buffer is used instead of water, first rinse thoroughly with buffer before rinsing with water.
21. Find a setting where the maximum number of particles is detected but no noise or scattering is misidentified as a particle. View a number of different frames before deciding on a particular setting by moving the slider in the main display.

References

1. Bachmann MF, Jennings GT (2010) Vaccine delivery: a matter of size, geometry, kinetics and molecular patterns. Nat Rev Immunol 10(11):787–796
2. Bachmann MF, Jennings GT (2010) Vaccine delivery: a matter of size, geometry, kinetics and molecular patterns. Nat Rev Immunol 10(11):787–796
3. Shah RR et al (2014) The impact of size on particulate vaccine adjuvants. Nanomedicine (Lond) 9(17):2671–2681
4. Xiang SD et al (2006) Pathogen recognition and development of particulate vaccines: does size matter? Methods 40(1):1–9
5. Yu Z, Reid JC, Yang YP (2013) Utilizing dynamic light scattering as a process analytical technology for protein folding and aggregation monitoring in vaccine manufacturing. J Pharm Sci 102(12):4284–4290
6. Filipe V, Hawe A, Jiskoot W (2010) Critical evaluation of Nanoparticle Tracking Analysis (NTA) by NanoSight for the measurement of nanoparticles and protein aggregates. Pharm Res 27(5):796–810
7. Jornada DS et al (2012) Lipid-core nanocapsules: mechanism of self-assembly, control of size and loading capacity. Soft Matter 8(24): 6646–6655
8. Malvern Instruments Limited (2015) Orthogonal and complementary nanoparticle characterization techniques, combining dynamic light scattering with nanoparticle tracking analysis. White Paper. Available from: http://www.malvern.com/en/support/resource-center/Whitepapers/WP151106OrthogonalComplementaryNanomaterialCharacterisationTechniques.aspx
9. Rahimian S et al (2015) Polymeric nanoparticles for co-delivery of synthetic long peptide antigen and poly IC as therapeutic cancer vaccine formulation. J Control Release 203: 16–22
10. Malvern Instruments Limited (2014) Dynamic light scattering: an introduction in 30 minutes. Technical Note. Available from: http://www.malvern.com/en/support/resource-center/technical-notes/TN101104DynamicLightScatteringIntroduction.aspx
11. Frisken BJ (2001) Revisiting the method of cumulants for the analysis of dynamic light-scattering data. Appl Opt 40(24): 4087–4091
12. Mailer AG, Clegg PS, Pusey PN (2015) Particle sizing by dynamic light scattering: non-linear cumulant analysis. J Phys Condens Matter 27(14):145102
13. Pecora R (1985) Dynamic light scattering: applications of photon correlation spectroscopy. Plenum Press, New York
14. Koppel DE (1972) Analysis of macromolecular polydispersity in intensity correlation spectroscopy: the method of cumulants. J Chem Phys 57(11):4814–4820
15. Burchard W (1992) Static and dynamic light scattering approaches to structure determination of biopolymers. In: Harding SE, Sattelle DB, Bloomfield DA (eds) Laser light scatter-

ing in biochemistry. Royal Society of Chemistry: Cambridge, UK. p 3–22

16. Malvern Instruments Limited (2015) Application of Dynamic Light Scattering (DLS) to protein therapeutic formulations: principles, measurements and analysis. Available from http://www.malvern.com/en/support/resource-center/Whitepapers/WP140404ApplicDLSprotein4FAQ.aspx
17. Malvern Instruments Limited (2013) Zetasizer Nano Series user manual. Cited Man0485 Issue 1.1 Available from http://www.malvern.com/en/support/resource-center/user-manuals/MAN0485EN.aspx
18. Malvern Instrument Limited (2015) NanoSight LM10 operating manual. Cited Man0510; Available from http://www.malvern.com/en/support/resource-center/user-manuals/MAN0510EN.aspx
19. Malvern Instruments Limited (2014) Zetasizer Nano Series accessories guide. Man0487 Issue 2.0; Available from http://www.malvern.com/en/support/resource-center/user-manuals/MAN0487EN.aspx
20. Standardization., G.I.O.f., ISO 22412, in Particle Size Analysis—Dynamic Light Scattering (DLS). 2008
21. Malvern Instruments Limited (2015) NanoSight syringe pump operating manual. [MAN0534-03-EN-00]. Available from http://www.malvern.com/en/support/resource-center/user-manuals/MAN0534EN.aspx

Chapter 18

Quantification of Multiple Components of Complex Aluminum-Based Adjuvant Mixtures by Using Fourier Transform Infrared Spectroscopy and Partial Least Squares Modeling

Quinton M. Dowling and Ryan M. Kramer

Abstract

Fourier transform infrared (FTIR) spectroscopy is widely used in the pharmaceutical industry for process monitoring, compositional quantification, and characterization of critical quality attributes in complex mixtures. Advantages over other spectroscopic measurements include ease of sample preparation, quantification of multiple components from a single measurement, and the ability to quantify optically opaque samples. This method describes the use of a multivariate model for quantifying a TLR4 agonist (GLA) adsorbed onto aluminum oxyhydroxide (Alhydrogel®) using FTIR spectroscopy that may be adapted to quantify other complex aluminum based adjuvant mixtures.

Key words Glucopyranosyl lipid adjuvant (GLA), Aluminum adjuvant, Vaccine adjuvants, FTIR, Absorption spectroscopy, Vaccines, Alhydrogel, Partial least squares modeling

1 Introduction

Vaccine adjuvants and their formulations present a significant analytical challenge. Adjuvants are chemically diverse; including such disparate compounds as inorganic aluminum salts, phosphorylated hexaacyl disaccharides, and saponins [1–3]. Aluminum salts are particularly analytically challenging; they are not compatible with most chromatographic techniques. Furthermore, adjuvants may be formulated as part of a colloidal suspension, for example liposomes, emulsions, and aluminum salts, rendering the sample opaque and not amenable to most spectrophotometric techniques. However, FTIR spectroscopy is a well-developed tool that is relatively inexpensive, simple to use, and is widely applicable to vaccine development. When coupled with an attenuated total reflectance (ATR)

Christopher B. Fox (ed.), *Vaccine Adjuvants: Methods and Protocols*, Methods in Molecular Biology, vol. 1494, DOI 10.1007/978-1-4939-6445-1_18, © Springer Science+Business Media New York 2017

accessory, FTIR is capable of measuring the absorbance spectrum of opaque samples. In addition, FTIR spectroscopy has a long history in pharmaceutical applications [4, 5]. FTIR spectroscopy is quantitative, directly measures the constituent of interest, and when coupled with an ATR accessory requires minimal sample preparation. A single FTIR spectrum provides extensive information, because measurements are taken across a wide wavelength range, typically reported as wave numbers (cm^{-1}), and because materials commonly included in vaccines absorb light in the IR region. There are a wide range of sample accessories available for FTIR spectroscopy. Accessory selection depends on sample type and the analytical needs of the user. ATR accessories are particularly useful for a wide range of sample types. An ATR accessory uses the property of total internal reflection where IR light is passed through a material at an angle such that the beam is reflected without attenuation at the inside surface. An evanescent wave forms at the point where the beam is reflected. When a sample is brought in close proximity to the surface of this material the sample interacts with the evanescent wave. In this way the totally reflected IR beam is attenuated, producing an absorbance spectrum. Zinc selenide, germanium, and diamond are common materials for FTIR-ATR spectroscopy.

Here we present a method using FTIR-ATR spectroscopy and a partial least squares (PLS) regression to quantify the components in an adjuvant system consisting of the synthetic TLR4 agonist GLA formulated as a nanoparticle with dipalmitoylphosphatidylcholine (DPPC) adsorbed to aluminum oxyhydroxide (Alhydrogel®). This is a more detailed version of the method described in Ref. [6]. Chemometric methods like PLS greatly extend the power of spectroscopic techniques by using the entire spectrum to create a regression rather than a single peak intensity or peak area. PLS was first introduced by the Swedish statistician Herman Wold and popularized by his son Svante Wold. To create a PLS regression, spectra of samples with known concentrations are collected. The relation between the concentration matrix and intensity matrix is then determined and used to calculate the concentration of spectra from unknown samples. Most modern spectroscopy software will include tools for performing PLS regressions.

Previous work has used FTIR methods to directly characterize both aluminum adjuvant alone and antigen adsorbed on aluminum adjuvant [6–9]. Here we describe a method for quantifying GLA, DPPC, and Alhydrogel® by FTIR-ATR spectroscopy. We generate a sample set containing independently varied concentrations of each component. The spectrum from each of those samples is then used to generate a PLS model for quantifying the concentration of each component in an unknown sample.

2 Materials

1. Software: OPUS 7.2 with the Quant package installed (Bruker, Billerica, MA, USA).
2. Instrument: Nicolet Magna 850 II (Thermo Scientific, Waltham, MA, USA).
3. ATR Accessory: ZnSe 6 bounce, 45° incident beam angle (Specac, Orpington, UK) (*see* **Note 1**).
4. GLA and DPPC (Avanti Polar Lipids, Alabaster, AL, USA).
5. Alhydrogel® (Brenntag, Langley, BC, Canada).
6. Chloroform, HPLC grade.
7. Ultrapure water.

3 Methods

3.1 Partial Least Squares Regression Calibration Set

1. Prepare a GLA stock and a DPPC stock in chloroform (*see* **Note 2**): Weigh out separately 3 mg GLA and 3 mg DPPC and dissolve separately in 3 ml chloroform to produce 1 mg/ml stock solutions.
2. Aliquot chloroform lipid mixtures according to Table 1 into a single vial.
3. Evaporate chloroform under reduced pressure overnight. This forms a thin film of evenly mixed lipid.
4. Add 500 μl ultrapure water to the lipid samples.
5. Heat and sonicate calibration set at 60 °C for 90 min to form a small particle suspension.
6. Meanwhile prepare Alhydrogel at 2× concentration in ultrapure water according to Table 1. Starting with stock Alhydrogel at 10 mg/ml aluminum ion, dilute the indicated volume with ultrapure water to a final volume of 500 μl.
7. Mix 400 μl of each sample from **step 4** of Subheading 3.1 with 400 μl from **step 6** of Subheading 3.1 to produce the final calibration set. Vortex briefly to mix.
8. Place 20 μl of the lipid mixture from **step 5** of Subheading 3.1 in triplicate HPLC vials and freeze at −80 °C for quantitation by HPLC at a later time.

3.2 Instrument Setup

1. Position the ZnSE ATR accessory in the sample compartment.
2. Fill the lnMCT detector coolant reservoir with liquid nitrogen.
3. Allow 30 min for the system to reach thermal equilibrium.

Table 1
List of volumes and final concentrations for calibration set

Sample	GLA stock volume (μl)[a]	DPPC stock volume (μl)[b]	Alhydrogel volume (μl)[b]	GLA final concentration (μg/ml)[c]	DPPC final concentration (μg/ml)[c]	Alhydrogel final concentration (mg/ml)[c]
1	26	13	100	26	13	1.0
2	97	35	250	97	35	2.5
3	138	84	300	138	84	3.0
4	142	21	350	142	21	3.5
5	42	70	400	42	70	4.0
6	100	61	75	100	61	0.8
7	133	147	375	133	147	3.8
8	185	112	275	185	112	2.8
9	235	56	125	235	56	1.3
10	208	50	225	208	50	2.3
11	187	206	120	187	206	1.2
12	211	127	175	211	127	1.8
13	197	120	150	197	120	1.5
14	63	25	200	63	25	2.0
15	119	43	75	119	43	0.8

[a]GLA and DPPC stock concentrations are 1 mg/ml in chloroform. Volumes of GLA and DPPC indicated are added together in Subheading 3.2 prior to chloroform evaporation
[b]Alhydrogel stock concentration is 10 mg/ml aluminum ion. Indicated volume is mixed with ultrapure water in Subheading 3.6 to for a total volume of 500 μl
[c]Final concentrations of calibration set samples after mixing lipid and Alhydrogel® samples in Subheading 3.7

3.3 Sample Cell Prep

1. Remove the ATR crystal from the instrument and clean in a fume hood.
2. Clean the ATR crystal by gently wiping with cotton swabs soaked in: chloroform, 20 mM Citrate buffer pH 6.0 (*see* **Note 3**), and then ultrapure water.
3. Rinse the crystal thoroughly with ultrapure water and wick water droplets away with a delicate task wiper (Kimwipes® or equivalent).
4. Place the crystal back in the sample compartment and wait for 30 min for the compartment environment to return to equilibrium.

3.4 Sample Measurement

1. Collect a background spectrum; Scans: 512; Region: 4000–650 cm^{-1}; Resolution: 2 cm^{-1}.

2. Load 100 μl of sample from **step 7** of Subheading 3.1 onto the ATR crystal. Samples are dried directly onto the ATR crystal in a dry air environment. Collect repeat measurements until a stable spectrum is achieved indicating that the water has fully evaporated (*see* **Note 4**); Scans: 512; Region: 4000–650 cm^{-1}; Resolution: 2 cm^{-1}
3. Wash the sample cell as in **steps 1–3** of Subheading 3.3.
4. Return the ATR crystal to the sample compartment and collect a few scans to confirm cell cleanliness.
5. Repeat **steps 1–4** for all of the samples described in Table 1 (*see* Fig. 1).

3.5 Data Processing

1. In OPUS 7.2 open the collected sample spectra.
2. Review the shape of the spectra visually to get a sense of the variability between samples.

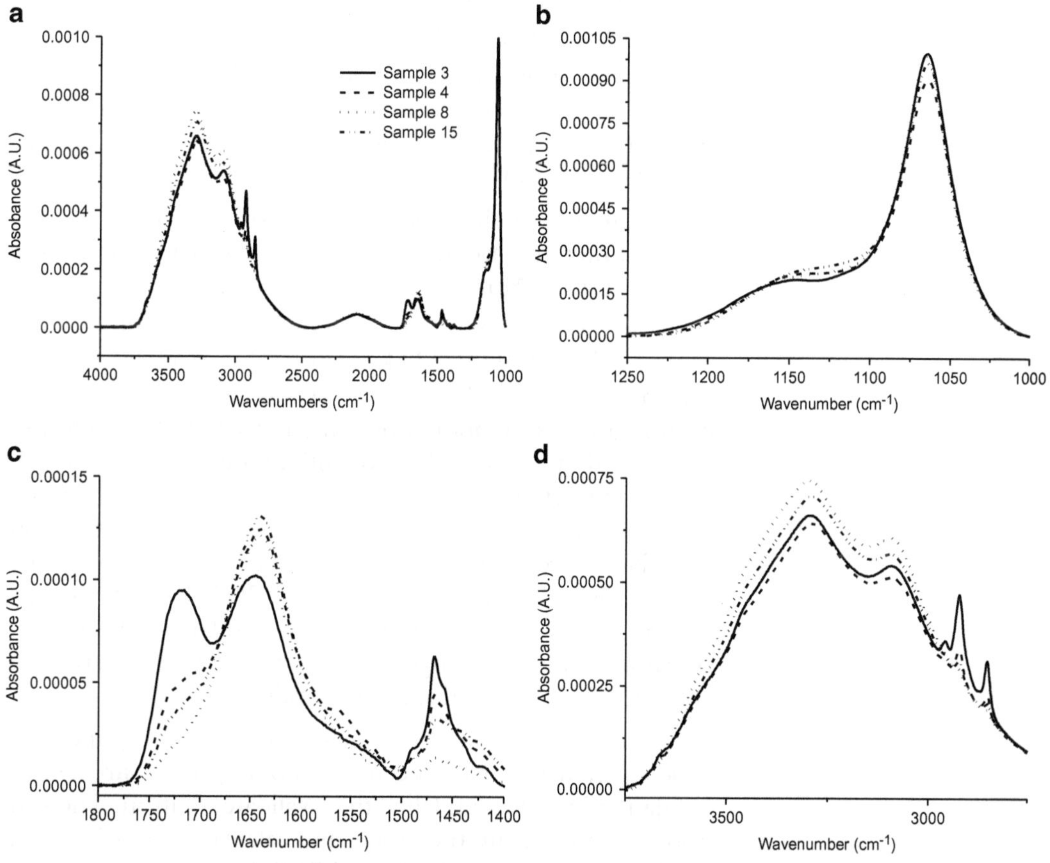

Fig. 1 Representative Fourier transform infrared spectra of GLA, DPPC, and aluminum oxyhydroxide containing samples. Spectra are of the samples indicated in the legend and were prepared according to Table 1 and as described in this chapter. The *panels* depict various spectral ranges of the same spectra including absorbance spectra from 4000 to 1000 cm^{-1} (**a**), 1250 to 1000 cm^{-1} (**b**), 1800 to 1400 cm^{-1} (**c**), and 3750 to 2750 cm^{-1} (**d**)

3. In the "Manipulate" menu select "Baseline Correction".
4. Click the "Start Interactive Mode". On the left side of the window select "Polynomes." Place baseline points by double-clicking on the spectrum (*see* **Note 5**). Points are placed above the OH stretching region, between 2450 and 1800 cm^{-1}, and around 1400, 1000, and 700 cm^{-1}. Click "Store" to apply the correction.
5. In the "Manipulate" menu select "Normalization." Select"Vector Normalization" and click "Normalize."

3.6 Multivariate Analysis Model Generation

1. If not already running, open the OPUS 7.2 software. Spectra do not need to be loaded into the Display window (*see* **Note 6**).
2. Select "Setup Quant 2 Method" from the Evaluate menu.
3. Under the Components tab click the "Add Component" button.
4. In the "Name" text box enter the name or identifier of the component. In the "Unit" text box type in the concentration units for that component (*see* **Note 7**).
5. Under the "Spectra" tab click the "Add Spectra" button. Browse to the directory containing the calibration data. Select the calibration spectra and click the "Open" button. The spectra will be listed in a table.
6. The right side of the table has text boxes for concentration values. Enter the appropriate concentrations for the calibration spectra (*see* **Note 8**).
7. Click on the Parameters tab (*see* **Note 9**). For DPPC quantification, select 2994.9–2324.8 cm^{-1} (the methylene stretch region) and 1990.2–1319.1 cm^{-1} (Carbonyl region and fingerprint region) as calibration regions, and select First Derivative preprocessing. For GLA quantification, select 3665.1–2324.8 cm^{-1} (the hydroxyl and methylene stretch region) and 1655.6–984.5 cm^{-1} (Carbonyl region and fingerprint region) as calibration regions, and select First Derivative preprocessing. For Alhydrogel quantification, select 3330.5–1989.2 cm^{-1} (the hydroxyl and methylene stretch region) and 1655.6–984.5 cm^{-1} (Carbonyl region and fingerprint region) as calibration regions, and select First Derivative preprocessing.
8. Click on the "Validate" tab. Select only the component for which parameters have been optimized. Make sure "Cross Validation" is selected. Click the "Validate" button. The software will now create the model and calculate regression diagnostics and will select the "Graph" tab for the user.
9. The graph in the "Graph" tab will show the Prediction/True graph. In the dropdown menu labeled "Prediction/True" select RMSECV/Rank to determine the appropriate rank

(also called component or factor depending on the software). The OPUS software will recommend a rank.

10. View the loadings by clicking on the "Loadings" button. Make sure that the primary loadings are rational, i.e., they reflect regions of the spectrum that are associated with the component of interest.
11. In the "Reports" tab from the drop-down menu labeled "True-Prediction" select "Spectral Residuals" and check for outliers. F Prob < 0.05. Outlier samples should be removed from the model. Go back to the "Spectra" tab, select the outlier spectrum and press the "Delete" keyboard key. Return to **step 7** and rebuild the model (*see* **Note 10**).
12. Select the Store Method tab. Click the Store Method button, select the appropriate validation name, and press Ok. Save the .Q2 file with an appropriate name.

3.7 Quantify Unknown with PLS Model

1. Collect spectra from unknown samples as described in Subheading 3.4.
2. Select "Quant 2 Analysis/File List" from the "Evaluate" menu.
3. In the "Methods" tab click the "Add Methods" button. Select the methods generated in Subheading 3.6 and click "Open."
4. Select the "Spectra" tab and click on the "Add Spectra" button. Select unknown sample spectra and click "Open."
5. Select the "Analysis Results" tab and click "Analyze". The software will calculate concentration predictions and will also calculate the Mahalanobis distance to determine if the sample is an outlier (exceeds the Mahalanobis distance limit, *see* **Note 10**). Concentrations outside of the Mahalanobis distance limit or outside of the limits of the calibration set should not be considered accurate.

4 Notes

1. Methods can be adapted for various sample cell accessories such as transmission cells or other ATR cells. The decision to work with a specific accessory and wet or dry samples should be evaluated on a case by case basis. All experiments should be carried out at a controlled temperature, or collection times kept below 10 min to minimize sample heating by the IR beam.
2. Avoid collinearity between constituents. If two components are collinear across the calibration samples, the PLS model will not be able to distinguish between the two.
3. The ZnSe crystal is not compatible with strongly acidic conditions.

4. Spectra do not need to be collected consecutively or on the same day as long as noise levels in unknown samples are in the same range as noise levels in the calibration set, i.e., the noise is fully described by the model. The same measurement parameters are used for each sample in the calibration set, as well as each unknown sample.
5. Zoom in on the region where each point is placed to make sure the point is accurately positioned. Place points minimally to reduce distorting spectral features related to components in the sample.
6. There are many software tools for constructing a PLS model; most modern spectrometers come with software to construct a PLS regression. Some examples of software include OPUS and Thermo Scientific GRAMS/AI. Alternatively there are packages available for R, a software environment for statistical computing, that can be used to perform a PLS regression.
7. These do not impact the values reported but are useful for keeping track of components, especially in complex samples.
8. Check that the components are not correlated for the calibration set by clicking on the "Comp. Correlations" button. Select each combination of components from the drop-down menu at the top of the "Components Correlation" window. Low r^2 values are desirable. Click exit to return to the Setup window.
9. Parameter selection is specific to the type of sample and component. Parameters are divided into two categories: Preprocessing and Calibration Regions. Preprocessing options provided by OPUS include options like "Straight line subtraction," "First derivative," "Second derivative," and "Vector normalization." These options are described in detail in the OPUS help file. If the contribution of each component of interest to the total spectrum is known, parameter selection may be performed manually. OPUS also provides a parameter optimization algorithm.
10. Ideally there should not be many outliers. Also, if when removing one outlier a second outlier is created the initial set of controls is probably too small. Some outliers may actually be influential observations that have a large impact on the regression. Either remove influential observations or add more samples to fill in between the bulk of the observations and the influential observation. If an outlier is observed consider recollecting the spectrum for that sample. Note also that the user can adjust the cutoff for an outlier. Using a small Mahalanobis distance cutoff will provide the best outlier detection. As long as the noise level and constituent identity of a sample spectrum is relatively constant one can use a cutoff of 2–3 and

obtain good results. The distance limit in the OPUS software is defined as follows:

$$MahDistCut = X * Rank / M$$

Where X is the cutoff coefficient selected by the user, M is the total number of samples in the calibration set, and Rank is the number of PLS latent variables determined by a one-sided F-test (95 % confidence interval) on Prediction Errors Sum of Squares.

References

1. Hem SL, HogenEsch H (2007) Aluminum-containing adjuvants: properties, formulation, and use. In: Singh M (ed) Vaccine adjuvants and delivery systems. John Wiley & Sons, Hoboken, NJ, pp 81–114
2. Anderson RC, Fox CB, Dutill TS, Shaverdian N, Evers TL, Poshusta GR, Chesko J, Coler RN, Friede M, Reed SG, Vedvick TS (2010) Physicochemical characterization and biological activity of synthetic TLR4 agonist formulations. Colloids Surf B: Biointerfaces 75(1):123–132
3. Kensil CR, Patel U, Lennick M, Marciani D (1991) Separation and characterization of saponins with adjuvant activity from Quillaja saponaria Molina cortex. J Immunol 146(2): 431–437
4. Salari A, Young RE (1998) Application of attenuated total reflectance FTIR spectroscopy to the analysis of mixtures of pharmaceutical polymorphs. Int J Pharm 163(1–2):157–166
5. Van Eerdenbrugh B, Taylor LS (2011) Application of mid-IR spectroscopy for the characterization of pharmaceutical systems. Int J Pharm 417(1–2):3–16
6. Agopian A, Ronzon F, Sauzeat E, Sodoyer R, El Habib R, Buchet R, Chevalier M (2007) Secondary structure analysis of HIV-1-gp41 in solution and adsorbed to aluminum hydroxide by Fourier transform infrared spectroscopy. Biochim Biophys Acta 1774(3):351–358
7. Dowling QM, Schwartz AM, Vedvick TS, Fox CB, Kramer RM (2014) Quantitative measurement of toll-like receptor 4 agonists adsorbed to alhydrogel by fourier transform infrared-attenuated total reflectance spectroscopy. J Pharm Sci 104(2):768–74
8. Johnston CT, Wang SL, Hem SL (2002) Measuring the surface area of aluminum hydroxide adjuvant. J Pharm Sci 91(7): 1702–1706
9. Rinella JV Jr, White JL, Hem SL (1995) Effect of anions on model aluminum-adjuvant-containing vaccines. J Colloid Interface Sci 172(1):121–130

Chapter 19

Determination of Protein Content in Alhydrogel®-Based Vaccines by *O*-Phthalaldehyde Assay

Kelly M. Rausch and Daming Zhu

Abstract

The quantification of antigens adsorbed to aluminum-based adjuvants (alum) typically involves a method that first extracts antigen from the alum followed by the quantification of the antigen available in the extract. Extraction procedures often result in less than 100% desorption of the antigen from the alum adjuvant and may alter the conformation of the antigen, reducing the accuracy of the subsequent method used for quantification. There is no generic method available for directly assessing the protein content when formulated on alum. Here we offer a method that can directly quantify protein adsorbed to Alhydrogel® using a simple fluorescence assay that is highly accurate and reproducible for Alhydrogel® formulations containing 25–400 μg/mL of antigen.

Key words OPA, *o*-phthalaldehyde, Alhydrogel, Aluminum hydroxide, Alum, Vaccine, Protein assay, Protein quantification

1 Introduction

Our lab routinely uses Alhydrogel® for formulating vaccines used both in research and clinical studies (cGMP). To monitor the antigen content on the formulations, we developed the *o*-phthalaldehyde (OPA) assay [1] to provide a consistent, reliable, and direct method for quantifying our antigens on Alhydrogel®. Alum adjuvants produce interference in the Lowry, BCA, and Bradford assays, and therefore, although often used for extracted antigens, are not suitable for the direct quantification of formulated antigens. OPA has been used since approximately 1959 to quantify submicron amounts of biogenic amines, peptides, and proteins in both tissues and solutions [2–11]. It produces a strong fluorescence signal after reacting with N-terminal (primary) amine groups, or amine groups in the side chains of lysine, in the presence of a thiol, usually 2-mercaptoethanol in alkaline conditions [12, 13]. As the OPA does not react with alum, or with other components used in typical buffering solutions, this offers a good option for quantifying

Christopher B. Fox (ed.), *Vaccine Adjuvants: Methods and Protocols*, Methods in Molecular Biology, vol. 1494,
DOI 10.1007/978-1-4939-6445-1_19, © Springer Science+Business Media New York 2017

antigens on Alhydrogel with extremely low background. The assay is accurate (87–100%), sensitive (25–400 μg/mL antigen), and not greatly affected by glycosylation, surface charge, pH of the buffering system in the range of 6.9–7.4 or different concentrations of Alhydrogel in the formulation [1].

The method described here uses a 96-well plate to analyze samples in triplicate against a freshly prepared standard. Fluorescence values derived from excitation/emissions at 340/455 nm are calculated by regression to a standard curve to determine quantity of overall antigen in the sample. Both supernatant and pelleted components as well as whole vaccine can be evaluated, providing a method to ascertain qualitatively both the bound and unbound quantities of antigen on the Alhydrogel.

2 Materials

1. o-phthalaldehyde (OPA) reagent (Pierce) (*see* **Note 1**).
2. Black microtiter plates, 96-well flat bottom (ThermoFisher).
3. Saline: 0.9% sodium chloride for injection, USP.
4. Alhydrogel, 2.0% (Brenntag Biosector).
5. Wallac VICTOR^3 1420 Multilabel Counter (PerkinElmer).
6. pH meter.
7. Vortex Genie 2 or similar benchtop vortex.
8. Multichannel pipettes, tips and solution basins.
9. Ultrathin pipette tips such as Multiflex Round tips (Sorenson Bioscience, Inc.).
10. 15-mL polypropylene tubes.
11. 1.5-mL microcentrifuge tubes.

3 Methods

For each vaccine sample type to be tested, one 96-well black, flat bottomed assay plate will be used. This method records how to run each set of standards in triplicate, and each vaccine test sample supernatant or pellet in up to six replicates. A control formulation or other standard sample can be added to the plate if desired. Placebo formulation samples (saline and Alhydrogel® formulation only) are run in replicates on the plate to record background responses for the OPA reagent. A schematic is provided (Figs. 1 and 2) as an example for loading the plate. Note that the Wallac Victor^3 or similar instrument should be allowed to warm up for at least 15 min prior to use. Total set up time should be approximately 2–3 h, with the plate being read within 5–10 min of loading. All preparations and assay reading occur at room temperature.

	1	2	3	4	5	6	7	8	9	10	11	12
A	Placebo Super 2	Placebo Super 2	Placebo Super 2	Placebo Super 2	Placebo Super 2	Placebo Pellet	Placebo Pellet	Placebo Pellet	Placebo Pellet	Placebo Pellet	Control PELLET	Control Super 2
B	OPA reagent only	400 μg/mL STD	200 μg/mL STD	100 μg/mL STD	50 μg/mL STD	25 μg/mL STD	12.5 μg/mL STD	6.25 μg/mL STD	3.125 μg/mL STD	1.5625 μg/mL STD	Control PELLET	Control Super 2
C	OPA reagent only	400 μg/mL STD	200 μg/mL STD	100 μg/mL STD	50 μg/mL STD	25 μg/mL STD	12.5 μg/mL STD	6.25 μg/mL STD	3.125 μg/mL STD	1.5625 μg/mL STD	Control PELLET	Control Super 2
D	OPA reagent only	400 μg/mL STD	200 μg/mL STD	100 μg/mL STD	50 μg/mL STD	25 μg/mL STD	12.5 μg/mL STD	6.25 μg/mL STD	3.125 μg/mL STD	1.5625 μg/mL STD	Control PELLET	Control Super 2
E	Vial 1 Super 2	Vial 2 Super 2	Vial 3 Super 2	Vial 4 Super 2	Vial 5 Super 2	Vial 6 Super 2	Vial 1 PELLET	Vial 2 PELLET	Vial 3 PELLET	Vial 4 PELLET	Vial 5 PELLET	Vial 6 PELLET
F	Vial 1 Super 2	Vial 2 Super 2	Vial 3 Super 2	Vial 4 Super 2	Vial 5 Super 2	Vial 6 Super 2	Vial 1 PELLET	Vial 2 PELLET	Vial 3 PELLET	Vial 4 PELLET	Vial 5 PELLET	Vial 6 PELLET
G	Vial 1 Super 2	Vial 2 Super 2	Vial 3 Super 2	Vial 4 Super 2	Vial 5 Super 2	Vial 6 Super 2	Vial 1 PELLET	Vial 2 PELLET	Vial 3 PELLET	Vial 4 PELLET	Vial 5 PELLET	Vial 6 PELLET
H	Vial 1 Super 2	Vial 2 Super 2	Vial 3 Super 2	Vial 4 Super 2	Vial 5 Super 2	Vial 6 Super 2	Vial 1 PELLET	Vial 2 PELLET	Vial 3 PELLET	Vial 4 PELLET	Vial 5 PELLET	Vial 6 PELLET

Fig. 1 Example of sample loading schema for OPA assay

	1	2	3	4	5	6	7	8	9	10	11	12
B	OPA reagent only	200 μg/mL STD	150 μg/mL STD	100 μg/mL STD	75 μg/mL STD	50 μg/mL STD	25 μg/mL STD	12.5 μg/mL STD	6.25 μg/mL STD	3.125 μg/mL STD	Control PELLET	Control Super 2

Fig. 2 Alternate standard row schema (*see* **Note 4**)

3.1 Preparation of Saline Solution

1. The vaccine of interest should contain between 25 and 400 μg/mL of antigen on Alhydrogel. The amount of Alhydrogel should also be known. This will be called the Vaccine Test sample.
2. Test the pH of the Vaccine Test sample at RT. Prepare approximately 200 mL of the same solution used to constitute the vaccine, and adjust the pH to match the pH of the Vaccine Test sample using sodium hydroxide or hydrochloric acid (for this procedure description, we use 0.9 % Saline for Injection as the buffer), (*see* **Note 2**).

3.2 Preparation of Vaccine Test and Control Formulation Samples

1. Use a minimum of at least three separate vials or aliquots containing at least 1.0 mL each of the vaccine to be tested. If a control formulation (for reference) is desired, obtain at least one vial/aliquot in 1.0 mL for this sample. Label each test sample numerically (i.e., 1–6 or "Control" according to the number of Vaccine Test samples or if a control formulation is used).
2. Vortex each vial for 1 min at a medium to medium low speed setting (~3) on a Vortex Genie 2 or similar vortex. This should not be a rapid vortex, but just enough to resuspend the Alhydrogel at the bottom of the vial/aliquot. Transfer 1.0 mL of each formulation into a new, sterile microcentrifuge tube labeled "Pellet" for the Vaccine Test samples 1–6, and label any control formulation as "Control" as appropriate.

3. Centrifuge the microcentrifuge tubes at 16,000 × *g* for 2 min. This will pellet the Alhydrogel in the Vaccine Test and Control samples.
4. Using a 200-μL ultrathin pipette tip carefully measure the volume of and transfer all supernatant from above the pellet to a new sterile microcentrifuge tube, labeled "Super 1" 1–6 or "Control" as appropriate. Be careful not to disturb the pellets. Record the volumes of the supernatants transferred. Store the tubes containing the pelleted Alhydrogel® at RT in a separate microcentrifuge tube rack.
5. Spin all "Super 1" tubes again at 16,000 × *g* for 2 min. Transfer the topmost 700 μL of each "Super 1" tube into a new sterile microcentrifuge tube labeled "Super 2" and 1–6 or "Control" as appropriate.
6. Set the "Super 2" samples aside. Just prior to loading the samples into the 96-well black microtiter plate, centrifuge the "Super 2" tubes as in **step 3** of Subheading 3.2. Use only the topmost portion of each "Super 2" tube as the supernatant sample loaded onto the plate.
7. Obtain the "Pellet" tubes reserved at RT in **step 4** of Subheading 3.2. Obtain the supernatant volumes recorded in **step 4** of Subheading 3.2.
8. Resuspend the "Pellet" samples individually by adding the same volume of pH-adjusted saline or solution prepared in **step 2** of Subheading 3.1 as the volume of supernatant that was initially recorded as transferred for each tube in **step 4** of Subheading 3.2. Resuspend by carefully pipetting the pellet up and down, then vortex at a medium setting (5.5 on a Vortex Genie 2) by just briefly pulsing ~3 times. The pellets should each be approximately 1.0 mL after resuspension, to match the original volume of the vaccine sample.

3.3 Preparation of Antigen/Alhydrogel® Standards

A freshly prepared vaccine formulation is made and used to generate a standard curve. For this example, we use 1600 μg/mL Alhydrogel® as the concentration of Alhydrogel® in the Vaccine Test samples, and we prepare the standards at the same Alhydrogel® concentration.

1. Vigorously mix the Alhydrogel® 2 % stock from Brenntag for at least 2 min to thoroughly resuspend the gel. Transfer 1 mL of the Alhydrogel® to an microcentrifuge tube labeled "Alhydrogel."
2. Into a new microcentrifuge tube labeled "10,000 μg/mL Alhydrogel for STD 1", transfer 100 μL of the Alhydrogel® from the 1 mL aliquot in **step 1** of Subheading 3.3. Add 100 μL of pH-adjusted saline from **step 2** of Subheading 3.1 and vortex at 5.5 (Vortex Genie 2) for 1 min. This tube now

contains 10,000 μg/mL Alhydrogel® in saline and will be used for preparing the standards.

3. Use the known amount of Alhydrogel® in the Vaccine Test sample to prepare a Placebo formulation, and the appropriate standards. Transfer 10.35 mL of the pH-adjusted saline from **step 2** of Subheading 3.1 into a 15-mL polypropylene tube labeled "Placebo: 1600 μg/mL Alhydrogel". Transfer the 0.9 mL remaining in the stock "Alhydrogel" tube from **step 1** of Subheading 3.3 into the 15-mL tube containing saline. Wash the "Alhydrogel" tube twice with 1 mL of the saline/ Alhydrogel® mixture in the "Placebo: 1600 μg/mL Alhydrogel" 15-mL tube and mix well to ensure all 0.9 mL of "Alhydrogel" was transferred to the 15-mL tube. The "Placebo: 1600 μg/mL Alhydrogel" tube will be added directly to the 96-well plate to prepare both the standards and to obtain background values for the assay.
4. Transfer 1 mL of "Placebo: 1600 μg/mL Alhydrogel" to a new sterile microcentrifuge tube, and process the sample in the same way as the Vaccine Test samples in **steps 2** through **8** of Subheading 3.2. Label these "Placebo Pellet" and "Placebo Super 2" samples.
5. In a new microcentrifuge tube labeled "STD1" add the appropriate amount of antigen, pH-adjusted saline and "10,000 μg/ mL Alhydrogel" to prepare the highest standard and Alhydrogel® concentration desired (*see* **Note 3**). This example will use a concentration of 400 μg/mL antigen (*see* **Note 4**). Prepare a minimum of 300 μL of formulation in order to run the standards in triplicate (80 μL of formulation per set of standards is required).

3.4 Preparing the Fluorescence Reader

1. Our lab uses the Wallac Victor³ 1420 basic bench top fluorescence reader for this assay. The instrument is allowed to warm up for at least 15 min prior to reading plates.
2. The plates should be read at ~1, 5, and 10 min by the same protocol, with 340 nm excitation/455 nm emission. Each plate should have all wells read in about 2 min (*see* **Note 5**).

3.5 Preparing the Assay Plate and Running the Assay

1. Using Figs. 1 and 2, and based on your own requirements, design the plate loading schema you will follow prior to loading any samples. From 4–6 vials can be analyzed per plate, depending on the number of replicates desired for each sample. We typically use 4–6 replicates of each sample. Figure 1 represents the use of four replicate samples for each of six Vaccine Test samples (vials) tested.
2. Mix the "Placebo: 1600 μg/mL Alhydrogel" tube from **step 3** of Subheading 3.3 well by inversion and vortexing. Transfer the contents of the tube into a sterile solution basin, and using

a multichannel pipette (12 channel), quickly mix and then add 40 μL of "Placebo: 1600 μg/mL Alhydrogel" to each well 3–10 in Rows B-D according to the provided schematics (see Figs. 1 and 2) (*see* **Note 6**).

3. Quickly and gently mix the "STD1" tube to ensure all Alhydrogel is resuspended thoroughly. Using a pipet, add 40 μL of "STD1" to each of wells 2 and 3 in rows B-D. Well 2 will contain 40 μL and well 3 will now contain 80 μL total volume.
4. To prepare the Standard sets on the plate, use a multichannel pipette (12 channel) with only three consecutive tips attached. Prepare serial dilutions by first mixing the 80 μL in well 3 of rows B-D gently by withdrawing and dispensing up and down ten times. Change tips, and transfer 40 μL from well 3 to well 4 and mix by withdrawing and dispensing up and down ten times. Change tips and transfer 40 μL from well 4 to 5. Repeat the mixing and transfer steps for Standard wells 5–10. After mixing well 10, remove 40 μL from well 10 and discard. There should now be 40 μL of each standard in wells 2–10 of 3 rows, B–D.
5. Obtain the Vaccine Test "Super 2" and "Pellet" samples tubes from **steps 6** and **8** of Subheading 3.2. Using Fig. 1 as an example, the wells in Column 1, Rows E–H, on the 96-well black microtiter plate will be the "Super 2" samples obtained from Vaccine Test sample vial 1, and Column 7, Rows E-H will be the "Pellet" samples from Vaccine Test sample vial 1. Remaining Vaccine, Control and Placebo samples are loaded into the plate as indicated. Samples will be loaded in 40-μL volumes with 4 or 5 (control or placebo) replicates of each "Super 2" or "Pellet" portion. Change tips after a single dispensing of any sample, and expel sample from tips completely into well.
6. Centrifuge the "Super 2" tubes as in **step 3** of Subheading 3.2, just prior to loading the samples into the plate. Use only the topmost portion of each "Super 2" tube as the supernatant sample. Load the number of replicates (4 in Fig. 1) of 40 μL each of "Super 2" to the appropriate wells as indicated in your schema.
7. Quickly vortex the "Pellet" samples to thoroughly resuspend the Alhydrogel® just prior to loading into the plate. Load the number of replicates (4 in Fig. 1) of 40 μL each of "Pellet" to the appropriate wells as indicated in the schema.
8. Any wells that remain empty (in Fig. 1, this is Column 1, Rows B–D) will be filled with OPA reagent only, and can be used to evaluate background level of the reagent.
9. Once all samples are loaded into the plate, prepare for using the OPA reagent. Dim the environment by reducing light (especially direct light sources), and have aluminum foil prepared to

cover both the solution basin that will hold the OPA reagent and the microtiter plate (*see* **Note 1**). Have 2 × 15-mL aliquots warmed to RT within 30 min. Do not allow the reagent to sit at RT for an extended period of time prior to use (over 2 h).

10. In the low-light environment, quickly add the 2 × 15-mL OPA reagent aliquots to the solution basin and cover with foil. Using a 12-channel pipette, draw up 200 μL of OPA reagent into the pipette tips and then dispense back into the solution basin to wet the tips. Then draw up 200 μL OPA reagent and transfer to the 12 wells in Row A. Work quickly to add the reagent, but work carefully to avoid introducing air bubbles to the wells by not expelling all reagent in the pre-wetted tips. Discard the tips, and repeat this process for each row. Keep the foil on the plate and the solution basin between transfers.
11. Immediately transfer the covered plate to the Wallac Victor[3] analyzer and gently shake the plate 5–10 times while it is in the plate holder to remove any air bubbles. Observe the wells and note if any air bubbles remain (*see* **Note 7**).
12. The plate should be analyzed at the time points that are determined for each vaccine to be most appropriate. Our lab records readings at ~1, 5, and 10 min, which is appropriate for our vaccines to obtain the strongest and most consistent mean fluorescence signal (*see* **Note 5**).

3.6 Calculating the Concentrations in the Samples Using Linear Regression

1. Remove any value that is 15 % different than the mean reading (*see* **Note 8**).
2. The average value of each set of replicates is obtained. For example, according to the Fig. 1 schema, the five replicates of the Placebo "Pellet" sample are averaged to obtain the Placebo "Pellet" fluorescence value. Once averages from all sample types are obtained, the average of the Placebo "Pellet" and Placebo "Super 2" samples is subtracted from the average of the "Pellet" and "Super 2" Vaccine Test and Control sets to eliminate background from Alhydrogel and buffer components (i.e., use the Placebo "Pellet" average to subtract for background of Vaccine Test "Pellet" samples and use the average of the Placebo "Super 2" samples to subtract from the Vaccine Test "Super 2" supernatant samples).
3. A standard curve is generated by linear regression using the average fluorescence values obtained from each standard concentration, subtracting the average Placebo "Pellet" value, then calculating the amount of antigen in each sample from the linear equation ($y = mx + b$, with the R^2 value for the curve at ≥ 0.98 to be considered valid). The fluorescence values obtained for each sample type are then converted into concentration values by fitting each average value to the curve generated by the standards.

4 Notes

1. The OPA reagent should be stored at 2–8 °C, and protected from light at all times. It is advised to prepare and store aliquots of 15 mL in polypropylene tubes (like Falcon or Corning). All aliquots should be wrapped or covered in aluminum foil. OPA reagent aliquots prepared in advance should be warmed to room temperature no more than 2 h prior to use. Only bring to room temperature the amount of reagent that will be needed for the assay(s). For each 96-well plate, 2 × 15 mL aliquots should be used. After being warmed, aliquots should be discarded if not used. Use only fresh aliquots (unopened) for each assay. Discard the original reagent bottle after it has been opened for more than 2 months.

   While working with the OPA reagent during the assay, it is advised to wrap or cover any tube, plate, or aliquot that will contain the OPA reagent with aluminum foil and to work quickly in a dimmed environment.

2. Buffers containing primary amines, such as Tris or glycine, will interfere with the assay. Adjusting the pH of the buffer is not necessary if the vaccine is formulated in PBS. You may wish to sterile filter the solution prior to use, but this is not necessary.
3. The antigen used should be, for best accuracy, the same lot of material used to prepare the vaccine sample, or a reference lot of antigen that is equivalent to that in the vaccine.
4. Standards are determined by directly evaluating each antigen in a series of these assays, to ascertain the most appropriate range for each product. In our experience, the assay is most sensitive and best used initially between 25 and 400 μg/mL antigen. One can also narrow the standard range by preparing two separate high standard stocks, for example, a 200 μg/mL and a 150 μg/mL stock, and then diluting them separately on the plate to obtain a tighter range than a 1:1 serial dilution of just the 200 μg/mL stock would provide. For example, the 200 μg/mL stock is diluted from well 2 to well 4, and the 150 μg/mL is diluted from well 3 to well 5, to produce a range that is 200, 150, 100, 75, 50, 25, 12.5, 6.25 μg, etc. on the plate. See Fig. 2.
5. Evaluations are performed by running the same plate at various time points and then analyzing the resulting fluorescence values. Suggested time points for initial investigation are 1, 5, and 10 min. At 5 min the overall accuracy and mean fluorescent response is the most consistent for our vaccine products. An analysis at 10 min is done as well and serves as a back-up in case of problems when running multiple plates on the same types of samples—if for some reason a delay beyond 5 min occurs for one plate, the 10 min analyses can be used to obtain

similar data sets between plates. As each analysis takes ~2–2.5 min, it is difficult to effectively read the plate at less than 2 min or between 5 and 10 min consistently. The fluorescence values decreased slightly as incubation time increases.

6. If more standards are desired, then additional wells/rows can be used, with other replicates reduced.
7. Air bubbles can alter the fluorescence values obtained. Often they can be eliminated by gently shaking the plate. If a bubble persists, a sterile ultrathin pipette tip can be used to remove it, but the well should still be noted in case the value appears vastly different from the other replicates in the sample set. This value should then be eliminated from the final analysis.
8. Air bubbles or other contaminants such as dust may infrequently contribute to outlying fluorescence readings.

Acknowledgement

This work was supported by the Intramural Research Program of the National Institute of Allergy and Infectious Diseases, National Institutes of Health.

References

1. Zhu D, Saul A, Huang S, Martin LB, Miller LH, Rausch KM (2009) Use of *o*-phthalaldehyde assay to determine protein contents of Alhydrogel-based vaccines. Vaccine 27(43):6054–6059
2. Shore PA, Burkhalter A, Cohn VH (1959) A method for the fluorometric assay of histamine in tissues. J Pharmacol Exp Ther 127:182–186
3. Cohn VH Jr, Shore PA (1961) A microfluorometric method for the determination of agmatine. Anal Biochem 2(3):237–241
4. Benson JR, Hare PE (1975) O-phthalaldehyde: fluorogenic detection of primary amines in the picomole range. Comparison with fluorescamine and ninhydrin. Proc Natl Acad Sci 72(2):619–622
5. Avarez-Coque MCG, Hernández MJM, Camañas RMV, Fernández CM (1989) Studies on the formation and stability of isoindoles derived from amino acids, o-phthalaldehyde and N-acetyl-cysteine. Anal Biochem 180: 172–176
6. Kang SL, Dennis GD (1978) Fluorometric amino-acid analysis with o-phthaldialdehyde (OPA). Int J Biochem 9(7):457–467
7. Molnár-Perl I (2001) Derivatization and chromatographic behavior of the o-phthaldialdehyde amino acid derivatives obtained with various SH-group-containing additives. J Chromatogr A 913(1–2):283–302
8. Church FC, Porter DH, Catignani GL, Swaisgood HE (1985) An o-phthalaldehyde spectrophotometric assay for proteinases. Anal Biochem 146(2):343–348
9. Hapuarachchi S, Janaway GA, Aspinwall CA (2006) Capillary electrophoresis with a UV light-emitting diode source for chemical monitoring of native and derivatized fluorescent compounds. Electrophoresis 27(20):4052–4059
10. Go K, Horikawa Y, Garcia R, Villarreal FJ (2008) Fluorescent method for detection of cleaved collagens using O-phthaldialdehyde (OPA). J Biochem Biophys Methods 70(6): 878–882
11. Frank MP, Powers RW (2007) Simple and rapid quantitative high-performance liquid chromatographic analysis of plasma amino acids. J Chromatogr B 852(1–2):646–649
12. Roth M (1971) Fluorescence reaction for amino acids. Anal Chem 7:880–8822
13. Wong OS, Sternson LA, Schowen RL (1985) Reaction of o-phthalaldehyde with alanine and thiols: kinetics and mechanism. J Am Chem Soc 107(22):6421–6422

Chapter 20

Staining and Transfer Techniques for SDS-PAGE Gels to Minimize Oil-in-Water Emulsion Adjuvant Interference

Alicia M. Schwartz, Michelle Y. Chan, Dawn M. Fedor, Sandra J. Sivananthan, and Ryan M. Kramer

Abstract

Adjuvants in modern vaccines boost and shape immune responses and allow for antigen dose-sparing. Analysis of protein antigens in the presence of adjuvants can prove challenging, especially if the adjuvant interferes with visualization of the protein band on an SDS-PAGE gel. In this chapter, a variety of different techniques are presented to mitigate the interference of a nanoemulsion adjuvant, GLA-SE, with different recombinant proteins of varying molecular weight by addressing sample preparation and staining methods.

Key words Antigen, Adjuvant, SDS-PAGE, PVDF membrane, Coomassie stain, Gold stain, Silver stain

1 Introduction

Adjuvants are a critical element of modern vaccine formulations with the ability to boost immune responses and allow antigen dose sparing [1–3]. Studying the interactions between antigens and adjuvants in vaccine formulations allows understanding of vaccine efficacy, stability, and mechanism of action [3–5]. While aluminum salt adjuvants are the most commonly used type of adjuvant [6], emulsion-based adjuvants are also widely used in vaccine development [7]. Both antigen–adjuvant systems have proven a challenge in gel electrophoresis. For an aluminum-based adjuvant mixture, where the quantity of adsorbed antigen requires direct measurement, a desorption may be used whereby the antigen–adjuvant solution is mixed with a desorption buffer, centrifuged, and the antigen-containing supernatant is analyzed [8, 9]. An extraction method can also be utilized in oil-containing adjuvants, allowing the protein to run on a gel unobstructed [10, 11]. However, extractions require sample manipulation and do not guarantee antigen integrity [8, 11], emphasizing the need for adjuvant-compatible electrophoretic methods.

Christopher B. Fox (ed.), *Vaccine Adjuvants: Methods and Protocols*, Methods in Molecular Biology, vol. 1494,
DOI 10.1007/978-1-4939-6445-1_20, © Springer Science+Business Media New York 2017

Described below are four different staining protocols for antigen–adjuvant mixtures, Coomassie stain on tris–glycine gel or polyvinylidene fluoride (PVDF) membrane [12, 13], gold stain on PVDF membrane and silver stain on tris–glycine gel [14]. Each of these protocols has advantages and disadvantages based on protein molecular weight and load mass. While these methods are not novel, they have been optimized to enhance band intensity of the antigen while minimizing interference by the nanoemulsion adjuvant, GLA-SE.

2 Materials

Make all solutions as directed by the manufacturer using ultrapure water for all dilutions. Use analytical grade or higher purity reagents for all reagents not included in kits. Always use clean vessels when preparing solutions. Mix all prepared solutions well and store at room temperature unless otherwise noted. Store all reagents as directed by manufacturer.

2.1 Coomassie Stain on Tris–Glycine Gel

1. Novex tris–glycine gels: 4–20% tris–glycine gel, 1.0 mm.
2. SDS-PAGE running buffer: 1× tris–glycine SDS running buffer.
3. Reducing sample buffer: 4× LDS sample buffer with 5% (v/v) β-mercaptoethanol (βME). Remove Novex NuPAGE 4× LDS sample buffer from 4 °C storage and equilibrate to room temperature. Vortex contents and test that solution is fully soluble by pulling 500 μL of buffer into pipette tip and looking for bubbles or obstructions in tip. If bubbles or an obstruction are visible, return as much of the buffer to the bottle as possible and allow to sit for several minutes longer. Vortex and repeat solubility check until the solution appears to be fully soluble. Remove 9.5 mL of the 4× buffer from the bottle and add into a 15 mL Falcon tube. Add 0.5 mL of βME. Vortex solution and aliquot 0.5 mL into microcentrifuge tubes. Freeze aliquots at −20 °C for storage up to 6 months. For an in-use aliquot, retain at 4 °C.
4. SDS solution: 20% (w/v) sodium dodecyl sulfate (SDS).
5. Stain: Coomassie stain for SDS-PAGE gels (Novex SimplyBlue SafeStain).
6. VWR rocking platform, model 200.

2.2 Coomassie Stain on PVDF Membrane

1. Transfer Buffer: 12 mM tris base, 10 mM glycine, and 20% (v/v) methanol. Transfer Chamber: Blotting chamber for membrane transfer such as XCell II™ Blot Module (Life Technologies).
2. Sponge Pads: Sponge Pads for Blotting (Life Technologies).

3. Membranes: 0.2-μm PVDF membrane with filter paper sandwich (Life Technologies).
4. Membrane Rinse 1: 0.1% (w/v) Tween 20 in PBS.
5. Membrane Rinse 2: 1× PBS (135 mM NaCl, 2.7 mM potassium chloride, 4.3 mM sodium phosphate, 1.4 mM potassium phosphate, pH 7.2)
6. Stain: 10% (w/v) Coomassie, 50% (v/v) methanol, 7% (v/v) acetic acid.
7. Destain: 50% (v/v) methanol, 7% (v/v) acetic acid.

2.3 Gold Stain on PVDF Membrane

1. Stain: Gold stain for PVDF membranes such as Colloidal Gold Total Protein Stain (Bio-Rad).

2.4 Silver Stain on Tris–Glycine Gel

1. Fix: 50% (v/v) ethanol, 10% (v/v) acetic acid.
2. Ethanol solution: 30% (v/v) ethanol.
3. Silver Stain: Sensitizing, staining, and developing solutions. The manufacturer's procedure outlined in the ProteoSilver™ Silver Stain Kit (Sigma) was followed to prepare the sensitizer, silver, and developer solutions.
4. Staining Tray: A tray for staining the gel with a plug that allows hands-free drainage.

3 Methods

Exact protein load masses are not specified here since different proteins will stain with different sensitivities and limits can be determined by experimentation. Generally, in our experience, a 0.5–2-μg protein load can be visualized easily with a Coomassie stained SDS-PAGE. When working with protein loads in the 5–50 ng range, silver stain works well (*see* Fig. 1). In cases where oil from the emulsion adjuvant is electrophoresed into the gel and interferes with the protein band, a membrane transfer is recommended. We have successfully stained PVDF-membranes using Coomassie stain for a 0.5–2-μg protein load and gold stain for a 10–100-ng protein load (*see* Figs. 2 and 3, respectively).

3.1 Coomassie Stain on Tris–Glycine Gel (See Note 1)

1. Dispense antigen–adjuvant solution into a 0.6-mL microcentrifuge tube in a sufficient volume for the desired load of protein. Add the 4× reducing sample buffer to achieve a 1× final concentration by pipetting up and down into solution to mix (*see* **Note 2**).
2. Heat prepared samples in a 90 °C water bath for 15 min. When done, remove from water bath and place in a room temperature water bath for 1 min.
3. Centrifuge samples for 30 s at 400 × *g* (*see* **Note 3**).

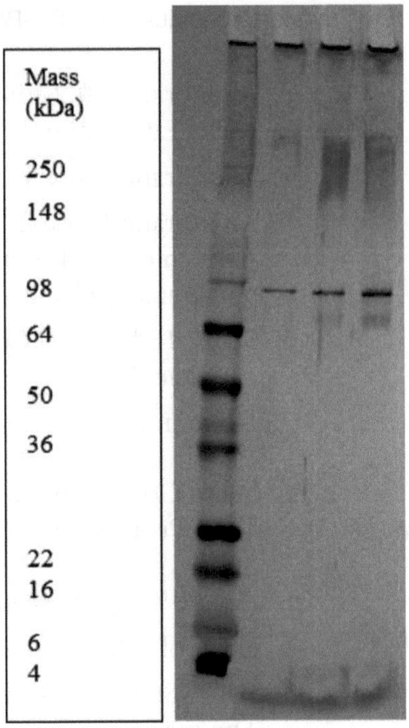

Fig. 1 93 kDa antigen and GLA-SE silver stained gel. Lane content from *left* to *right*: SeeBlue Plus2 prestained standard (*lane 1*), 5.5 ng antigen (*lane 2*), 11.25 ng antigen (*lane 3*), 22.5 ng antigen (*lane 4*)

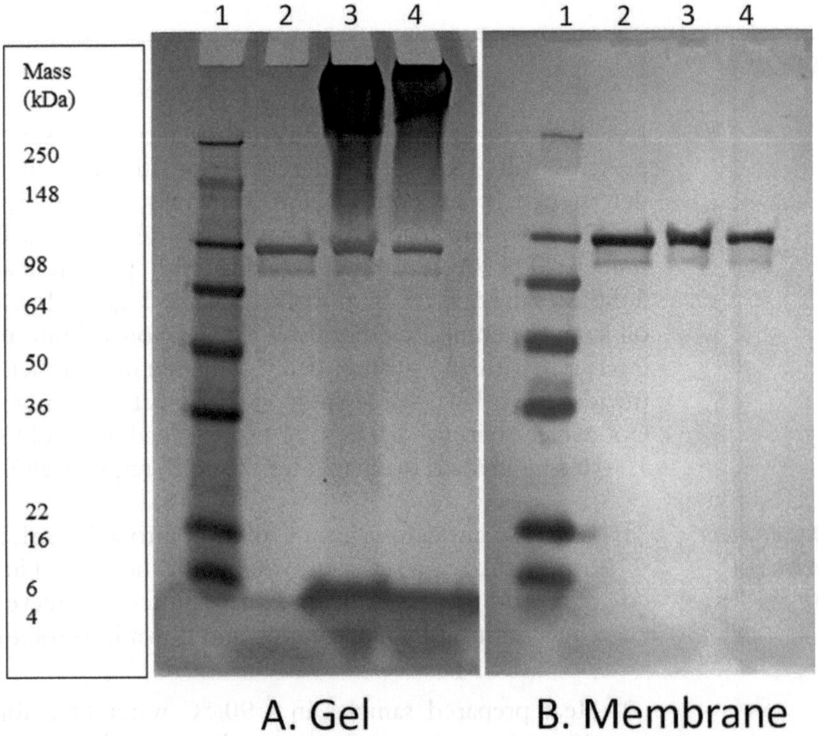

Fig. 2 93 kDa antigen and GLA-SE Coomassie-stained gel (**a**) and Coomassie-stained PVDF membrane (**b**) using SimplyBlue SafeStain. Gels were loaded with SeeBlue Plus2 prestained standard (*lane 1*), 1 μg antigen alone (*lane 2*), 1 μg antigen in presence of GLA-SE (*lane 3*), and 0.5 μg antigen in presence of GLA-SE (*lane 4*)

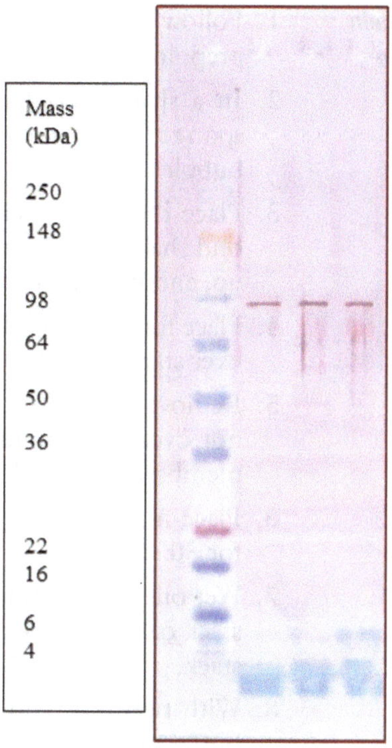

Fig. 3 93 kDa antigen and GLA-SE gold stained PVDF membrane. Lane content from *left* to *right*: SeeBlue Plus2 prestained standard (*lane 1*), 5.5 ng antigen (*lane 2*), 11.25 ng antigen (*lane 3*), 22.5 ng antigen (*lane 4*)

4. Into an XCell SureLock™ Mini-Cell, place tris–glycine gel into chamber. Lock gel in with plastic lock and fill central chamber completely with running buffer. Fill the back chamber with enough running buffer so that the level of buffer is lower than the central chamber by approximately 1 in.
5. Pipette 200 μL of running buffer into each lane of the gel to rinse lanes prior to loading protein.
6. Load 10 μL of SeeBlue Plus2 Prestained Standard into one lane of the gel, followed by full volume of prepared samples in remaining lanes. Place lid on cell.
7. Attach 4 mm PowerPac™ adaptor to cell electrodes and plug into PowerPac™ Basic power supply. Turn voltage up to 180 V and run time to 65 min. Press run.
8. When electrophoresis is complete, crack open case and use a spatula to remove gel foot. Place gel in water-filled dish and rock for 5 min.
9. Decant water and fill dish with enough SimplyBlue SafeStain to cover gel. Cover the dish and rock overnight to stain. Destain by decanting stain and filling dish with water. Exchange water out every couple of hours until the gel is adequately destained.

3.2 Coomassie Stain on PVDF Membrane (See Note 4)

1. Follow the method in **steps 1–7** of Subheading 3.1 for sample prep, load, and run of SDS-PAGE (*see* **Note 5**).
2. In a shallow container filled with transfer buffer, soak 8–9 sponge pads, pressing and submerging fully to remove bubbles.
3. Place the positive electrode of the transfer chamber in a second shallow container, so that the inside of the chamber faces up, and fill container with an inch of transfer buffer.
4. Place four sponges down on electrode and pour transfer buffer over stack.
5. Remove membrane from filter sandwich by squirting methanol over the membrane to hydrate it, then gently pull the membrane off the filter with tweezers.
6. Place membrane in container with methanol and gently rock for 30 s.
7. Wet one filter in transfer buffer and immediately add it to the stack of sponges on the electrode. Pour transfer buffer on the stack.
8. With tweezers, add membrane on top of filter. Pour transfer buffer on the stack.
9. Remove gel from cell and break open casing (*see* **Note 6**). Remove the foot and wells of the gel and remove the gel from the plastic case.
10. Gently place the gel on the membrane, pushing out any bubbles that might form between the gel and the membrane. Pour transfer buffer on the stack.
11. Wet remaining filter in transfer buffer and immediately place on top of gel. Pour transfer buffer on the stack.
12. Add final five sponges to the stack, place negative electrode on top of stack, and sandwich chamber together (*see* **Note** 7).
13. Place chamber in XCell SureLock™ Mini-Cell and fill chamber with transfer buffer. Place plastic lock behind the chamber and lock into place. Fill chamber and cell with transfer buffer and place lid on cell.
14. Attach 4 mm PowerPac™ adaptor to cell electrodes and plug into PowerPac™ Basic power supply. Turn voltage up to 60 V until small bubbles are visible, then turn the voltage down to 30 V and run the transfer for 90 min.
15. Upon completion of transfer, remove membrane from stack and place transfer-side up (same orientation as used for packing) in dish filled with Membrane Rinse 1 (PBS/Tween) and rock for 15 min (*see* **Note 8**).
16. Decant and rinse membrane with three exchanges of Membrane Rinse 2 (PBS), rocking each rinse in hand for several seconds prior to decanting liquid.

17. Rinse the membrane with water, decant, and pour enough 10% Coomassie stain in the dish to fully cover the membrane.
18. Allow to rock for 2.5 min, decant the stain and add enough destain to fully cover the membrane.
19. Rock in destain for 1.5 min. Decant destain and allow membrane to rock in water for 10 min (*see* **Note 9**).
20. Remove from water and place on Kimwipes®. Allow membrane to fully dry (*see* **Note 10**).

3.3 Gold Stain on PVDF Membrane (See Note 11)

1. Follow the method in **steps 1–7** of Subheading 3.1 for sample prep, load, and run of SDS-PAGE (*see* **Note 12**).
2. Follow the method in **steps 2–14** of Subheading 3.2 for membrane transfer.
3. Upon completion of transfer, remove membrane from stack and place transfer-side up in dish filled with Membrane Rinse 1 (PBS/Tween) and rock for 15 min (*see* **Note 13**).
4. Decant and rinse membrane with 3 exchanges of Membrane Rinse 2 (PBS), rocking each rinse in hand for several seconds prior to decanting liquid.
5. Rinse the membrane with water, decant, and pour enough Colloidal Gold stain over the membrane to fully submerge the membrane in the stain. Allow the membrane to rock until the bands are clearly visible (*see* **Note 14**).
6. Decant gold stain and rinse the membrane with water. Place the membrane on a Kimwipes® and allow it to fully dry (*see* **Note 15**).

3.4 Silver Stain on Tris–Glycine Gel (See Note 16)

1. Follow the method in **steps 1–7** of Subheading 3.1 for sample prep, load, and run of SDS-PAGE (*see* **Note 17**).
2. When electrophoresis is complete, crack open case and remove gel foot. Place gel in water-filled staining tray and rock for 5 min.
3. Decant water and fill dish with 100 mL of fix solution (*see* **Note 18**).
4. Allow to rock overnight (*see* **Note 19**).
5. Starting with the ethanol wash step, all staining steps are followed exactly as described in the ProteoSilver™ Silver Stain Kit directions from the manufacturer (*see* **Note 20**).

4 Notes

1. This is a standard SDS-PAGE sample preparation and run time for both antigen alone and antigen–adjuvant combination samples. The appropriate staining method to use is dependent on sample concentration, molecular weight of the

antigen, and the identity of the antigen itself. Point to consider: For long term stability studies where protein is expected to degrade to below the detectable limits for Coomassie staining, consider using gold and silver staining which will detect lower concentrations of protein if the same format and stain is preferred for all time points in the study.

2. Be aware of the minimum and maximum load volume per well for the gel being used. Load a volume that completely fills the bottom of the well without exceeding the max load volume. Additional sample modification may be required. For example, if the sample volume is under 10 μL, the remaining volume to 10 μL is made up with the protein buffer and 10 μL of 2× reducing buffer is added to the protein. The 4× reducing buffer is diluted to 2× with water.

3. An alternative sample prep method that mitigates some of the adjuvant interference is as follows (*see* Fig. 4): Dispense 20 μL antigen–adjuvant solution into a 0.6-mL Eppendorf tube. Add 40 μL of 20% SDS to the tube, followed by 20 μL of 4× reducing sample and thoroughly mix with a pipette. Heat prepared samples in a 90 °C water bath for 15 min. Heating the samples for the entire duration is critical to adequately disperse the oil interference at the top of the gel. Even when 20% SDS is not added to the sample, proper heating increases resolution of the band against the adjuvant smear. After 15 min, remove the samples from the water bath and place in room temperature water for 1 min. Centrifuge samples for 30 s at 400×*g*. Run gel and choose a staining method that can be used to detect the final concentration after dilution.

4. This staining method is particularly useful for antigens in the 120–250 kDa range, which will be obstructed by the oil smear of the GLA-SE. This method is better than the Coomassie-stained tris–glycine gel for less concentrated antigen solutions, as it does not require further dilution with 20% SDS. However, it is still inferior to gold and silver stains for antigen detection.

5. In our lab, protein bands have been detected on a Coomassie-stained PVDF-membrane transfer down to 0.1 μg, but a load between 0.5 and 2 μg is recommended for optimum visualization.

6. While not ideal, a gel stored overnight at 4 °C in a plastic-wrapped plastic case was determined to be suitable for transfer. Prior to opening the case, the gels were soaked in water for 10 min to assure they were fully hydrated to minimize tearing.

7. If transferring two membranes, place three sponges on electrode followed by membrane sandwich, two more sponges, another membrane sandwich, and a final 3 sponges. A carefully and fully packed chamber increases chances for a successful transfer.

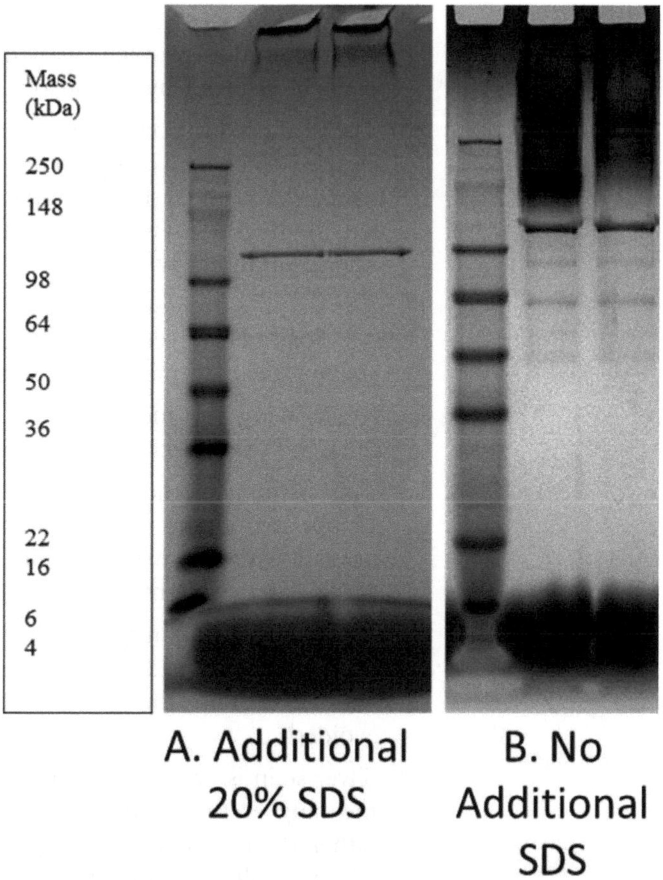

Fig. 4 110 kDa antigen and GLA-SE Coomassie-stained gels. (**a**) Sample preparation included addition of 20 % SDS to the sample for a final SDS concentration of 10 % and a protein load of 0.5 μg (*duplicate lanes shown*). (**b**) Sample preparation excluded addition of 20 % SDS, and had a 2 μg load (same protein, *separate samples shown*)

8. The membrane can also be left in the Membrane Rinse 1 solution to rock overnight with no impact on integrity.
9. For the first 30 s or so of the staining and destaining of the membrane, rock the dish by hand until the liquid appears uniform in color. Without this step stain will diffuse out of the membrane, but settle on the surface, resulting in an uneven background color when the membrane dries.
10. By allowing the membrane to dry fully (2–3 h minimum), lines and other background interferences are minimized.
11. This staining method is ideal for higher molecular weight proteins that are low in concentration. The background for this method, however, tends to be higher than the other methods shown here.

12. A 5.5-ng load of antigen is detectable with this method. A more common problem with this method is an overload of protein. Under 1 μg has proven a reasonable load.
13. The dish used to contain the membrane should be thoroughly cleaned and wiped out prior to use to minimize any contaminants attaching to the membrane. The membrane can also be left in the PBS/Tween solution to rock overnight with no impact on integrity.
14. The staining process can take up to 2 h depending on the antigen load. However, the background increases with longer staining time, so minimizing staining time is ideal.
15. By allowing the membrane to dry fully (2–3 h minimum), lines and other background interferences are minimized.
16. This staining method is ideal for low concentration samples. Unlike membrane transfers, the adjuvant interference is still present with this method, but only minimal staining occurs, making it a viable method for antigen–adjuvant solutions.
17. A 5.5-ng load of antigen is detectable with this method. The same mass-overload problem seen with gold stain is present with silver stain; for best results, a load over 1 μg should be avoided.
18. Silver stain is particularly sensitive to contamination, so using the plug at the bottom of the tray to empty the solutions rather than restraining the gel with a hand is important. In addition, all trays are rinsed with water, sprayed down with IPA, wiped out, and rinsed with water again prior to use.
19. The ProteoSilver™ directions indicate a 20 min rock is sufficient to fix the gel, but advise fixing overnight to reduce background.
20. During the development step, the development of the gel is stopped just before the desired band intensity as the gel will continue to develop for a short time after addition of the stop solution. Stopping the development at this point prevents over-development, as well as minimizes adjuvant staining.

Acknowledgments

We are grateful to Kelly Rausch from the Laboratory of Malaria Immunology and Vaccinology, National Institute of Allergy and Infectious Disease, National Institutes of Health for originally suggesting the 20% SDS-based sample preparation described in **Note 3**.

References

1. Kenney RT, Edelman R (2003) Survey of human-use adjuvants. Expert Rev Vaccines 2(2):167–188
2. Reed SG et al (2009) New horizons in adjuvants for vaccine development. Trends Immunol 30(1):23–32
3. Fox CB et al (2013) Working together: interactions between vaccine antigens and adjuvants. Ther Adv Vaccines 1(1):7–20
4. Kool M, Fierens K, Lambrecht BN (2012) Alum adjuvant: some of the tricks of the oldest adjuvant. J Med Microbiol 61(Pt 7):927–934
5. O'Hagan DT et al (2012) The mechanism of action of MF59 – an innately attractive adjuvant formulation. Vaccine 30(29):4341–4348
6. Petrovsky N, Aguilar JC (2004) Vaccine adjuvants: current state and future trends. Immunol Cell Biol 82(5):488–496
7. Mbow ML et al (2010) New adjuvants for human vaccines. Curr Opin Immunol 22(3): 411–416
8. Zhu D et al (2012) Efficient extraction of vaccines formulated in aluminum hydroxide gel by including surfactants in the extraction buffer. Vaccine 30(2):189–194
9. Rinella JV et al (1998) Elutability of proteins from aluminum-containing vaccine adjuvants by treatment with surfactants. J Colloid Interface Sci 197(1):48–56
10. Lai RP et al (2012) Mixed adjuvant formulations reveal a new combination that elicit antibody response comparable to Freund's adjuvants. PLoS One 7(4):e35083
11. Miles AP, Saul A (2005) Extraction and characterization of vaccine antigens from water-in-oil adjuvant formulations. Methods Mol Biol 308:293–300
12. Millipore (1997) Protein blotting applications guide
13. Pryor JL, Xu W, Hamilton DW (1992) Immunodetection after complete destaining of Coomassie blue-stained proteins on immobilon-PVDF. Anal Biochem 202(1): 100–104
14. Schuchard M, Mehigh R, Kappel W (2003) ProteoSilver™: High Sensitivity Silver Stain for SDS-PAGE. Sigma-Aldrich Corporation https://www.sigmaaldrich.com/content/dam/sigma-aldrich/docs/Sigma/General_Information/vol4-issue1-proteosilver.pdf.

Chapter 21

Interactions Between Antigens and Nanoemulsion Adjuvants: Separation and Characterization Techniques

Michelle Y. Chan, Dawn M. Fedor, Tony Phan, Lucien Barnes V, and Ryan M. Kramer

Abstract

Determining the association of vaccine components in a formulation is of interest for designing and optimizing well characterized vaccines. Three methods are described to assess interactions between protein antigens and oil-in-water nanoemulsion adjuvants. The methods include (1) ultracentrifugation to measure free versus adjuvant-associated protein, (2) size exclusion chromatography (SEC) to qualitatively assess existing interactions, and (3) Native PAGE as a means to visualize the formulation run in its native state on a polyacrylamide gel. As with many techniques, the methods alone are not definitive, but data from multiple orthogonal assays can provide a more complete picture of protein–adjuvant interactions.

Key words Antigen, Adjuvant, Nanoemulsion, Interactions, Association, Separation

1 Introduction

The addition of adjuvants to vaccines significantly increases the potency of protein antigens and allows for shaping of the desired immune response [1–3]. When combining protein antigens with adjuvants, such as aluminum salts and oil-in-water nanoemulsions, insight into the interactions between the two components is useful for optimizing vaccine stability and antigenicty. For example, it has been shown that electrostatic interactions, hydrophobic attraction, and/or ligand exchange [4, 5] drive adsorption of proteins onto aluminum hydroxide [6–8]. Many variables, including protein molecular weight, pH, buffer, and excipients, can significantly affect the degree of adsorption and stability of a formulation [6, 8–10]. Percent of antigen adsorbed can be determined by centrifugation of the formulation followed by the analysis of unbound protein in the supernatant by UV, BCA assay, ELISA, or other standard protein quantitation methods [4, 11]. This information can be useful in designing and optimizing an effective vaccine, since antigen

Christopher B. Fox (ed.), *Vaccine Adjuvants: Methods and Protocols*, Methods in Molecular Biology, vol. 1494,
DOI 10.1007/978-1-4939-6445-1_21, © Springer Science+Business Media New York 2017

adsorption to aluminum salts may or may not be required for efficacy [8, 12]. Methods have also been developed for direct analysis of protein without separation from the aluminum adjuvant. One example is the *o*-phthalaldehyde assay with fluorescence detection for protein quantitation in the presence of aluminum [13]. Another example is Fourier transform infrared spectroscopy to determine changes in the secondary structure of proteins while adsorbed to aluminum adjuvants compared to unbound protein [11, 14, 15].

While multiple methods have been described to examine protein interactions with aluminum compounds, less instruction is published for analyzing protein interactions with nanoemulsions [16, 17]. The lack of methods can be attributed to the difficulty of analyzing a protein in a turbid nanoemulsion solution since spectroscopic methods generally require samples that are transparent. In this chapter, we present three methods to help understand interactions between protein and nanoemulsions. The first method uses ultracentrifugation to separate unbound protein from protein associated to an oil-in-water nanoemulsion by density. The second method uses gravity flow chromatography in a Sepharose column for separation. The third method uses Clear Native PAGE to qualitatively assess protein–nanoemulsion interactions on a gel. The limitations of these methods are that they are generally qualitative, although more quantitative approaches can be developed. All methods shown in this chapter were developed using a 93 kDa protein and a glucopyranosyl lipid adjuvanted stable nanoemulsion (GLA-SE).

2 Materials

2.1 Ultracentrifugation

1. Ultracentrifuge: OptimaTM MAX-XP (Beckman Coulter, Brea, CA, USA).
2. Rotor for 1.5-mL microcentrifuge tubes (Beckman Coulter, Brea, CA, USA).
3. 1.5-mL microcentrifuge tubes.
4. 1-mL syringe needles with 18 G needle.

2.2 SEC by Gravity Flow Gel Filtration

1. Empty Chromatography Columns: 1.5 × 12-cm polypropylene Econo-Pac® columns, 20-mL bed volume (Bio-Rad, Hercules, CA, USA).
2. Female Luer Plugs (Bio-Rad, Hercules, CA, USA).
3. Sepharose CL-4B: 4 % cross-linked agarose gel filtration media, 45–165-μm bead size range (GE Healthcare Life Sciences, Pittsburgh, PA, USA).

2.3 Clear Native PAGE

1. Neat Glycerol.
2. XCell SureLock™ Mini-Cell (Life Technologies, Grand Island, NY, USA).

3. PowerPac™ Basic Power Supply (Bio-Rad, Hercules, CA, USA).
4. NativePAGE™ 4–16% Bis–Tris Protein Gels, 1.0 mm, 10-well (Life Technologies, Grand Island, NY, USA).
5. 1× NativePAGE™ anode buffer is prepared by adding 50 mL of 20× NativePAGE Running Buffer (Life Technologies, Grand Island, NY, USA) to 950 mL of water. Mix well. Note that the cathode buffer containing coomassie dye that is typically used with NativePAGE is not used here.
6. SimplyBlue SafeStain (Life Technologies, Grand Island, NY, USA).
7. 30% (v/v) ethanol solution is prepared by adding 30 mL of 200-proof ethanol to 70 mL of water.

3 Methods

3.1 Ultracentrifugation

Ultracentrifugation can be used to separate components of a protein and emulsion mixture by density (*see* **Note 1**). After ultracentrifugation, since the squalene oil phase is less dense than water, protein associated with the emulsion can be found in the oil phase in the top layer of the sample. The unbound protein will remain in solution below the oil. Fractions of the sample are collected using a pipette or syringe needle and then analyzed for content using SDS-PAGE. Protein alone and emulsion alone controls should also be run for comparison.

1. Add 0.5 mL of sample to a 1.5-mL microcentrifuge tube and load into the ultracentrifuge. Balance the rotor with a mock sample if appropriate.
2. Spin at 186,000 × *g* for 2 h at 4 °C (*see* **Notes 2** and **3**).
3. Carefully remove the sample from the rotor. Examine the tube. If sufficient separation has been achieved, the sample will contain an oil phase at the liquid–air interface and an aqueous phase as the subnatant.
4. Carefully open the tube and place on a stand that allows for the entire tube to be visible (*see* **Note 4**). Place a finger on the top edge of the tube to hold it in a secure position for fraction collection.
5. Collect fractions as follows (*see* Fig. 1a) and dispense into new tubes. Follow safe practices when working with sharps and do not place fingers directly in the path of a needle during collection.
6. Subnatant: Using a syringe held parallel to the benchtop, pierce the lower (approximately 2/3) end of the tube. Bore a hole using the needle and slowly collect approximately 100 μL of subnatant. When performing this step, be consistent with hole placement for all samples. This can be done by using the graduations on the tubes.

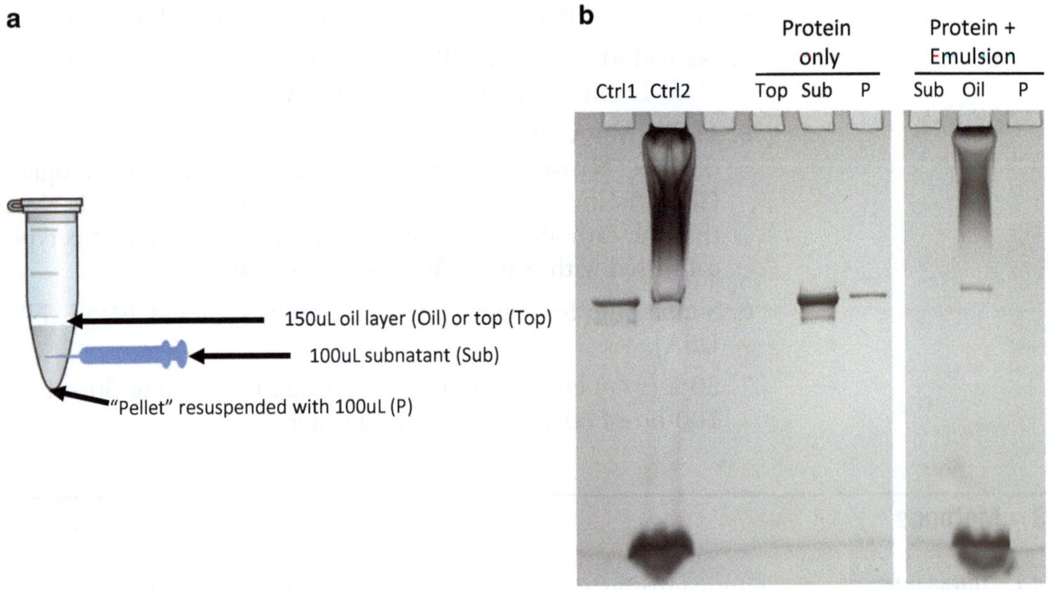

Fig. 1 (**a**) Illustration of sample collection after ultracentrifugation. (**b**) Example reducing SDS-PAGE gel containing sample fractions after ultracentrifugation. The samples run in this example were protein alone and protein + GLA-SE. Control 1 (Ctrl 1) and 2 (Ctrl2) are protein alone and protein + GLA-SE without ultracentrifugation using a 1 μg load. The protein alone sample shows that the protein migrates to the bottom of the tube with some possible pelleting (however, as described in **Note 5**, the "pelleted" protein is 5× concentrated for enhanced visualization). The protein + emulsion sample suggests that the protein is associated with the emulsion since protein is only found in the oil phase and is not found in the subnatant or pellet

7. Oil: Using a pipette, carefully collect the oil layer in 150 μL. Some oil may be left behind and some subnatant may inadvertently be collected. A clean collection is ideal but is not always possible.
8. Remove the remaining sample and discard. This contains a mixture of remaining oil and aqueous subnatant phases.
9. "Pellet" (referring to material that may be pelleted or left behind at the bottom of the tube): Using a pipette, add 100 μL of buffer to the tube and pipette up and down rigorously to resuspend the pellet (*see* **Note 5**).
10. Run collected fractions on an SDS-PAGE gel. Refer to the chapter by Schwartz et al. in this monograph regarding an SDS-PAGE method with samples that contain oil-in-water emulsions.
11. Assess antigen–adjuvant interaction by determining if protein is found within the oil phase of an ultracentrifuged sample. *See* Fig. 1b.

3.2 SEC by Gravity Flow Gel Filtration

This method can be used to separate a formulation containing protein and emulsion using a Sepharose column (*see* **Note 6**). The resulting fractions are run on an SDS-PAGE gel to assess interactions indicated by co-elution. Protein alone and emulsion alone controls should be run for comparison.

1. Equilibrate all materials to room temperature before use.
2. Vigorously shake the container with the Sepharose beads for several minutes to ensure a homogenous mixture.
3. Pour approximately 100 mL into a beaker and let the slurry sit on the benchtop for 5–10 min to degas prior to packing the column (*see* **Note 7**).
4. Snap off the tip at the bottom of the column.
5. Set up the column so that it stands vertically, using a ring stand or rack that allows the bottom of the column to be accessible for flow-through and sample collection. Place an empty container underneath the column to collect flow-through while packing the column.
6. To pack the column, carefully pour approximately 25 mL of slurry into the column in a single pouring motion (*see* **Note 8**). Minimize the introduction of air bubbles by pouring the slurry down a glass rod with the end held against the inside wall of the column.
7. Fill the reservoir with eluent buffer. The eluent should be the same as the buffer used in the sample which will be run through the column.
8. Carefully flush the column with at least three complete column volumes (3 × 20 mL) of eluent (*see* **Note 9**). The column has been properly packed once the packing level stabilizes. If the packing level has not stabilized, continue flushing the column. Do not let the column run dry (*see* **Notes 10** and **11**).
9. When ready to load the sample, allow the buffer in the reservoir to fully enter the column. Then gently add 1 mL of sample (*see* **Note 12**). All additions to the column should be gentle in order to minimize the disturbance of the column surface.
10. Immediately after the sample has fully entered the column, add 1 mL of buffer.
11. Immediately after the 1 mL buffer has fully entered the column, add 2 mL of buffer.
12. Add an additional 1 mL of buffer after the 2 mL of buffer has entered the column and start collecting 1-mL fractions. This fraction is labeled as fraction #4.
13. Continue adding buffer, 1 mL at a time, while collecting 1-mL fractions, ending after fraction #20.
14. These collected fractions can be run on an SDS-PAGE gel to qualitatively assess the interaction of protein and emulsion. Refer to the chapter by Schwartz et al. in this monograph regarding an SDS-PAGE method with samples that contain oil-in-water emulsions.
15. Compare results to protein alone and emulsion alone using this method. To assess antigen–adjuvant interactions, look for changes in protein elution profile and evidence of antigen–adjuvant co-localization. *See* Fig. 2.

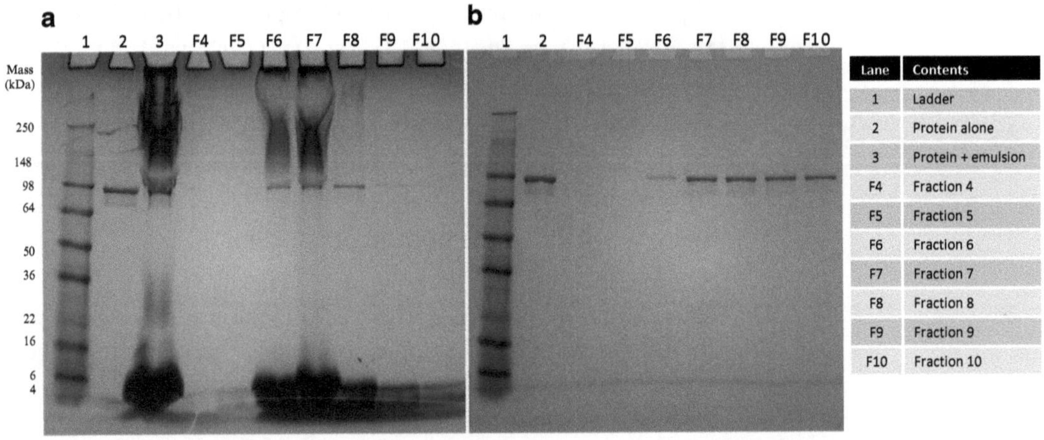

Fig. 2 (**a**) A reducing SDS-PAGE gel containing fractions collected from a protein and emulsion sample (0.1 mg/mL 93 kDa protein + 2 % GLA-SE) separated using a Sepharose column. *Lanes 2* and *3* are protein alone and protein + emulsion controls (without chromatography) loaded at 1 μg of protein per well. The protein co-elutes with the emulsion in fractions 6–8 suggesting protein–emulsion interaction. (**b**) A reducing SDS-PAGE gel containing fractions collected from a protein alone control separated using a Sepharose column. *Lane 2* is protein alone (without chromatography) loaded with 1 μg. The protein starts to elute in fraction 6 and continues to elute strongly through fraction 15 (not shown). Compared to Fig. 2a, a clear shift in protein elution is seen, suggesting interaction between the protein and the emulsion

3.3 Clear Native Page

Clear native PAGE is a useful way to visualize the protein in a protein and nanoemulsion formulation in its native state. In this method, the sample is mixed with glycerol (to increase sample density for gel loading) and then loaded on a Bis–Tris native gel without the addition of any charge modifying agents such as a Coomassie dye, which is used for blue-native PAGE. The Coomassie dye is avoided in this method since protein and emulsion interactions can be altered by its addition. Without an added negative charge shift, the protein migrates according to size, shape, and intrinsic charge in relation to the pore sizes in the gel matrix [18]. Protein alone and emulsion alone controls should also be run for comparison.

1. Assemble the gel cassette in the gel box: remove the gel cassette from its pouch, remove the white tape and comb from the cassette, and lock into place in the gel box.
2. Using 1× NativePAGE anode buffer, completely fill the upper (inner) chamber of the gel box and fill the lower (outer) chamber to a level approximately 1 in. below the inner chamber fill level.
3. Rinse out wells by gently pipetting 1× NativePAGE anode buffer in and out of each well.
4. Prepare sample in 5 % (v/v) glycerol. For example, mix 4 μL of neat glycerol with 76 μL of sample (*see* **Notes 13** and **14**).

5. Load sample for a protein load mass of approximately 3–5 μg. The volume will depend on the sample concentration, taking caution not to exceed the maximum load volume of the well (*see* **Note 15**).
6. Place lid on gel box, turn on power supply, and run gel at 150 V for 4 h or an amount of time optimized for the sample (*see* **Note 16**). Start electrophoresis immediately after loading the gel.
7. Turn off power supply and remove the gel cassette from the gel box. Crack open cassette and carefully transfer gel to a plastic dish containing deionized water. Cut off the foot of the gel using a spatula. Rock for 5 min.
8. Decant water and add enough SimplyBlue SafeStain to generously cover the gel. Rock overnight at room temperature.
9. To destain, decant stain and add enough 30 % ethanol solution to generously cover the gel. Rock at room temperature for 30 min.
10. To assess antigen–adjuvant interactions, compare results against lanes containing protein alone and emulsion alone. For a sample where the protein interacts with the emulsion, less (or no) protein will electrophorese into the gel as compared with protein alone (*see* **Note 17**). *See* Fig. 3.

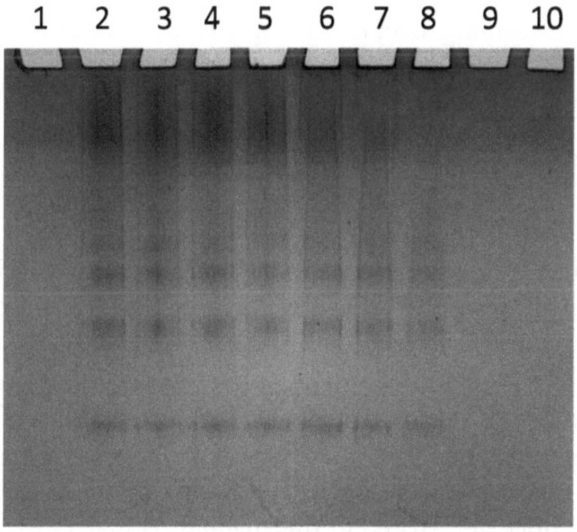

Lane	Contents
1	Buffer Blank
2	Protein alone
3	Protein + 0.01% emulsion
4	Protein + 0.05% emulsion
5	Protein + 0.1% emulsion
6	Protein + 0.5% emulsion
7	Protein + 1.0% emulsion
8	Protein + 2.0% emulsion
9	2.0% emulsion alone
10	Buffer Blank

Fig. 3 A clear-native PAGE containing 0.1 mg/mL protein mixed with 0–2 % emulsion (GLA-SE). Wells were loaded with 2.85 μg protein/lane. *Lane 9* shows that the emulsion does not enter the gel (the oil and lipid components of GLA-SE are stained by Coomassie in reducing SDS-PAGE), so only unbound protein is expected to be electrophoresed into the gel. While fixing protein concentration and increasing emulsion content, the unbound protein becomes less apparent indicating association of protein and adjuvant

4 Notes

1. An alternative to using a standard ultracentrifuge is using an air driven ultracentrifuge (Airfuge®, Beckman Coulter, Brea, CA). Samples can easily be extracted from their Open-Top, Thinwall tubes (Beckman Coulter, Brea, CA) since a syringe needle can more easily pierce these tubes. 175 and 450-μL maximum volume tubes are available so volumes will differ from this method.
2. 186,000 × *g* was chosen for this method based on instrument/rotor maximum speed. Samples can be centrifuged at higher speeds and for a shorter or longer period of time depending on the sample and sample volume used.
3. Rotor may be chilled at 4 °C prior to loading samples.
4. An empty 10–200-μL pipette tip box works well as a stand. Place the bottom of the microcentrifuge tube in one of the holes used for a single tip. The top of the tube is held down by a finger at all times without fully covering the top of the tube.
5. Use the same buffer as used for the protein. A 100-μL resuspension volume will enhance concentration of protein seen on a gel since the original sample volume was 0.5 mL. Alternatively, it may be preferable to use a 0.5-mL resuspension volume to equally evaluate samples in all lanes.
6. See the manufacturer's instructions (GE Healthcare Instructions 71-7098-00 AD) for additional tips on the selection of beads and running samples on Sepharose columns.
7. The beaker can be covered with Parafilm and then sonicated to accelerate the degassing step.
8. The reservoir at the top of the column has a 10-mL capacity. Pouring 5 mL above the 20-mL graduation mark will yield a final pour level just above the reservoir ridge.
9. When adding eluent, be careful to add slowly and evenly around the diameter of the reservoir. The top layers of the beads are very easily disturbed. A flat or upward meniscus is ideal.
10. Make sure that there is always eluent in the reservoir so that the column does not run dry. Attach a Luer plug to the bottom of the column to stop the flow and cover the top of the reservoir if the column is to be left unattended. Columns can be packed in advance and stored in this manner.
11. The flow rate of the gravity fed column can be measured using a graduated cylinder and timer. The flow rate should be stable for an equilibrated column.
12. Volume will depend on concentration of sample. The vendor recommends 2–5 % of the total volume bed (equivalent to 0.4–1.0 mL of sample for a 20-mL column). The sample will be

diluted (approximately threefold) when eluted from the column. Be sure that the eluted concentration is detectable on SDS-PAGE for detection.

13. Positive displacement pipettes can be used to accurately dispense viscous liquids such as glycerol.
14. Concentration and volume can be varied with a target protein load of approximately 3–5 μg per lane. The concentration of glycerol mixed with the sample may also need to be increased (for example, up to 10–20% v/v) depending on the density of the sample, in order to prevent sample migration out of well.
15. When loading the gel, pipette slowly, starting with the tip towards the bottom of the well, and moving the tip up as more volume is added. Keep the gel box containing the loaded samples as stationary as possible after loading. While glycerol is present to allow samples to sink in the well, emulsions can be very buoyant and too much agitation before electrophoresis can result in sample loss.
16. Time will need to be adjusted depending on the protein of interest. Since there is no dye front to help estimate run time, a preliminary experiment varying run time can first be performed.
17. Quantitation of protein band intensity can be performed using ImageJ or similar software. Pixel intensities can be compared between different lanes to more quantitatively assess gel results.

References

1. Kool M, Fierens K, Lambrecht BN (2012) Alum adjuvant: some of the tricks of the oldest adjuvant. J Med Microbiol 61(7):927–934
2. O'Hagan DT, Ott GS, De Gregorio E, Seubert A (2012) The mechanism of action of MF59—an innately attractive adjuvant formulation. Vaccine 30(29):4341–4348
3. Oleszycka E, Lavelle EC (2014) Immunomodulatory properties of the vaccine adjuvant alum. Curr Opin Immunol 28:1–5
4. Iyer S, Robinett RS, HogenEsch H, Hem SL (2004) Mechanism of adsorption of hepatitis B surface antigen by aluminum hydroxide adjuvant. Vaccine 22(11–12):1475–1479
5. Marrack P, McKee AS, Munks MW (2009) Towards an understanding of the adjuvant action of aluminium. Nat Rev Immunol 9(4):287–293
6. al-Shakhshir RH, Regnier FE, White JL, Hem SL (1995) Contribution of electrostatic and hydrophobic interactions to the adsorption of proteins by aluminium-containing adjuvants. Vaccine 13(1):41–44
7. Brewer JM (2006) (How) do aluminium adjuvants work? Immunol Lett 102(1):10–15
8. Huang M, Wang W (2014) Factors affecting alum–protein interactions. Int J Pharm 466(1–2):139–146
9. Peek LJ, Martin TT, Elk Nation C, Pegram SA, Middaugh CR (2007) Effects of stabilizers on the destabilization of proteins upon adsorption to aluminum salt adjuvants. J Pharm Sci 96(3):547–557
10. Salnikova MS, Joshi SB, Rytting JH, Warny M, Middaugh CR (2008) Preformulation studies of Clostridium difficile toxoids A and B. J Pharm Sci 97(10):4194–4207
11. Dowling QM, Schwartz AM, Vedvick TS, Fox CB, Kramer RM (2014) Quantitative measurement of toll-like receptor 4 agonists adsorbed to alhydrogel by fourier transform infrared-attenuated total reflectance spectroscopy. J Pharm Sci 104(2):768–774
12. Romero Mendez IZ, Shi Y, HogenEsch H, Hem SL (2007) Potentiation of the immune response to non-adsorbed antigens by aluminum-containing adjuvants. Vaccine 25(5):825–833

13. Zhu D, Saul A, Huang S, Martin LB, Miller LH, Rausch KM (2009) Use of o-phthalaldehyde assay to determine protein contents of Alhydrogel-based vaccines. Vaccine 27(43):6054–6059
14. Agopian A, Ronzon F, Sauzeat E, Sodoyer R, El Habib R, Buchet R, Chevalier M (2007) Secondary structure analysis of HIV-1-gp41 in solution and adsorbed to aluminum hydroxide by Fourier transform infrared spectroscopy. Biochim Biophys Acta 1774(3):351–358
15. Fox CB, Kramer RM, Barnes VL, Dowling QM, Vedvick TS (2013) Working together: interactions between vaccine antigens and adjuvants. Ther Adv Vaccines 1(1):7–20
16. Fox CB, Barnes VL, Evers T, Chesko JD, Vedvick TS, Coler RN, Reed SG, Baldwin SL (2013) Adjuvanted pandemic influenza vaccine: variation of emulsion components affects stability, antigen structure, and vaccine efficacy. Influenza Other Respir Viruses 7(5):815–826
17. Fox CB, Moutaftsi M, Vergara J, Desbien AL, Nana GI, Vedvick TS, Coler RN, Reed SG (2013) TLR4 ligand formulation causes distinct effects on antigen-specific cell-mediated and humoral immune responses. Vaccine 31(49):5848–5855
18. Wittig I, Schagger H (2005) Advantages and limitations of clear-native PAGE. Proteomics 5(17):4338–4346

Chapter 22

Screening Vaccine Formulations in Fresh Human Whole Blood

Jalil Hakimi, Sepideh Aboutorabian, Frederick To, Salvador F. Ausar, Nausheen Rahman, and Roger H. Brookes

Abstract

Monitoring the immunological functionality of vaccine formulations is critical for vaccine development. While the traditional approach using established animal models has been relatively effective, the use of animals is costly and cumbersome, and animal models are not always reflective of a human response. The development of a human-based approach would be a major step forward in understanding how vaccine formulations might behave in humans. Here, we describe a platform methodology using fresh human whole blood (hWB) to monitor adjuvant-modulated, antigen-specific responses to vaccine formulations, which is amenable to analysis by standard immunoassays as well as a variety of other analytical techniques.

Key words hWB human whole blood, Whole-blood assay, Vaccine formulation screening, Adjuvant modulation, Vaccine, Functionality, Immunomodulation, Cytokine signature

1 Introduction

Understanding the complexity of immunity to vaccine formulations that include potent new adjuvants is a major hurdle to vaccine development. Currently, the only way to truly understand the complex processes has been to inject the vaccine into an animal model, usually mouse, and monitor the response. However, there are known challenges with the use of animal models, one being whether the response in an animal can truly translate to humans [1–4]. This is particularly so when new adjuvants, such as TLR agonists that are known to be species specific, are used [5]. In addition the precise and detailed biochemical analysis used to characterize the vaccine formulation is not complemented with the relatively crude and variable immune response elicited in animal models.

Although there have been enormous efforts towards improving animal models, the development of a robust human-based approach, whether ex vivo or in vitro, would be a major step forward in understanding how vaccine formulations might

Christopher B. Fox (ed.), *Vaccine Adjuvants: Methods and Protocols*, Methods in Molecular Biology, vol. 1494, DOI 10.1007/978-1-4939-6445-1_22, © Springer Science+Business Media New York 2017

behave in humans. A human cell-based assay offers numerous advantages over using live animals, including measurement of responses with physiological relevance to humans, as well as ease in manipulation with a convenient assay format (i.e., in microtiter plates) [6]. Fresh human whole blood (hWB) is ideal to use in such an assay as it retains all of the components in blood and does not require significant sample manipulation [7–13]. This allows the hWB to be cultured in simple culture media almost immediately after withdrawal, maintaining the blood under more physiologically relevant conditions. More importantly, in addition to peripheral blood mononuclear cells (PBMC), which are known to be critical for innate immunity, other cell types such as polymorphonuclear leukocytes (PMNL) are within hWB and these have been found to play a profound role in cellular function and cytokine production (e.g., neutrophils [14–16]); this gives a more comprehensive model of the immune response.

The following protocol describes a simple root methodology to perform a fresh hWB assay to monitor an adjuvant-modulated, antigen-specific response to vaccine formulations over a 6–12-day culture period. This extended culture duration allows monitoring of memory T cell responses (e.g., IFN-γ), and allows for the study of slower-onset adjuvant immunomodulation effects [8]. This is an important feature of the assay as such information can contribute significant insight into an adjuvant's mechanism of action, which is crucial for the discovery and development of new adjuvants and vaccine formulations [17, 18]. In addition, we have found that results from the hWB assay are complementary to those obtained using animals [8]. This protocol can be used for a variety of different formulation screening projects, for example vaccine candidate screening, dose response studies, formulation stability studies, and excipient screening [7, 8]. Alternatively, the assay could also be used to study differences in immunological responses to a particular vaccine formulation using different donor samples.

While the protocol is relatively simple, there are a number of key components that are discussed in the notes section. We do not go into detail on how to monitor the hWB supernatants; however, a basic cytokine immunoassay (such as ELISA) can be broadened to become as complex or detailed as desired. The approach is amenable to '-omics' technologies and the possibilities around the root methodology are therefore enormous. While the mechanisms behind the hWB assay are yet to be fully understood, it represents a new method to complement animal data, providing added assurance for a vaccine's function in humans and therefore de-risking transition to clinical trials.

2 Materials

2.1 General Equipment

1. Sterile U-bottom tissue culture 96-well microtiter plates (BD® Falcon) or equivalent (*see* **Note 1**).
2. Flat-bottom 96-well microtiter plates, low cell binding (Nunc®) or equivalent.
3. BD Vacutainer® blood collection tubes, with heparin (*see* **Note 2**).
4. Single-channel and multichannel pipettes.
5. Sterile Dualfilter T.I.P.S.® SealMax, different sizes (Eppendorf) (*see* **Note 3**).
6. Humidified incubator set at 37 °C and 5 % CO_2.
7. Laminar flow bio-hood.
8. Microplate centrifuge, or benchtop centrifuge equipped with microplate rotor.
9. Laboratory freezers (−20 and −80 °C).

2.2 Human Whole-Blood Assay Reagents

1. Antigen(s), adjuvant(s), and other formulation components.
2. Human whole blood (hWB) collected from healthy donors (*see* **Note 4**) in a BD Vacutainer® blood collection tube with heparin.
3. Serum-free culture medium for human blood cells such as AIM-V® (Thermo Fisher Scientific), or alternative (*see* **Note 5**).
4. Phytohemagglutinin (PHA): 1 mg/mL Stock solution in phosphate-buffered saline (pH 6.8), stored at −20 °C. To be used as a positive control after diluting a fresh aliquot to 10 μg/mL with serum-free media.
5. Recombinant human serum albumin (rHSA): 1 mg/mL Stock solution in 10 mM Tris (pH 7.4), 0.22 μm filtered, stored at 2–8 °C. To be used as a negative control.

2.3 Analytical Items

1. Cytokine analysis kit, either single-cytokine assays (e.g., enzyme-linked immunosorbent assay (ELISA) kit for interferon gamma (IFN-γ)) or multiplex assays (e.g., Luminex) (*see* **Note 6**).

3 Methods

The steps in this procedure should be performed at room temperature in a laminar flow bio-hood using aseptic technique, unless otherwise noted. Persons performing this procedure should follow the appropriate safety guidelines for working with human blood samples (*see* Ref. [19]). Ensure that all waste materials (e.g., unused blood in BD Vacutainer® tubes and harvested whole-blood culture plates) are disposed appropriately.

An overview of the method is shown in the schematic below (Fig. 1) [7]. There are four major steps in the protocol:

1. Preparation of the formulations to be screened.
2. Preparation of human whole-blood cultures.
3. Harvesting culture supernatants after overnight cultures and analyzing cytokine profiles (*see* **Note 7**).
4. Harvesting culture supernatants after 6–12-day cultures and analyzing cytokine profiles (*see* **Note 7**).

3.1 Preparation of Formulations

It is helpful to map out the 96-well plate(s) and determine the volume of formulations that will be required for blood stimulation prior to preparing the formulations.

1. Allow the formulation components, media, and equipment to thermally equilibrate to room temperature.
2. Prepare all formulations at 2× the concentration to be tested, using serum-free media as the diluent (*see* **Note 8**).
3. Prepare all controls (*see* **Note 9**) at 2× the concentration to be tested, using serum-free media as the diluent (*see* **Note 8**).
4. Ensure that all samples are mixed well by gently inverting the samples.
5. Dispense 100 μL of each sample per well in the U-bottom tissue culture 96-well microtiter plate(s). Each sample should be dispensed into at least six wells (*see* **Note 10**). The samples may be dispensed up to a day before blood stimulation, in which case the plates should be sealed with parafilm around the edges, and stored at 2–8 °C until ready for blood stimulation (*see* **Note 11**).

3.2 Fresh Human Whole-Blood Cultures and Blood Stimulation

This protocol only describes the approach using extended 6–12-day cultures. A standard overnight culture can also be performed and this technique is already well described in the literature (e.g., Refs. [9, 13]) (*see* **Note 7**).

1. Allow the prepared U-bottom tissue culture 96-well microtiter plates to thermally equilibrate to room temperature (*see* **Note 12**).
2. Obtain fresh hWB sample(s) that have been heparinized in a BD Vacutainer® blood collection tube (*see* **Note 13**).
3. Dilute the heparinized hWB tenfold (1:10) with pre-warmed (room temperature) serum-free media.
4. Dispense 100 μL of the diluted hWB to each sample well in the U-bottom tissue culture 96-well microtiter plate(s). Note that this will dilute the formulation samples to their target concentrations in the wells, and gives a final blood dilution of 1:20 (*see* **Note 14**).

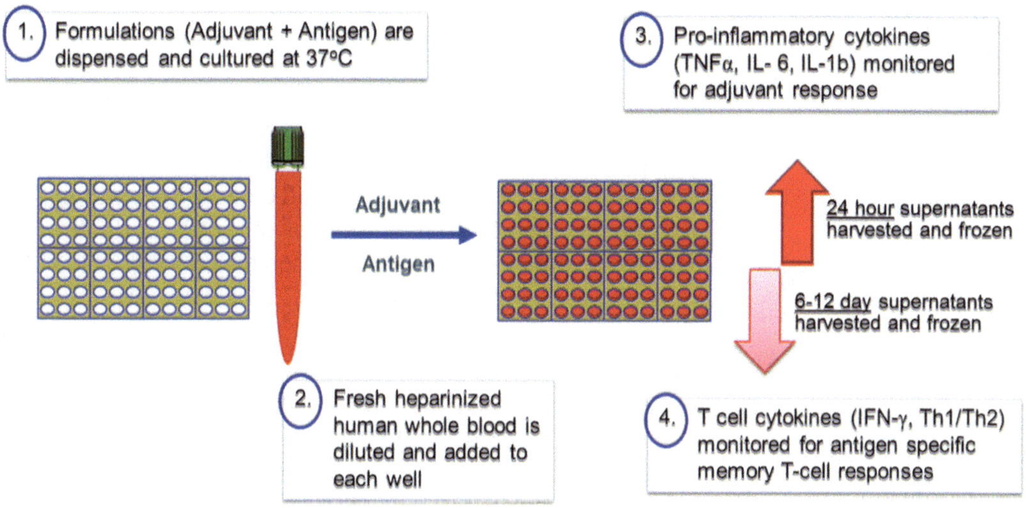

Fig. 1 Schematic overview of the human whole-blood assay. Reproduced from Brookes et al. (2014) with permission from Taylor and Francis [7]

5. Incubate the plate(s) at 37 °C with 5 % CO_2 for 6–12 days in a humidified incubator (*see* **Note 15**).

3.3 Harvesting and Analyzing the hWB Culture Supernatants

1. Remove the tissue culture plate(s) from the incubator. Examine the wells for any signs of red blood cell hemolysis (*see* **Note 16**).
2. Centrifuge the plate(s) at 1100 rpm (218 × *g*) for 1 min.
3. Harvest 130 μL of culture supernatant from each well and transfer it to a new flat-bottom 96-well plate. Be very careful not to disturb the cell pellet; the supernatants should not contain any blood cells.
4. Dispose the hWB U-bottom culture plate(s) following appropriate guidelines for biological waste disposal (*see* **Note 17**).
5. If performing single-well analysis for each individual culture supernatant (*see* **Note 18**), close the plate(s), seal with parafilm around the edges, and store at −20 °C until analysis (**step 7** of Subheading 3.3); otherwise, proceed with **step 6** of Subheading 3.3 for a pooled analysis.
6. To perform a pooled analysis for each formulation (*see* **Note 19**), combine 30 μL of harvested supernatant from each well corresponding to the same formulation into a pooled well in a new flat-bottom 96-well plate. Prepare these pooled wells in triplicate. Ensure that the supernatants are mixed well by pipetting up and down a few times. Close the plate(s), seal with parafilm around the edges, and store at −20 °C until analysis.
7. Analyze the supernatants (single-well (*see* **Note 18**) or pooled wells (*see* **Note 19**)) using a cytokine analysis kit such as an ELISA kit for IFN-γ.

4 Notes

1. U-bottom tissue culture 96-well microtiter plates are highly recommended for culturing the hWB cells. The U-bottom wells provide an optimal surface for cell growth and cell-to-cell contact, compared to flat-bottom and conical-bottom wells. In addition, the depth/volume ratio of the wells in the 96-well plate format may provide optimal aeration to the cells when compared to larger well formats (i.e., 24-well plates).
2. Heparin is a widely used anticoagulant; however, it could potentially cause interferences with some adjuvants or excipients in a formulation [20]. If this occurs, other anticoagulants should be considered. Avoid calcium chelating anticoagulants (e.g., EDTA and citrate) as calcium is required for cell activation and signaling.
3. These pipette tips or equivalent dual filter tips are highly recommended for cell culture preparations to prevent cross-contamination and to reduce the risk of aerosol contamination.
4. The hWB is collected at an on-site health center. All volunteers completed an informed consent form permitting the use of their blood in these studies. Donors were screened for infectious diseases. Blood samples can be selected based on the donor's prior exposure to certain vaccines/antigens relevant to the vaccine formulation under investigation (e.g., for candidate TB vaccine formulations, BCG-vaccinated or tuberculin skin test (TST) positive donors can be chosen) as this allows for the study of memory T cell responses. If available, point-of-care screening devices can be used to quickly identify a donor's prior exposure before blood withdrawal. If subjects are naïve (i.e., no memory T cell response expected) then there is no benefit in analyzing the 6–12-day time point.
5. The use of simple cell culture media is highly recommended as the fresh hWB is already nutrient-rich, precluding the need for additives such as serum, plasma, or enrichment factors. Any medium appropriate for culturing blood cells can be used, such as RPMI-1640 and IMDM.
6. The supernatants collected from the hWB cultures are amenable to analysis by a variety of analytical techniques. Standard immunoassays such as ELISA can be performed to analyze the response of single cytokines, or a panel of cytokines. The supernatants can also be analyzed by multiplex assay kits. Alternatively, other analytical methods could be considered, depending on the study.
7. The overnight and 6–12-day cultures are to be prepared in parallel (i.e., in separate culture plates). This protocol only describes the 6-12-day culture; overnight hWB cultures are

already well described in the literature (e.g., Refs. [9, 13]). As shown in Fig. 1, overnight cultures are useful for monitoring innate immune responses to the formulation by measuring the pro-inflammatory cytokines produced in the supernatant. In contrast, the 6–12-day cultures are useful for monitoring memory T cell cytokines (e.g., IFN-γ) as well as monitoring slower onset adjuvant-modulated responses.

8. Alternatively, 20× concentrated samples can be prepared using standard formulation buffers and reagents, which can then be diluted tenfold (to 2×) using culture media. This may be helpful for samples that are sensitive to the media or require special preparation steps (e.g., dissolution in a particular solvent). Depending on their stability, the samples may be prepared up to a day before blood stimulation, in which case they should be stored at 2–8 °C.

9. PHA (5 μg/mL per well) can be used in extended cultures as a positive control for T cell stimulation. Other positive controls should be considered depending on the formulation(s) being studied. A recommended negative control is rHSA at similar target concentrations as those used for the antigen (i.e., mock formulations with rHSA in place of the antigen). Other controls include formulations with no antigen (i.e., adjuvant only, with or without rHSA); formulations with no adjuvant (i.e., antigen only and rHSA only); and blank controls (i.e., media or buffer only).

10. The number of replicate wells to use per formulation depends on the type of study and the number of formulations being screened. We recommend using at least 6 wells per formulation as this gives enough sample to perform a representative pooled analysis (*see* **Note 18**) in triplicate. For single-well analysis (*see* **Note 17**), 10–30 wells should be used to capture the distribution of lower frequency precursor memory T cells possibly at a semi-clonal dilution. The number of wells needs to be gauged against the frequency of responding T cells in preliminary studies.

11. Depending on the stability of the samples to be screened, it is recommended to prepare the culture plate(s) well in advance of obtaining the hWB samples. This will give the experimenter ample time to obtain the hWB sample, bring it back to the working area, and dispense the hWB. The hWB should be dispensed within 2 h of it being drawn and can be applied to preloaded plates in just a few minutes.

12. Ensure that the plate(s) are pre-warmed to room temperature before the blood is scheduled to be dispensed, especially if they were stored at 2–8 °C. If necessary, the plate(s) and media can be placed in a 37 °C incubator to accelerate this.

13. The hWB samples should be maintained at room temperature and used immediately. Do not warm, refrigerate or freeze the blood samples. It is highly advisable to coordinate the blood withdrawals and sample pick-up with the local hospital or health center to facilitate this process. Having a clinical facility close to the laboratory is required for hWB work.
14. Traditional whole blood cultures use a final 1:10 dilution of hWB rather than a 1:20 dilution [10]. We have found that using a 1:20 dilution provides an equivalent response in cytokine production, but with lower background in comparison to 1:10 dilutions. The 1:20 dilution also facilitates the extension of culture durations beyond 6 days which is necessary to observe slower onset responses induced by some adjuvants (e.g., IC31®) [8]. In addition, this dilutes the serum in the hWB which may be more optimal for extended cultures as the cells are grown in autologous serum.
15. If the culture duration is to be greater than 10 days, we recommend including a media replenishing step at Day 6 to supplement the culture. To do this, remove 30 μL of culture supernatant from each well and replenish the cultures by adding 30 μL of fresh pre-warmed media, being careful not to disturb the cell layer. The harvested supernatants can be kept for a mid-point analysis of the cultures (store at -20 °C until analysis). Note that this replenishing step introduces some dilution of the final culture supernatant (i.e., 15%) that needs to be accounted for during the final analysis.
16. As red blood cells are retained in the hWB used in the assay, any signs of hemolysis can be detected by visually inspecting the cell cultures. This is a particularly useful feature of using whole blood, as vaccine formulations and formulation components can be assessed for hemotoxic and necrotic effects which would otherwise be missed with PBMC cultures. In effect the presence of erythrocytes serves as a control to confirm there is a healthy culture. We never see hemolysis in regular control wells of medium alone or positive controls. While we expect much cell death in the culture we suspect it is apoptotic (or non-inflammatory), since background activity is always low (at least for IFN-γ).
17. The cultured cells can be retained for further analysis and characterization (e.g., by flow cytometry or mass cytometry [21]). This is especially useful after a single-well analysis as the cells involved in each population can be characterized to better understand the quality of the immune response observed.
18. A single-well analysis of each individual culture supernatant can be a powerful tool when the precursor frequency of memory T cells is low for the antigen being studied. In

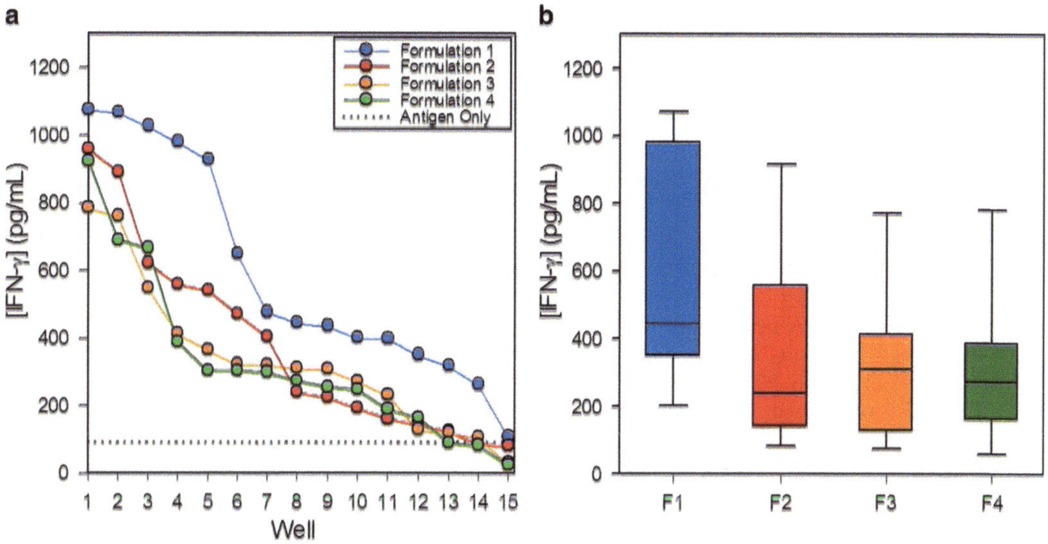

Fig. 2 Analysis of IFN-γ response from 10 day hWB cultures in the presence of different vaccine formulations. (**a**) shows the single-well responses for each formulation ordered from highest to lowest, with the antigen only control shown as the *dotted line* (94 pg/mL); (**b**) shows a boxplot representation of the single-well responses for each formulation, with whiskers representing the 10th and 90th percentiles. No response was observed for the adjuvant-only control. The Wilcoxon-Mann-Whitney *U* test was used to evaluate the differences between responses to different formulations and a statistically significant difference was found between responses to F1–F3 and F1–F4 ($p = 0.016$ and $p = 0.006$, respectively)

these cases the response in each well is quite distinct from the next; as a result, the response in each individual well can vary greatly. By performing a single-well analysis, subtle differences in immune responses can be identified, giving a measure of the quality of the T cell response which may otherwise be missed in a pooled analysis. The immune response profile across multiple wells for different formulations can then be accurately compared by performing statistical tests (e.g., the Wilcoxon-Mann-Whitney *U* test) to show a difference in the quality of response to different formulations (e.g., Fig. 2). The cells in each well can be analyzed to further characterize the quality of each response (*see* **Note 17**).

19. A pooled well analysis provides an average result from all wells that is reflective of the overall hWB response. Pooled well analyses are useful for initial broad formulation screening to identify lead candidates inducing the greatest immune response, as well as other studies where the overall immune response is the primary result being studied.

References

1. Rice J (2012) Animal models: not close enough. Nature 484:S9
2. Cook N, Jodrell DI, Tuveson DA (2012) Predictive in vivo animal models and translation to clinical trials. Drug Discov Today 17:253–260
3. Greek R, Menache A, Rice MJ (2012) Animal models in an age of personalized medicine. Personal Med 9:47–64
4. Davis MM (2008) A prescription for human immunology. Immunity 29:835–838
5. Duthie MS, Windish HP, Fox CB, Reed SG (2011) Use of defined TLR ligands as adjuvants within human vaccines. Immunol Rev 239:178–196
6. Higbee RG, Byers AM, Dhir V, Drake D, Fahlenkamp HG, Gangur J, Kachurin A, Kachurina O, Leistritz D, Ma Y, Mehta R, Mishkin E, Moser J, Mosquera L, Nguyen M, Parkhill R, Pawar S, Poisson L, Sanchez-Schmitz G, Schanen B, Singh I, Song H, Tapia T, Warren W, Wittman V (2009) An immunologic model for rapid vaccine assessment – a clinical trial in a test tube. Altern Lab Anim 37:19–27
7. Brookes RH, Hakimi J, Ha Y, Aboutorabian S, Ausar SF, Hasija M, Smith SG, Todryk SM, Dockrell HM, Rahman N (2014) Screening vaccine formulations for biological activity using fresh human whole blood. Hum Vaccin Immunother 10(4):1129–1135
8. Aboutorabian S, Hakimi J, Boudet F, Montano S, Dookie A, Roque C, Ausar SF, Rahman N, Brookes RH (2015) A high ratio of IC31 adjuvant to antigen is necessary for H4 TB vaccine immunomodulation. Hum Vaccin Immunother 11(6):1449–1455
9. Damsgaard CT, Lauritzen L, Calder PC, Kjaer TM, Frokiaer H (2009) Whole-blood culture is a valid low-cost method to measure monocytic cytokines – a comparison of cytokine production in cultures of human whole-blood, mononuclear cells and monocytes. J Immunol Methods 340:95–101
10. Weir RE, Morgan AR, Britton WJ, Butlin CR, Dockrell HM (1994) Development of a whole blood assay to measure T cell responses to leprosy: a new tool for immune-epidemiological field studies of leprosy immunity. J Immunol Methods 176:93–101
11. Silva D, Ponte CGG, Hacker MA, Antas PRZ (2013) A whole blood assay as a simple, broad assessment of cytokines and chemokines to evaluate human immune responses to Mycobacterium tuberculosis antigens. Acta Trop 127:75–81
12. Chen J, Bruns AH, Donnelly HK, Wunderink RG (2010) Comparative in vitro stimulation with lipopolysaccharide to study TNFalpha gene expression in fresh whole blood, fresh and frozen peripheral blood mononuclear cells. J Immunol Methods 257:33–37
13. Fox CB, Sivananthan SJ, Duthie MS, Vergara J, Guderian JA, Moon E, Coblentz D, Reed SG, Carter D (2014) A nanoliposome delivery system to synergistically trigger TLR4 and TLR7. J Nanobiotechnol 12:17
14. Nauseef WM, Borregaard N (2014) Neutrophils at work. Nat Immunol 15(7):602–611
15. Davey MS, Morgan MP, Liuzzi AR, Tyler CJ, Khan MWA, Szakmany T, Hall JE, Moser B, Eberl M (2014) Microbe-specific unconventional T cells induce human neutrophil differentiation into antigen cross-presenting cells. J Immunol 193(7):3704–3716
16. Mantovani A, Cassatella MA, Costantini C, Jaillon S (2011) Neutrophils in the activation and regulation of innate and adaptive immunity. Nat Rev Immunol 11:519–531
17. O'Hagan DT, Fox CB (2015) Are we entering a new age for human vaccine adjuvants? Expert Rev Vaccines 14:909–911
18. Reed SG, Orr MT, Fox CB (2013) Key roles of adjuvants in modern vaccines. Nat Med 19:1597–1608
19. Centers for Disease Control and Prevention (2012). Guidelines for safe work practices in human and animal medical diagnostic laboratories. http://www.cdc.gov/mmwr/pdf/other/su6101.pdf. Accessed 11 Nov 2015
20. Coch C, Luck C, Schwickart A, Putschli B, Renn M, Holler T, Barchet W, Hartmann G, Schlee M (2013) A human in vitro whole blood assay to predict the systemic cytokine response to therapeutic oligonucleotides including siRNA. PLoS One 8:e71057
21. Bandura DR, Baranov VI, Ornatsky OI, Antonov A, Kinach R, Lou X, Pavlov S, Vorobiev S, Dick JE, Tanner SD (2009) Mass cytometry: technique for real time single cell multitarget immunoassay based on inductively coupled plasma time-of-flight mass spectrometry. Anal Chem 81:6813–6822

Chapter 23

Analysis of the Innate Response to Adjuvants: Characterization of the Draining Lymph Node by Fluorescence-Activated Cell Sorting

Anthony L. Desbien

Abstract

A clear index for a response to adjuvants is a change in the cellular composition of lymph nodes draining the site of adjuvant injection (Didierlaurent et al., J Immunol 183:6186–6197, 2009; Caproni et al., J Immunol 188:3088–98, 2012; Desbien et al., Eur J Immunol 1–11, 2014). During the steady state, lymph nodes (LNs) are composed of a fixed ratio of innate and adaptive cells awaiting activation signals from tissue draining lymph. Upon exposure to innate stimulants, lymph nodes undergo dramatic changes. The most apparent change to the lymph node is an increase in size. Antigen-independent activation of naïve T cells and B cells, as a consequence of type I interferon signaling, results in upregulation of CD69 (Sun and Zhang, J. Exp. Med 188:2335–2342, 1998), causing increased retention of cells in the lymph node and transient lymphopenia in the blood (Shiow et al., Nature 440:540–544, 2006). In addition tissue-resident dendritic cells, macrophages, as well as circulating inflammatory monocytes will migrate into draining LNs and display maturation markers associated with activation. Such features can provide powerful discrimination of adjuvant potencies.

Key words Innate immune response, Lymph nodes, Cell recruitment, Lymphopenia, Fluorescence-activated cell sorting

1 Introduction

Vaccines represent one of the most successful and cost-effective medical technologies in existence but their exact mechanisms of action are still unclear. But what is clear is that the majority of, if not all, vaccines contain components that engage the innate immune system [6]. Those components can be intrinsic to the antigen preparation, such as contaminants from bacterial cell walls or nucleic acids from viruses which are recognized by germline-encoded receptors like toll-like receptors (TLRs). When antigen preparations alone are not sufficiently immunogenic, extrinsic adjuvants are added. Current extrinsic adjuvants include molecules known to engage the TLRs and those with unknown targets like

Christopher B. Fox (ed.), *Vaccine Adjuvants: Methods and Protocols*, Methods in Molecular Biology, vol. 1494,
DOI 10.1007/978-1-4939-6445-1_23, © Springer Science+Business Media New York 2017

alum or MF59. Due to the complexity of the immune response, which incorporates an array of cell subsets and means of recognition, the analysis of adjuvants requires in vivo analysis. Indeed we have observed that in vitro systems fail to faithfully report in vivo adjuvant activities [7]. Additionally, formulation of ligands can greatly alter their activity; ostensibly inert components can themselves induce responses [8].

The lymph node is at the center of the innate and adaptive responses to adjuvants. Concordant with the increase in size of lymph nodes due to re-localization of naïve B cells and T cells from the blood, the activated lymph node can contain new cell types, arriving from periphery. The composition of recruited cells can vary dependent upon the nature of the adjuvant and the time after injection examined. This can include skin resident macrophages, inflammatory macrophages and neutrophils [1, 3]. And while such cells are relatively few in number, they are generally absent in steady-state lymph nodes, providing a distinct signature of adjuvant induced events. Upon direct engagement with adjuvants or via secondary activation by secreted factors, antigen-presenting cells will increase costimulatory molecules like CD80 and CD86, MHC I and II. These cells can also carry particles from the periphery as evident by studies with fluorescently labeled materials [9] .

The analysis of draining lymph node for the evaluation of the innate response to adjuvants offers several advantages:

1. Lymph nodes are easily isolated. With experience popliteal, inguinal, and axillary lymph nodes can all be harvested from a single mouse in under a minute of hands-on time.
2. Injection site draining lymph nodes contain soluble material including cytokines generated in peripheral tissue as well as analytes generated in the lymph node as a result of direct interaction with the adjuvant.
3. Lymph nodes are a site where adaptive immune responses are initiated.

The activation status of these cells can be assessed by staining for surface marker and intracellular cytokines for analysis by flow cytometry.

2 Materials

2.1 Injection Materials

1. Needle: 27 gauge, 200 μl tuberculin syringe.
2. Adjuvant of interest at predetermined dose (*see* **Note 1**).
3. Negative control (*see* **Note 2**).
4. Positive control (*see* **Note 3**).

2.2 Supplies for Sample Collection

1. Scissors.
2. Forceps.
3. 24-well tissue culture plate (low cell binding) for collection of organs.
4. 3 ml disposable syringe.
5. 30–40 μM cell strainers.

2.3 Supplies for Fluorescent Antibody Staining

1. Tissue digestion buffer: RPMI, 10 % FBS (prevents proteolytic activity to preserve cell surface proteins), 0.2 % collagenase IV (Worthington), benzonase at 25 units/ml.
2. FACS buffer: phosphate-buffered saline [1.54 mM potassium phosphate monobasic, 2.71 mM sodium phosphate dibasic, 155 mM sodium chloride, pH 7.2], 1 % fetal bovine sera or 0.5–1 % bovine serum albumin and 2 mM EDTA.
3. Fc receptor blocking antibody (CD16/32 specific).
4. Fluorochrome-conjugated antibodies for cell surface markers and intracellular targets.
5. BD fixation and permeabilization buffer.
6. BD perm/wash buffer.
7. 96-well round-bottom plate (low attachment) for staining.

3 Methods

3.1 Injection and Collection of Samples

1. Determine post-injection sampling schedule. Many responses peak and return to baseline within hours of adjuvant administration (*see* **Note 4**). Cell surface marker induction like CD69 and co-stimulatory markers like CD80/86 and MHC molecules are relatively more stable.
2. Inject adjuvant via parenteral route (*see* **Note 5**).
3. Euthanize animals via IACUC-approved methods according to schedule determined in **step 1** of Subheading 3.1. Alternatively, an early, sublethal bleed can be performed to assess serum cytokine levels. This carries the caveat that not all responses to adjuvant will induce systemic cytokine production. In fact localized responses can be more productive for generation of adaptive immunity [10]. Simultaneously, peripheral blood cell counts can be performed to analyze changes in cellularity.

3.2 Harvesting of Tissues

1. Extract lymph nodes into a buffered solution such as PBS. The relevant lymph nodes for lower extremity injections include the popliteal, inguinal, iliac, and axillary lymph nodes [11]. If cell culturing is to be employed, a complete media composed of RPMI, 10 % heat-inactivated fetal calf serum, antibiotics, supplemented with HEPES to maintain pH in ambient air

should be used. Cytokine transport blockers like monensin or brefeldin A can be added to help with cytokine staining [12]. A convenient method for harvesting is to use a 24-well plate (low binding, non-tissue culture-treated plate) containing a minimal volume of PBS (300–400 μl is sufficient to cover tissue). This allows minimal dilution of targets for secreted cytokine analysis as well as easy collection and transfer for downstream processing.

2. Homogenize tissue into single cell suspensions. Mechanical disruption is accomplished by pressing the lymph node against the bottom of the 24-well dish with the plastic end of a 3 ml syringe. The goal is to rupture the outer capsule of the lymph node. Enzymatic digestion of lymph nodes can be employed to enrich for macrophages and dendritic cells as well as endothelial cells (*see* **Note 6**).
3. Filter and transfer to 96-well U-bottom, low-attachment plate. 96-well 30–40 μM filters are available that allow quick processing. Otherwise samples should be passed through filters individually and then transferred to a plate.
4. Pellet cells by centrifuging in swinging bucket rotor at $500 \times g$ for 3 min. At this point, relative cell pellet sizes can be determined. FACS staining can tolerate a wide range of cell concentrations but it is not recommended to exceed a staining concentration of 20 million cells per ml. For plate-based staining this means six million cells as the maximum volume per well is roughly 300 μl. Considering that adjuvants can greatly increase the numbers of cells in draining lymph nodes (mostly naïve B cells and T cells), it may be necessary to count cells and dispense accordingly. Typically an unstimulated inguinal lymph node contains 5×10^4 cells but after immunization can have more than 1×10^7 cells. Collect supernatant if cytokine levels are to be determined; otherwise decant the solution by "flicking" the plate into a sink.
5. Wash cells by first vortexing the "flicked plate" high, with lid for a few seconds until the pellet is disrupted. Resuspend cells in 200 μl of FACS buffer and pellet as above.
6. Decant plate and suspend in Fc receptor blocking antibody diluted in FACS buffer. Incubate on ice for at least 10 min or transfer to 4 °C.
7. Proceed to FACS staining or pause here for overnight. As long as cells are maintained at 4° only a limited loss of viability will occur.

3.3 FACS Staining

1. For initial experiments stain for cell surface markers that define major cell populations: CD19 for B cells, CD3 (CD90) for T cells, CD11b for granulocytes, CD11c for dendritic cells and Ly-6G for neutrophils, as well as a combination of markers to

identify monocytes and macrophages including Ly-6C, CD11c and MHCII F4/80 is used extensively for identification of macrophages, although its fidelity to do so may be questionable [13]. Further refinement of subpopulations includes staining for CD169 and SIGNR-1, markers that define sinusoidal and medullary macrophages, which are critical to early encounters with adjuvant and microorganisms [14, 15]. Activation of subsets can be assessed by staining for CD69, CD80, CD86, CD40, MHCI, MHCII, all which have direct impact on T cell and B cell priming. Combine surface-marker-specific fluorescently labeled antibodies. Generally a 1:200 dilution of commercially prepared anti-mouse antibodies is a good starting dilution. Add sufficient diluted antibody cocktails to cells such that the concentration of cells does not exceed 4×10^7/ml. For example, add 50 μl of cocktail to 2×10^6 cells.

2. Incubate on ice for 10–15 min for the majority markers. Be aware that some optimization of staining conditions may be required. For example, the chemokine receptor CXCR5 absolutely requires room temperature incubation.
3. Wash cells twice by pelleting cells at $500 \times g$ for 3 min and resuspending in FACS buffer.
4. Fix cells in PBS and 2% paraformaldehyde or commercially available fixatives like BD Fixation and Permeabilization Solution. Incubate on ice for 20 min. Fixation allows cells to be stored for up to 72 h (more adventurous souls will push this time to a week) but carries the caveat that fluorescent proteins like GFP will be partially denature and lose their signal.
5. Wash cells twice in FACS buffer as above.
6. If intracellular targets are of interest, e.g., IFN-γ and TNFa, wash cells twice with a 0.1% saponin permeabilization buffer like BD perm/wash buffer.
7. Dilute anti-intracellular target antibodies in permeabilization buffer (this is required for saponin permeabilization since it is a transient perm buffer). Add to cells at similar concentrations as detailed above.
8. Incubate for at least 10 min on ice. Alternatively antibodies can left on overnight.
9. Wash cells twice in permeabilization buffer. Extended incubation in the permeabilization buffer may reduce background issues.
10. Wash cells in FACS buffer.
11. Filter cells using 96-well 30–40 μm plate filter by "pulsing" plate at 100 g for 10 s. Pelleting should be avoided as this will cause cells to clump to some degree and undue the purpose of filtration. Cells are ready for acquisition.

4 Notes

1. Many adjuvants targeting germline-encoded receptors are active in the picogram to microgram range upon injection. GLA, which is a synthetic TLR4 agonist, induces protective responses when administered as an aqueous formulation at a 1 μg dose [16]. Formulation of GLA as an squalene oil-in-water emulsion (arguably a combination of two independent adjuvants) enhances innate and anamnestic responses to vaccination [3, 17]. Therefore it is critical and unavoidable to incorporate a range of doses when evaluating adjuvants. Ideally, a functional dose would be determined through adaptive response evaluations. That dose would be used as a center point for innate mechanistic studies.
2. Controls for injection should include the vehicle used to deliver the adjuvant. Unanticipated vehicle effects can occur and therefore it is crucial to include a separate group [18]. Further, trauma from the injection can have inflammatory effects which is controlled by injection of an isotonic solution such as phosphate buffered saline.
3. In order to demonstrate that detection reagents and processing are functional, it is important to include a positive control. Ideally, one would use a vetted compound known to induce innate responses such as a toll-like receptor agonist (e.g., polyinosinic-polycytidylic acid).
4. The innate response to adjuvants occurs rapidly after injection and results in both primary and secondary responses, those elicited directly by adjuvant-cell interactions and responses induced by cytokines secreted from adjuvant-interacting cells. Primary responses associated with first contact between surveying innate cells and tissue can occur within minutes after injection [22]. Some adjuvant will travel directly to draining lymph nodes within minutes of injection, and, dependent on the size of particles, can penetrate into the cortex of the lymph node or be restricted to the subcapsular region for smaller and larger particles respectively [23]. This can lead to rapid, transcription-independent release of cytokines. For example, IL-18, which exists in lymph nodes constitutively as a pro-form [12], can be detected in lymph node fluid as quickly as an hour after adjuvant administration in an inflammasome-dependent manner, presumably through cleavage and secretion [3]. An example of secondary response includes the antigen-independent activation T cells and B cells manifesting in increased CD69 surface expression. Some subsets of memory CD8 T cells behave in an innate-like manner, producing IFN-γ in the absence of TCR stimulation, as a result of cytokine stimulation

[3, 12, 24, 25]. Residual material that does not travel to the LN directly, can be phagocytosed at the injection site and carried to the LN, leading to a second wave of adjuvant deposition in the LN mediated by cellular transport. Considering the multiphasic nature of the innate response to adjuvants, it is necessary to sample tissues at several time points, on the scale of minutes for immediate responses and hours to days for targets that require processing and or nascent synthesis.

5. Most preclinical studies examining adjuvant responses utilize parenteral injection methods. There are extensive guidelines for injection routes and volumes available [19, 20]. The most commonly used parenteral injection methods include: subcutaneous: base of tail injection 1000 μl, scruff of neck; 100 μl; Intramuscular injection: the hind leg quadriceps; 10–50 μl; Footpad: 30–50 μl. The use of footpad injections should evaluated on a substance to substance basis contingent upon degree of irritation expected. Footpad injections of the model adjuvants like complete Freund's adjuvant are largely no longer permitted due to the resultant inflammation and, consequently, the immobilization of the leg. The desirable feature of constrained drainage to the popliteal node can be recapitulated with alternative injection such and administration via injection to the hock [21].
6. For isolation of antigen-presenting cell subsets, which are more integrated into the stroma of LNs, tissue digestion buffer should be used. LN's can be harvested directly in this media and mechanically disrupted using two small-gauge needles to tear open LN

References

1. Didierlaurent AM et al (2009) AS04, an aluminum salt- and TLR4 agonist-based adjuvant system, induces a transient localized innate immune response leading to enhanced adaptive immunity. J Immunol 183:6186–6197
2. Caproni E et al (2012) MF59 and Pam3CSK4 boost adaptive responses to influenza subunit vaccine through an IFN type I-independent mechanism of action. J Immunol 188: 3088–3098
3. Desbien AL et al (2014) Squalene emulsion potentiates the adjuvant activity of the TLR4 agonist, GLA, via inflammatory caspases, IL-18, and IFN-γ. Eur J Immunol 1–11. doi: 10.1002/eji.201444543
4. Sun S, Zhang X, Tough DF, Sprent J (1998) Type I interferon-mediated stimulation of T cells by CpG DNA. J Exp Med 188:2335–2342
5. Shiow LR et al (2006) CD69 acts downstream of interferon-alpha/beta to inhibit S1P1 and lymphocyte egress from lymphoid organs. Nature 440:540–544
6. McKee AS, Munks MW, Marrack P (2007) How do adjuvants work? Important considerations for new generation adjuvants. Immunity 27:687–690
7. Misquith A et al (2014) In vitro evaluation of TLR4 agonist activity: formulation effects. Colloids Surf B Biointerfaces 113:312–319
8. Hagan DTO et al (2012) The mechanism of action of MF59 - an innately attractive adjuvant formulation. Vaccine 30:4341–4348
9. Morel S et al (2011) Adjuvant system AS03 containing α-tocopherol modulates innate immune response and leads to improved adaptive immunity. Vaccine 29:2461–2473

10. Smirnov D, Schmidt JJ, Capecchi JT, Wightman PD (2011) Vaccine adjuvant activity of 3M-052: an imidazoquinoline designed for local activity without systemic cytokine induction. Vaccine 29:5434–5442
11. Harrell MI, Iritani BM, Ruddell A (2009) Lymph node mapping in the mouse. J Immunol Methods 332:170–174
12. Kastenmüller W, Torabi-Parizi P, Subramanian N, Lämmermann T, Germain RN (2012) A spatially-organized multicellular innate immune response in lymph nodes limits systemic pathogen spread. Cell 150:1235–1248
13. Rose S, Misharin A, Perlman H (2012) A novel Ly6C/Ly6G-based strategy to analyze the mouse splenic myeloid compartment. Cytometry A 81:343–350
14. Junt T et al (2007) Subcapsular sinus macrophages in lymph nodes clear lymph-borne viruses and present them to antiviral B cells. Nature 450:110–114
15. Barral P et al (2010) CD169(+) macrophages present lipid antigens to mediate early activation of iNKT cells in lymph nodes. Nat Immunol 11:303–312
16. Clegg CH et al (2014) GLA-AF, an emulsion-free vaccine adjuvant for pandemic influenza. PLoS One 9:e88979
17. Anderson RC et al (2010) Physicochemical characterization and biological activity of synthetic TLR4 agonist formulations. Colloids Surf B Biointerfaces 75:123–132
18. Walter A et al (2013) Aldara activates TLR7-independent immune defence. Nat Commun 4:1560
19. Turner PV, Brabb T, Pekow C, Vasbinder MA (2011) Administration of substances to laboratory animals: routes of administration and factors to consider. J Am Assoc Lab Anim Sci 50:600–613
20. Picazo Guillen J (2004) Routes of administration. Med Cir Guerra 16:435–451
21. Kamala T (2007) Hock immunization: a humane alternative to mouse footpad injections. J Immunol Methods 328:204–214
22. Vono M et al (2013) The adjuvant MF59 induces ATP release from muscle that potentiates response to vaccination. Proc Natl Acad Sci U S A 110:21095–21100
23. Gretz JE, Norbury CC, Anderson AO, Proudfoot AE, Shaw S (2000) Lymph-borne chemokines and other low molecular weight molecules reach high endothelial venules via specialized conduits while a functional barrier limits access to the lymphocyte microenvironments in lymph node cortex. J Exp Med 192:1425–1440
24. Berg RE, Crossley E, Murray S, Forman J (2003) Memory CD8+ T cells provide innate immune protection against Listeria monocytogenes in the absence of cognate antigen. J Exp Med 198:1583–1593
25. Soudja SM et al (2014) Memory-T-Cell-Derived Interferon-γ Instructs Potent Innate Cell Activation for Protective Immunity. Immunity 40:974–988

Chapter 24

Assessment of Antigen-Specific Cellular Immunogenicity Using Intracellular Cytokine Staining, ELISpot, and Culture Supernatants

Elyse A. Beebe and Mark T. Orr

Abstract

Quantification of cytokine production by CD4 and CD8 T cells after in vitro recall stimulation with the immunizing antigen is a powerful approach to characterize the cellular immune responses to immunization. Here we describe three complementary methods for such quantification including flow cytometric analysis of cytokine production by intracellular staining, ELISpot determination of the numbers of cytokine-producing cells, and generation of secreted cytokines and chemokines in culture supernatants for analysis by ELISA and/or cytometric bead arrays.

Key words Intracellular cytokine staining, ELISpot, ELISA, Immunogenicity, T cell, Flow cytometry

1 Introduction

Assessment of the immunogenicity of vaccines includes quantification of both humoral and cellular immune responses specific to the vaccine antigen(s). Characterization of antigen-specific cellular immune responses typically focuses on one or more of (1) production of effector/signaling molecules such as chemokines and cytokines, (2) characterization of antigen-specific cells and characteristics by combinations of MHC I or II tetramer binding, surface markers, and transcription factors (e.g., T-bet or Bcl6 for T_H1 and T_{FH} populations, respectively) [1, 2], and (3) cellular function especially cytotoxicity in vitro and/or in vivo [3]. For production of effector/signaling molecules integration of multiple orthogonal assays to measure the (1) the frequency of cytokine-producing cells (ELISpot), (2) amount of cytokine produced (culture supernatant assays), and (3) identity and characteristics of cytokine-producing cells (intracellular cytokine staining(ICS)) provides a highly dimensional image of the product of vaccination. This wealth of information allows for a

Christopher B. Fox (ed.), *Vaccine Adjuvants: Methods and Protocols*, Methods in Molecular Biology, vol. 1494,
DOI 10.1007/978-1-4939-6445-1_24, © Springer Science+Business Media New York 2017

more informed down-selection of vaccine candidates based on a desired immunogenicity target profile. For example we have used this approach to develop vaccine adjuvants and regimens that preferentially elicit multi-functional T_H1 cells (capable of simultaneously producing CD154, IFN-γ, TNF, IL-2, and GM-CSF), T_H17 cells (capable of simultaneously producing CD154, TNF, and IL-17A), or T_H2 cells (producing IL-5 to the exclusion of IFN-γ) [1, 4, 5].

Herein we describe a streamlined work flow that employs all three assays using the same biological sample. These assays have been optimized for murine splenocytes, but can be adapted to other cell sources such as lymph nodes or lung tissue by employing tissues-specific methods for isolation of lymphocytes including mechanical disruption protocols and/or enzymatic digestion [1, 2, 5]. Similarly these assays and work flow can be adapted to other species using similar protocols by employing species-specific immune assay reagents, including but not limited to guinea pigs, nonhuman primates, and human samples. The choice of which assays to use will depend on both the objectives of the experiment and the availability of assay specific detection equipment including flow cytometers, ELISpot readers, plate readers, and cytometric bead analyzers. Of note the selection of fluorophore combinations for flow cytometry depends on the configuration (lasers and detectors) of the cytometer to be used. Optimization of flow cytometry panels and analysis of multi-functional T cells by flow cytometry has been reviewed elsewhere [6–8].

2 Materials

2.1 General Lab Supplies

1. 70 μm Strainer (BD Falcon).
2. 3 mL Syringes.
3. Sterile distilled water (Gibco).
4. Phosphate-buffered saline (PBS, Gibco): 1.54 mM Potassium phosphate monobasic, 2.71 mM sodium phosphate dibasic, 155 mM sodium chloride, pH 7.2.
5. RBC lysis buffer (eBioscience).
6. Complete media (cRPMI): Add heat-inactivated fetal bovine serum (FBS) (10%) and penicillin/streptomycin (1%; Life Technologies) to RPMI 1640 with GlutaMAX and 25 mM Hepes (Gibco).
7. PBS (*see* **item 4** of Subheading 2.1) with 1% bovine serum albumin (BSA).
8. Omni Prep Multi-Sample Homogenizer (Omni International).
9. Soft Tissue Black Tips (Omni International).

2.2 Flow Cytometry Reagents

1. Phorbol 12-myristate 13-acetate (PMA) (Sigma).
2. Ionomycin (Sigma).
3. BD GolgiPlug (BD Biosciences).
4. Perm/wash buffer, 10× stock (BD Biosciences) diluted 1:10 in distilled H_2O.
5. Cytofix/Cytoperm (BD Biosciences).
6. Fluorophore-conjugated antibodies for flow cytometry.
7. Fc block Anti-mouse CD16/32 Clone 24G2.
8. 96-Well cell strainer plates (Pall AcroPrep Advanced).
9. Ultracomp beads (eBiosciences).

2.3 ELISpot Reagents

1. Concanavalin A (ConA) (Sigma).
2. Sterile Multiscreen-IP plates (Millipore).
3. ELISA/ELISPOT Coating Buffer Powder (eBioscience #00-0044-59). Re-suspended in 1 L dH_20 and filtered through a 0.22 μm filter.
4. Wash buffer: 0.05% Tween 20 in PBS (*see* **item 4** of Subheading 2.1).
5. Peroxidase substrate kit (AEC) (Vector Laboratories).
6. ELISPOT Ready-Set-Go Kits, e.g., IFN-γ (eBioscience) and IL-5 (eBioscience).

3 Methods

3.1 Preparing Lymphocytes

1. Harvest spleens into 5 mL of cold cRPMI in 15 mL conical tube and keep on ice to maintain highest viability possible.
2. Homogenize spleen using Omni multi-prep homogenizer and soft tissue black tips or crushing the organ with the back of a 3 mL syringe plunger through a cell strainer.
3. Centrifuge for 5 min at 440 ×*g*.
4. Decant supernatant.
5. Add 1 mL RBC lysis buffer to each tube to lyse red blood cells.
6. Pipette up and down to break pellet and incubate for 2–3 min.
7. Add 5 mL cRPMI to wash and centrifuge for 5 min at 440 ×*g*.
8. Decant supernatant
9. Resuspend cells to 2×10^7 Cells/mL in cRPMI for ICS or 2×10^6 Cells/mL for ELISPOT and Culture Supernatant.

3.2 Stimulation and Staining for ICS

3.2.1 Stimulation

1. Plate out stimulations (e.g., immunizing antigens or PMA + Ionomycin) at a 2× concentration and media alone for negative control in 100 μl/well of cRPMI in a U-bottom 96-well plate (*see* **Notes 1** and **2**).
2. Add 100 μL of the cell suspension onto the stimulations for 2E6 cells/well in 200 μL total and 1× final concentration of stimulation in each well.
3. If degranulation is to be measured, fluorescently labeled antibodies to CD107a (LAMP1) can be included in the stimulation (*see* **Note 3**)
4. Incubate for 1–2 h at 37 °C for cells to respond to stimulation and release cytokines.
5. Add 10 μL/well of BD GolgiPlug (diluted 1:50 in cRPMI) for a 1:1000 final concentration. BD GolgiPlug contains brefeldin A which will block the intracellular protein transport processes which results in an accumulation of cytokines and/or proteins in the Golgi complex.
6. Incubate for 6–12 h at 37 °C to let the cytokines accumulate for enhanced detection capability during staining. (*see* **Note 4**).
7. Move to 4 °C until ready to stain.

3.2.2 Staining (See Note 5)

1. Make surface staining cocktail for 50 μL per well with optimized dilutions of surface stains and Fc block in PBS with 1 % BSA. Fc block will stop nonspecific binding of antibodies by Fc receptors. 1 % BSA will help with pelleting during centrifugation to ensure minimal cell loss. Surface stains might include CD4 (RM4-5), CD8 (53-6.7), and CD44 (IM7) (*see* **Notes 6** and **7**).
2. Centrifuge plates for 2 min at 780 × *g* to pellet cells.
3. Decant supernatant (*see* **Note 8**).
4. Resuspend cells in surface staining cocktail and incubate in the dark at 4 °C for at least 10 min up to overnight at 4 °C.
5. Dilute cells with 150 μL PBS with 1 % BSA to wash out stain and centrifuge for 2 min at 780 × *g*.
6. Decant supernatant.
7. Resuspend cells in 50 μL of BD Cytofix/Cytoperm and incubate in the dark for 20 min at RT. This step crosslinks antibodies to their cognate antigens from the previous steps and permeabilizes the cell to allow the staining antibodies to reach the cytokines located inside the cell.
8. Make intracellular staining cocktail for 50 μL per well with optimized dilutions of intracellular stains in 1× BD perm/wash. Intracellular stains might include IFN-γ (XMG1.2), TNF (MP6-XT22), IL-2 (JES6-5H4), CD154 (MR1) [9, 10], IL-5 (TRFK5), and/or IL-17A (TC11-18H10.1) depending on the goal of the experiment (*see* **Notes 3, 6, 7** and **9**).

9. Dilute cells with 150 μL of 1× BD perm/wash to wash out the Cytofix/Cytoperm buffer.
10. Centrifuge plates for 2 min at 780 ×*g* to pellet cells.
11. Decant supernatant.
12. Resuspend cells in intracellular staining cocktail and incubate in the dark at RT for at least 10 min up to overnight at 4 °C.
13. Wash cells with 150 μL of 1× BD perm/wash and centrifuge for 2 min at 780 ×*g* to pellet cells.
14. Decant supernatant.
15. Resuspend cells in 200 μL PBS with 1 % BSA and filter through Pall 96-well cell strainer plates into a new 96-well plate using a quick spin up to 300 ×*g*. Filtration is necessary to ensure that the stained cells are able to easily pass through the SIP on the cytometer without producing clogs. A quick spin will allow the cells to pass through the filter without pelleting in the bottom of the plate.
16. Keep samples in the dark until ready to acquire to ensure photo-bleaching does not occur to the light sensitive fluorophores used in flow cytometry.

3.2.3 Preparing Compensation Beads

1. To make single-stain controls add 0.5 μL of a fluorophore-conjugated antibody to one drop of compensation beads and repeat for as many fluorophores as are in the panel. Single-stained controls are needed for compensation of the cytometer to account for spectral overlap that occurs when using multiple fluorophores in the same panel.
2. Pipette up and down in each well to mix the beads with the stain.
3. Incubate at RT in the dark for at least 5 min.
4. Dilute with 150 μL of PBS with 1 % BSA.
5. Centrifuge for 2 min at 780 ×*g*.
6. Decant supernatant.
7. Resuspend wells in 200 μL PBS with 1 % BSA.
8. Keep beads in the dark until ready to acquire.

3.3 ELISPOT

3.3.1 Capture

1. Dilute the capture antibody in sterile coating buffer according to the manufacturer's instructions and add 100 μL to each well of Multiscreen-IP plate to coat the plates with the desired antibody.
2. Incubate at 4 °C overnight.
3. Decant liquid and wash thrice with 200 μL of coating buffer to prepare the plates for blocking.

3.3.2 Blocking

1. Add 200 µL cRPMI and incubate at RT for at least 2 h to block nonspecific protein binding with excess FBS protein.
2. Decant blocking buffer.

3.3.3 Incubation

1. Add 100 µL of 2× stimulations protocol (e.g., immunizing antigens, media alone as a negative control or ConA as a positive control). (*see* **Notes 1** and **10**).
2. Add 100 µL of 2×10^6/mL cell suspension to each well for a total of 2×10^5 cells/well and for a final concentration of 1X stimulation in every well.
3. Incubate plate at 37 °C with 5 % CO_2 for 48 h.

3.3.4 Detection

1. Decant cells from plate and wash wells 4X with 200 µL of wash buffer.
2. Dilute the detection antibody in reagent diluent according to the manufacturer's instructions.
3. Add 100 µL of detection antibody and incubate at 4 °C overnight.

3.3.5 Development

1. Decant the detection antibody and wash wells thrice with 200 µL of wash buffer to remove unbound detection antibody.
2. Dilute avidin-horseradish peroxidase (Av-HRP) per the manufacturer's instructions.
3. Add 100 µL of Av-HRP and incubate at room temperature for 45 min to bind to antibody coated protein via interaction with streptavidin on the detection antibody.
4. Decant and wash wells thrice with wash buffer and then at least twice with PBS to ensure that all the Tween is washed out.
5. Prepare fresh AEC substrate according to the manufacturer's instructions.
6. Add 100 µL of AEC to each well and incubate for 5–30 min until spots are clearly visible in positive control wells and before spots begin to appear in negative control wells.
7. Stop reaction by decanting AEC substrate and washing plates at least 4× with 200 µL DI water or under DI faucet for 2 min.
8. Peel off back of plates during wash and ensure both sides of the filter are adequately washed and so the filters can adequately dry for reading.
9. Allow plates to air-dry in the dark as the spots are light sensitive after development (*see* **Note 11**).
10. Read plates on ELISPOT reader after fully dry.

3.4 Culture Supernatant

1. Plate desired stimulations at 2× concentration and media as a negative control in a 96-well U-bottom plate (*see* **Note 1**).
2. Add 100 μL of 2×10^6cells/mL to appropriate wells for a total of 2×10^5 cells/well and 1× final concentration of the stimulations in each well.
3. Incubate in 37 °C incubator with 5% CO_2 for 48–72 h.
4. Centrifuge plates for 2 min at 780 × *g* to pellet cells.
5. Transfer 170 μL of supernatant into clean 96 well U-bottom plate without disturbing the cell pellet to save supernatant only for future analysis.
6. Cover plate with a plate sealer and store in a −20 °C freezer until ready to use for detection of secreted cytokines or chemokines by ELISA or cytometric bead array (e.g., Luminex).

4 Notes

1. Optimal stimulation concentrations for each antigen must be empirically determined for each assay. We recommend using a 5-point 5-fold dilution series starting at 50 μg/mL.
2. Recommended stimulation with PMA and Ionomycin as a positive control is 1 μg/mL final for each.
3. CD107a staining during stimulation rather than at the completion of the assay is recommended as this will reveal a higher frequency of transiently degranulating cells. This process is not inhibited by Brefeldin A (the active chemical in GolgiPlug) and thus can be used in conjunction with detection of intracellular cytokines. CD107a should not be used as an intracellular stain as it will label lysosomes present in all cells regardless of antigen specificity.
4. Stimulating cells for more than 12 h in the presence of Brefeldin A can lead to excessive cell death.
5. For flow cytometry cells should be kept in the dark as much as possible after starting to stain.
6. Optimal fluorophores for flow cytometry will depend on the individual experiment and cytometer configuration thus cannot be universally recommended.
7. Optimal antibody concentrations for flow cytometry staining must be empirically determined.
8. When decanting supernatant during ICS staining ensure that the flick is quick enough and hard enough to empty the wells without mixing the contents, but not so hard as to dislodge the cell pellet.

9. Once cells are permeabilized it is important to keep them in the detergent containing-perm/wash solution while staining intracellularly.
10. Recommended stimulation with ConA as a positive control is 0.75 μg/mL final.
11. Do not let ELISpot plates dry out until the development is finished and the backing is peeled off.

Acknowledgments

This project has been funded with Federal funds from the National Institute of Allergy and Infectious Diseases, National Institutes of Health, Department of Health and Human Services, under Contract No. HHSN272201400041C.

References

1. Orr MT, Fox CB, Baldwin SL, Sivananthan SJ, Lucas E et al (2013) Adjuvant formulation structure and composition are critical for the development of an effective vaccine against tuberculosis. J Control Release 172:190–200
2. Desbien AL, Reed SJ, Bailor HR, Dubois Cauwelaert N, Laurance JD et al (2015) Squalene emulsion potentiates the adjuvant activity of the TLR4 agonist, GLA, via inflammatory caspases, IL-18, and IFN-gamma. Eur J Immunol 45:407–417
3. Coler RN, Hudson T, Hughes S, Huang PW, Beebe EA et al (2015) Vaccination produces CD4 T Cells with a Novel CD154-CD40-dependent cytolytic mechanism. J Immunol 195:3190–3197
4. Baldwin SL, Bertholet S, Reese VA, Ching LK, Reed SG et al (2012) The importance of adjuvant formulation in the development of a tuberculosis vaccine. J Immunol 188:2189–2197
5. Orr MT, Beebe EA, Hudson TE, Argilla D, Huang PD et al (2015) Mucosal delivery switches the response to an adjuvanted tuberculosis vaccine from systemic TH1 to tissue-resident TH17 responses without impacting the protective efficacy. Vaccine In press
6. Roederer M, Nozzi JL, Nason MC (2011) SPICE: exploration and analysis of post-cytometric complex multivariate datasets. Cytometry A 79:167–174
7. Perfetto SP, Chattopadhyay PK, Wood J, Nguyen R, Ambrozak D et al (2014) Q and B values are critical measurements required for inter-instrument standardization and development of multicolor flow cytometry staining panels. Cytometry A 85:1037–1048
8. Nguyen R, Perfetto S, Mahnke YD, Chattopadhyay P, Roederer M (2013) Quantifying spillover spreading for comparing instrument performance and aiding in multicolor panel design. Cytometry A 83:306–315
9. Chattopadhyay PK, Yu J, Roederer M (2006) Live-cell assay to detect antigen-specific CD4+ T-cell responses by CD154 expression. Nat Protoc 1:1–6
10. Frentsch M, Arbach O, Kirchhoff D, Moewes B, Worm M et al (2005) Direct access to CD4+ T cells specific for defined antigens according to CD154 expression. Nat Med 11:1118–1124

Chapter 25

Eliciting Epitope-Specific CD8$^+$ T Cell Response by Immunization with Microbial Protein Antigens Formulated with α-Galactosylceramide: Theory, Practice, and Protocols

Pavlo Gilchuk, Frances C. Knight, John T. Wilson, and Sebastian Joyce

Abstract

CD8$^+$ cytotoxic T lymphocytes confer protection against infectious diseases caused by viruses, bacteria, and parasites. Hence, significant efforts have been invested into devising ways to generate CD8$^+$ T cell-targeted vaccines. Generation of microbe-free protein subunit vaccines requires a thorough knowledge of protective target antigens. Such antigens are proteolytically processed peptides presented by MHC class I molecules. To induce a robust antigen-specific CD8$^+$ T cell response through vaccination, it is essential to formulate the antigen with an effective adjuvant. Here, we describe a versatile method for generating high-frequency antigen-specific CD8$^+$ T cells through immunization of mice using the invariant natural killer T cell agonist α-galactosylceramide as the adjuvant.

Key words Adjuvant, α-Galactosylceramide, Antigen-specific CD8$^+$ T cells, Microbial protein antigens, Mouse immunization

1 Introduction

Vaccination is one of medical science's greatest achievements; it has led to the eradication of several infectious diseases and to a reduction in morbidity and mortality from many others [1]. The majority of licensed vaccines consist of live, live-attenuated, or inactivated pathogens that were developed by empirical approaches [2]. Understanding vaccine-mediated correlates of immunity is critical for rational design of novel pathogen-free vaccines against infectious diseases for which no effective vaccine currently exists, or to improve the safety and/or efficacy of existing vaccines [2–6].

It is generally thought that the most effective vaccines confer protection via mediation of neutralizing antibodies, which are readily detectable by in vitro assays. Hence, most effort continues to be invested in designing vaccines that induce antibody-mediated

Christopher B. Fox (ed.), *Vaccine Adjuvants: Methods and Protocols*, Methods in Molecular Biology, vol. 1494, DOI 10.1007/978-1-4939-6445-1_25, © Springer Science+Business Media New York 2017

protective immunity [6, 7]. In recent years, however, the focus on developing T cell-targeted vaccines has increased, as it has become clear that successful vaccination relies on both antibody- and T cell-mediated immunity (reviewed in Ref. [3, 8]).

The indispensable role of cellular immunity was observed even prior to modern advances in microbiology and immunology, from the historically recorded cases known as "experiments of nature." As early as the nineteenth century, Jenner and colleagues observed that a smallpox-immune mother had brought forth an infant who died a few days after birth owing to an infection contracted in utero, as the baby was born with pocks/pustules [9, 10]. Given that the mother's antibody repertoire circulates within the fetus and babies are born with underdeveloped cellular immunity [11–13], we can now surmise that protection from smallpox requires cellular immunity. Another example of the critical role of cellular immunity includes a case report for progressive vaccinia virus (VACV) infection in a subject with normal anti-viral antibody responses [14].

Immune $CD8^+$ T cells recognize infected cells via short microbial peptide epitopes presented by the host's major histocompatibility complex (MHC)-encoded class I molecules. Of note, MHC class I molecules present cytoplasmic antigens because their assembly with peptides predominantly occurs within the endoplasmic reticulum, though under inflammatory conditions it can occur within vacuoles as well (reviewed in Refs. [15, 16]). Recent studies have shown that $CD8^+$ T cells play a critical role in conferring protective immunity against a variety of infectious diseases, including those caused by respiratory viruses [17–21], poxviruses [22], cytomegalovirus [23], human immunodeficiency virus (HIV; [24]), *Plasmodium* species [25, 26], and *M. tuberculosis* [27]. Hence, T cell epitope-based vaccines can complement current efforts in developing safe and effective antibody-targeted subunit vaccines.

The challenge impeding the development of T cell-targeted subunit vaccines is identifying which of the microbe's peptide epitopes confer protective immunity amongst the many that are presented [28]. Such epitopes can be discovered by indirect approaches that can ascertain protein subunit immunogenicity and protective capability in surrogate animal models [29, 30]. Accordingly, there is a need for the design and implementation of an effective vaccination strategy that will elicit sufficiently high-frequency, antigen-specific $CD8^+$ T cells to allow thorough characterization of the response to subunit antigens. Unlike replicative microbial vaccines, heterologous proteins and peptides are poorly immunogenic when administered alone. Therefore, to induce a robust antigen-specific $CD8^+$ T cell response without the use of infectious agents or antigen-loaded exogenous dendritic cells (DCs) [31–33], it is essential to formulate the antigen with an effective adjuvant [34]. Successful $CD8^+$ T cell-targeted immunization has been demonstrated for peptide epitopes that are formulated with various toll-like receptor

(TLR) ligands [31, 35]. High-frequency $CD8^+$ T cells can be induced by peptides formulated with polyinosinic-polycytidylic acid (poly(I:C); TLR3 agonist) and co-stimulatory anti-CD40 antibody [36]. Peptide immunogenicity can be improved via chemical engineering of peptides and adjuvants with amphiphilic albumin-binding tags [37]. The immunogenicity of peptides can also be modulated through engineered delivery systems; these are discussed elsewhere [38, 39] and, hence, not reviewed here.

It should be noted that full-length protein antigens are typically more desirable for vaccination studies than peptide epitopes. This is because immunization with proteins allows elicitation of both antibody- and T cell-mediated immune responses [28, 40–42]. In addition, one protein may contain several immune epitopes, which is a desirable feature for human vaccines [43]. Because MHC class I molecules present cytoplasmic antigens, the priming of naïve $CD8^+$ T cells requires cross-presentation of exogenous antigens by antigen-presenting cells (APCs) that have taken up the administered protein. Small subsets of DCs—the tissue-resident, generally non-migratory, $CD103^+$ as well as splenic $CD8^+$ DCs in mice, or $CD1c^+$ and $CD141^+$ DCs in humans—play critical roles in cross-presentation of exogenous antigens (reviewed in Refs. [15, 16]). Antigen cross-presentation requires the activation and licensing of the appropriate DC subsets; $CD4^+$ T cells are the classical helper cells for DC activation and licensing (reviewed in Ref. [44]). So also, $CD4^+$ T cell help is essential for the differentiation of effector and memory $CD8^+$ T cells (reviewed in Ref. [44]). Because MHC class II molecules—which also present processed peptide antigens generated in vacuolar compartments to control the functions of $CD4^+$ T cells—are highly variable, vaccine design requires the identification of helper epitopes and their inclusion in $CD8^+$ T cell-targeted vaccines. Hence, harnessing a non-polymorphic antigen-presenting molecule and invariant T cells as vaccine targets that can provide help can be a viable option for enhancing $CD8^+$ T cell responses to subunit antigens. CD1d and the restricted semi-invariant natural killer T (NKT) cells have shown significant promise as experimental vaccine targets [44]; their biology has been recently reviewed elsewhere [45].

Immunogenicity of whole-protein antigens formulated with the NKT cell agonist α-galactosylceramide (αGalCer) as the adjuvant has demonstrated that this formulation stimulates robust antigen-specific T cell and antibody responses in mice [41, 46–48]. αGalCer is a synthetic glycolipid that closely resembles the marine sponge *Agelas mauritianus*-derived agelasphin 9b as well as self and bacterial glycolipid antigens (*see* Table 1 and references therein). Upon immunization, professional APCs, such as DCs, macrophages, and B cells, take up the administered protein antigen and αGalCer. Antigens undergo processing to short peptide epitopes that are presented by MHC class I molecules expressed

Table 1

Structure and properties of selected synthetic, microbial, and self NKT cell agonists

Lipid (class)[a]	Chain length[b]	Structure	Agonist[c]	References
αGalCer (GSL)	C18 C24:1	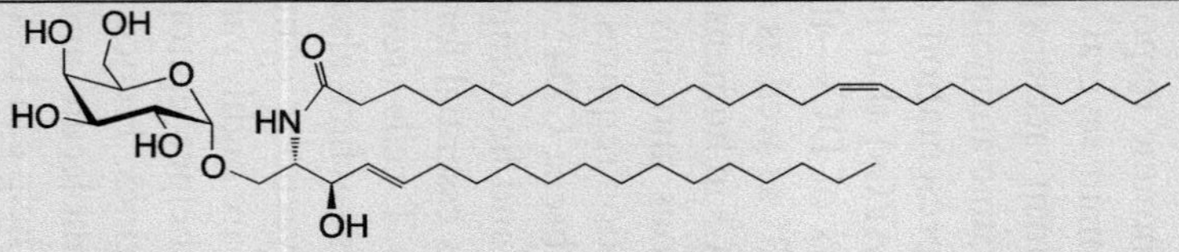	IFN-γ, IL-4 Self	[67]
Agel 9b (GSL)	C17 (C_{16}-Me) phyto C24	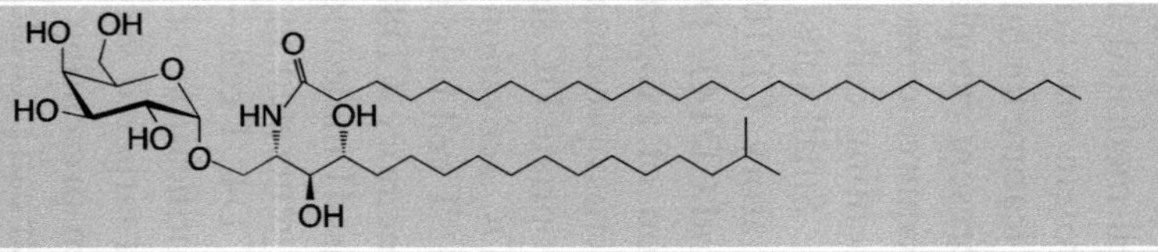	Anti-tumour; *Agelas mauritianus*	[68, 69]
αGalCer (GSL)	C18-phyto C26 *Common form used in functional studies (this is the molecule used in this chapter)*	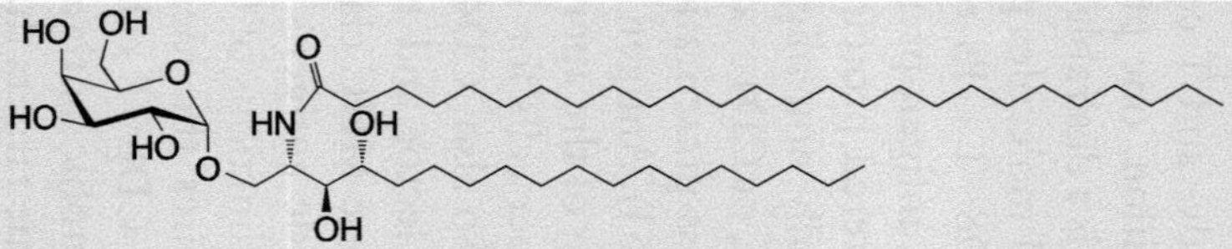	Very strong Robust IFN-γ, IL-4, and other cytokines; synthetic analogue of Agel 9b (KRN7000)	[70]
DB06-1 (GSL)	C18-phyto C26 (C_2S)	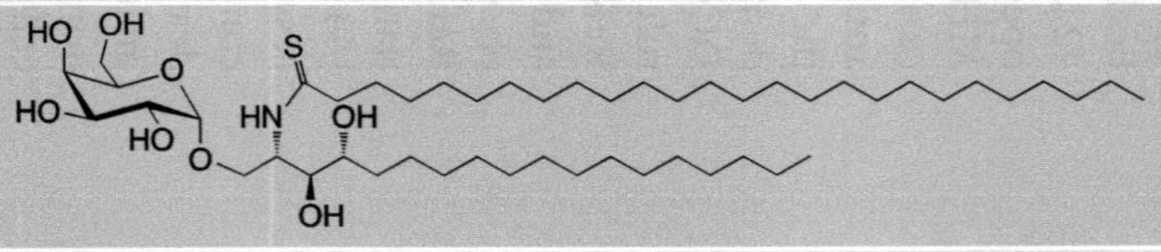	Strong; strong IFN-γ; IL-10 upon re-activation	[71]
α-*C*-GalCer (GSL)	C18-phyto C26 1,1′-*C*-glycoside	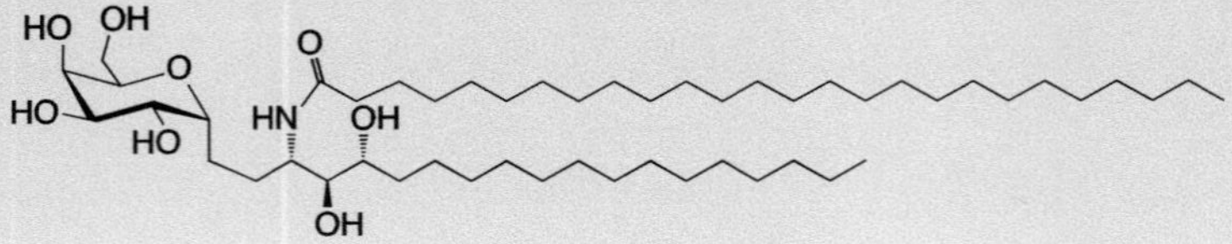	Weak (mo[d])-to-none (hu); IFN-γ; synthetic	[72]

FPh-αGalCer (GSL)	C18-phyto C10-fluoro-phenyl	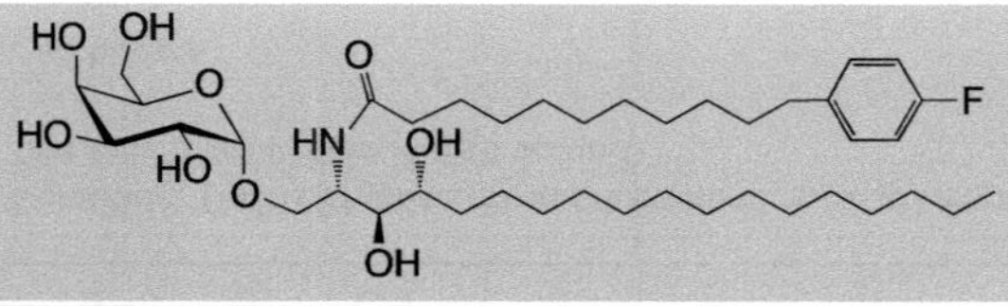	Very strong IFN-γ; synthetic	[73]
NU-αGalCer (GSL)	C18-phyto C26 C6″-naphthylurea	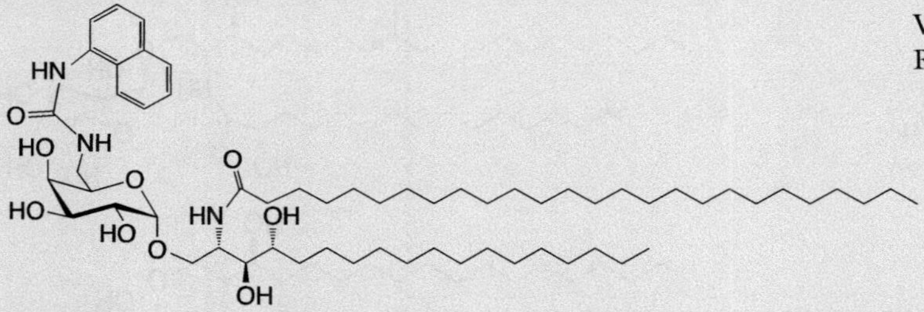	Very strong Robust IFN-γ; synthetic	[74]
PyrC-αGalCer (GSL)	C18-phyto C26 C6″-(pyridin-4-yl)-carbamate	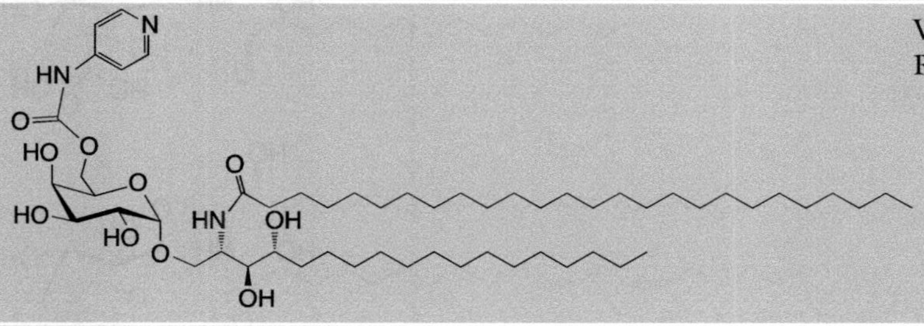	Very strong Robust IFN-γ, IL-12; synthetic	[75]
SMC124 (GSL)	C22-C_{11}cyclo-propyl C26	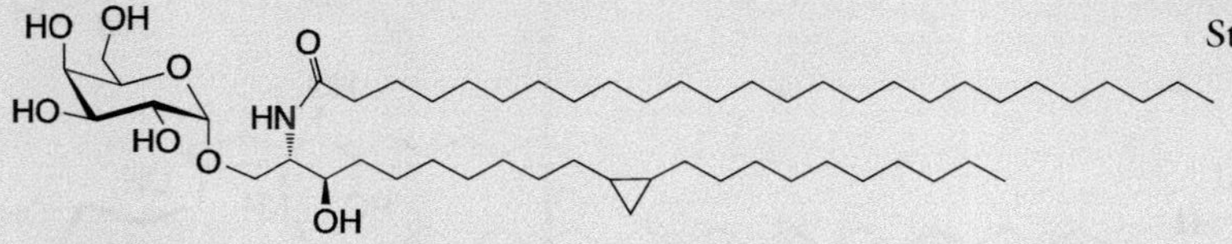	Strong IFN-γ; synthetic	[76]
EF77 (GSL)	C18-phyto C21:1-C_{10}-cyclo-propyl	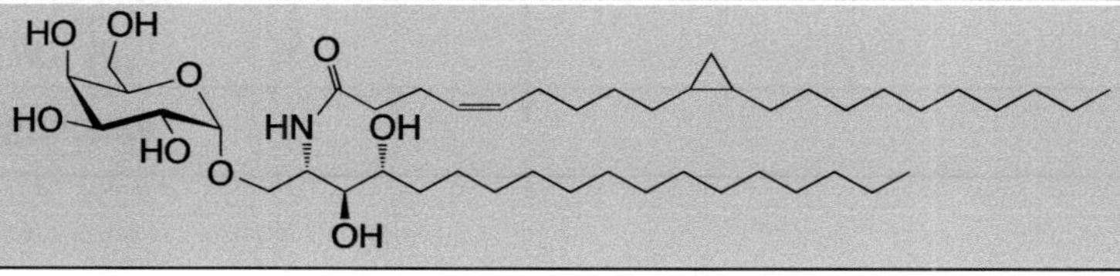	Strong IFN-γ; synthetic	[76]

(continued)

Table 1
(continued)

Lipid (class)[a]	Chain length[b]	Structure	Agonist[c]	References
OCH (GSL)	C9-phyto C24	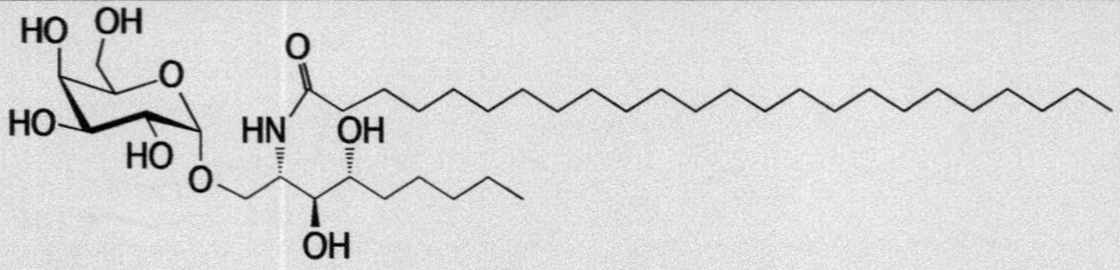	Weak (mo)-to-none (hu) IL-4 (low-to-no IFN-γ); synthetic	[77]
C20-diene (GSL)	C18-phyto C20:2	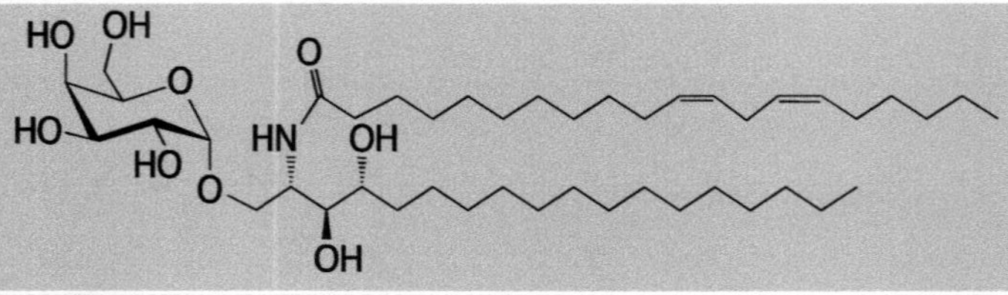	Strong IL-4 (low-to-no IFN-γ); synthetic	[78]
αGalACer (GSL)	C18-phyto C14	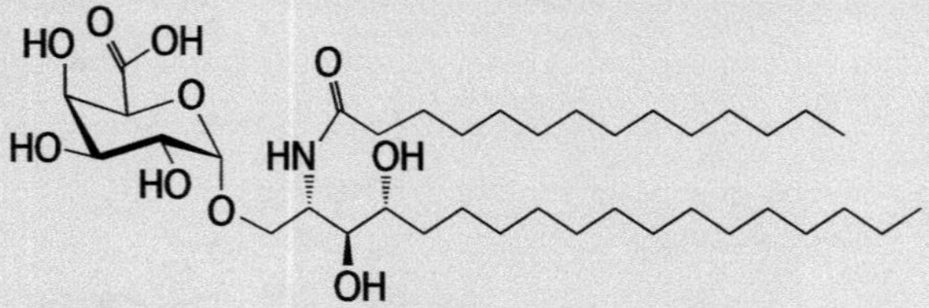	Weak; *Sphingomonas* spp.	[79, 80]
Asp B (GSL)	C20:2-C_9 Me C16-C_2OH	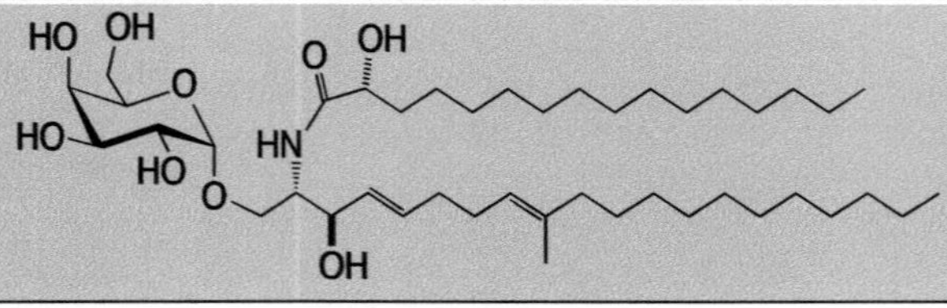	Weak *Aspergillus fumigatus*	[81]

[a] *Agel* agelasphin, *Asp B* asparamide B, *GalCer* galactosylceramide, *GalACer* galacturonosylceramide, *GSL* glycosphingolipid, *IL* interleukin
[b] Sphingosine/phytosphingosine chain length indicated first and *N*-acyl chain length second
[c] Agonist strength based on Ref. [82]
[d] Relative potency in comparison to αGalCer; ***mo*** mouse, ***hu*** human

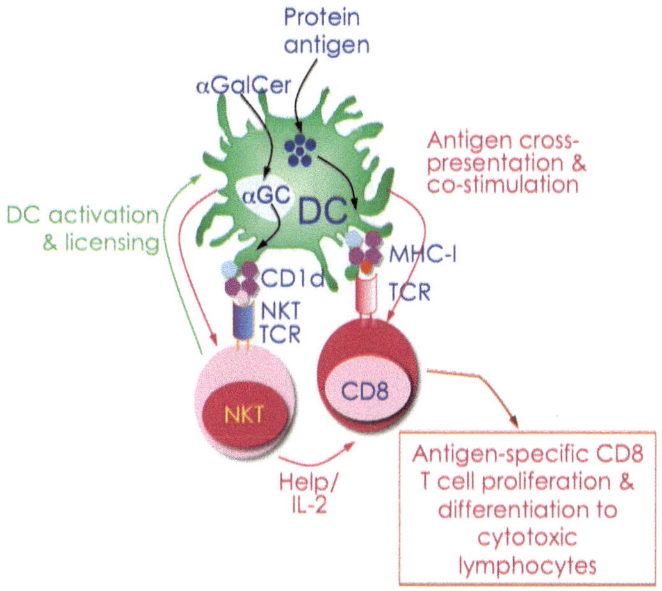

Fig. 1 Strategy by which a robust antigen-specific CD8+ T cell response is elicited in mice immunized with antigenic protein formulated with the glycolipid adjuvant αGalCer. Upon immunization, professional antigen-presenting cells, such as dendritic cells (DCs), endocytose administered protein antigen and αGalCer. The antigen undergoes processing into short peptide epitopes that are presented by MHC class I molecules on DCs for recognition via the T cell receptor (TCR) of antigen-specific CD8+ T cells. αGalCer is presented by MHC class I-like CD1d molecules and recognized by the TCR of semi-invariant NKT cells. Recognition of αGalCer rapidly activates NKT cells, which produce cytokine/chemokine messengers, thereby trans-activating DCs and initiating a cross talk between members of the innate and adaptive immune systems. NKT cell licensing of DCs facilitates antigen cross presentation by a less well-understood mechanism(s) [42, 44, 65]. Together, this provides stimulus to naïve antigen-specific CD8+ T cell precursors that then proliferate and differentiate into effector and memory CD8+ T cells [45]

by APCs for recognition via the T cell receptor (TCR) of antigen-specific CD8+ T cells. The MHC class I-like, lipid antigen-presenting CD1d molecules present αGalCer and the TCR of NKT cells recognize the co-complex. Recognition of αGalCer rapidly activates NKT cells. Activated NKT cells produce cytokine/chemokine messengers, thereby trans-activating DCs and initiating a crosstalk between cells of the innate and adaptive immune systems. Activated NKT cells and DCs together stimulate naïve antigen-specific CD8+ T cell precursors, which then proliferate and differentiate into effector and memory CD8+ T cells (Fig. 1; [28, 44, 45, 49, 50]). By virtue of its ability to communicate to virtually all cell types of the immune system, αGalCer has proven to be a potent adjuvant that enhances antibody and CD4 T cell responses to foreign antigens (reviewed in Ref. [45]).

Several studies have reported that αGalCer is an effective adjuvant for the elicitation of epitope-specific $CD8^+$ T cells against the model protein antigen ovalbumin [41, 51–53], or for enhancing antigen-specific $CD8^+$ T cell responses upon immunization with live viral vaccines [49, 54]. We recently demonstrated the potency of αGalCer as a $CD8^+$ T cell adjuvant for in vivo immunogenicity and protection studies which exploited pathogen-derived protein antigens ([28] and unpublished data). It is noteworthy that the activation of NKT cells by αGalCer results in the production of proinflammatory as well as immunoregulatory cytokines and chemokines (reviewed in [45]). Since DC activation and licensing as well as $CD8^+$ T cell differentiation require proinflammatory cytokines and chemokines, efforts to synthesize and identify αGalCer analogues that elicit proinflammatory activity are being sought but are not discussed here (*see* Table 1; reviewed in Ref. [55]). Herein, we describe protocols for the preparation of protein antigens and αGalCer adjuvant, mouse immunization, and assessment of antigen-specific $CD8^+$ T cell response, while analysis of antigen-specific antibody response and protective immunity is not described.

Experiments that assess immunogenicity require a large quantity of pure protein antigens, which, unlike model antigens, are not typically available commercially. Instead, the desired proteins are produced by recombinant DNA methods in *Escherichia coli* and then purified to a high degree of purity through engineered tags with the use of affinity resin. We designed, cloned, and produced nine recombinant VACV-derived protein subunits ($rA3L_{62-319}$, $rD1R_{565-844}$, $rD5R_{330-470}$, $rE2L_{26-301}$, $rF4L_{1-319}$, $rJ6R_{188-466}$, and $rL4R_{33-249}$, as well as epitope-engineered subunits $L4R/B8R_{70-79}$ and $L4R/A34R_{32-90}$), all of which contain a C-terminal histidine-tag to facilitate purification (Fig. 2; [28]). Upon immunization of mice, αGalCer-formulated antigens induced robust epitope-specific $CD8^+$ T cell and antibody responses that were detectable in blood and in various tissues (Fig. 3a–c). Vaccination with adjuvant and microbial antigen induced protective immunity against subsequent microbial challenge (Fig. 4 and unpublished data). Our immunization approach is suitable for elicitation of antigen-specific $CD8^+$ T cell and antibody responses to recombinant proteins that are produced as insoluble inclusion bodies (IB). Results that have emerged from the use of approaches described herein demonstrate the efficacy of the proposed immunization strategy for generating high-frequency antigen-specific $CD8^+$ T cells against microbial protein antigens that can be exploited for immunologic and vaccine studies.

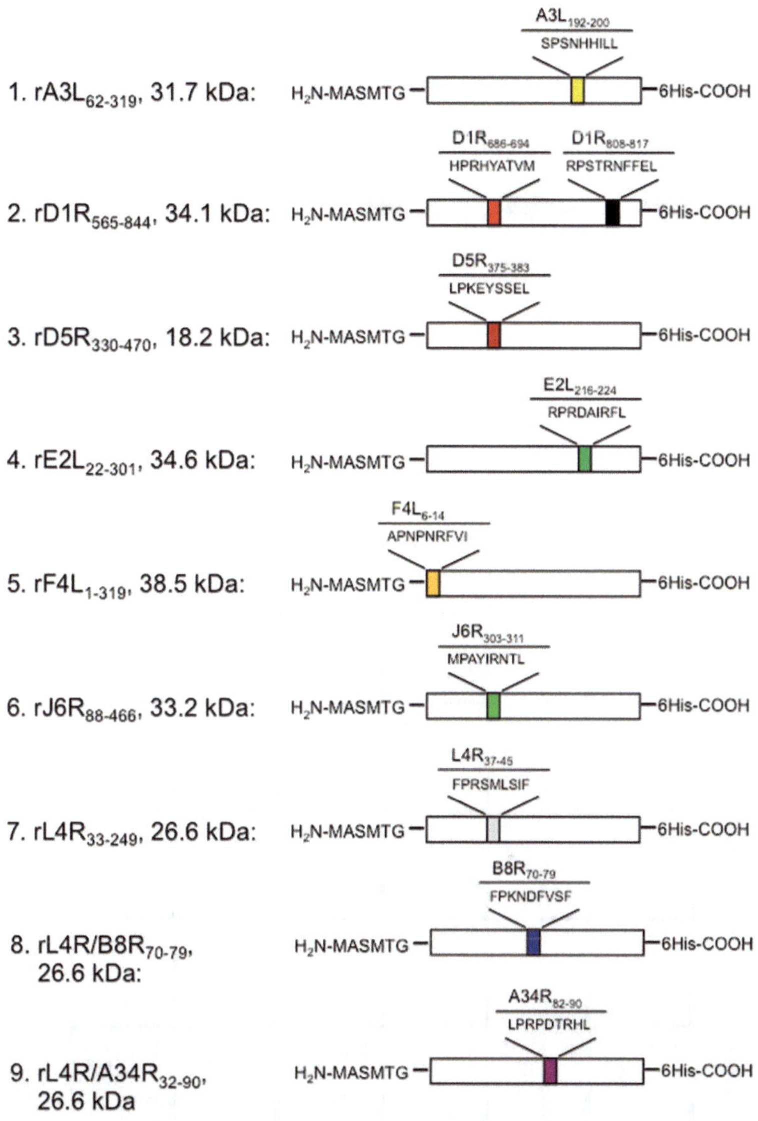

Fig. 2 Design of recombinant VACV-derived protein antigen subunits that contain immune CD8$^+$ T cell epitopes. Schematic chart of engineered proteins showing nine VACV antigens with amino acid positions selected for the design of a truncated recombinant subunit. Shown are the location and sequences of immune CD8$^+$ T cell epitopes, and their N- and C-terminal tag sequences introduced to facilitate expression and purification of recombinant proteins in *E. coli.* Soluble protein rL4R$_{33–249}$ was engineered with B8R$_{70–79}$ and A34R$_{82–90}$ immune epitopes to facilitate expression of soluble antigens by *E. coli.* All CD8$^+$ T cell epitopes are restricted to the HLA-B*07;02 (B7.2) molecules. This figure is adapted from our previous publication with permission from the Journal of Clinical Investigation [28]

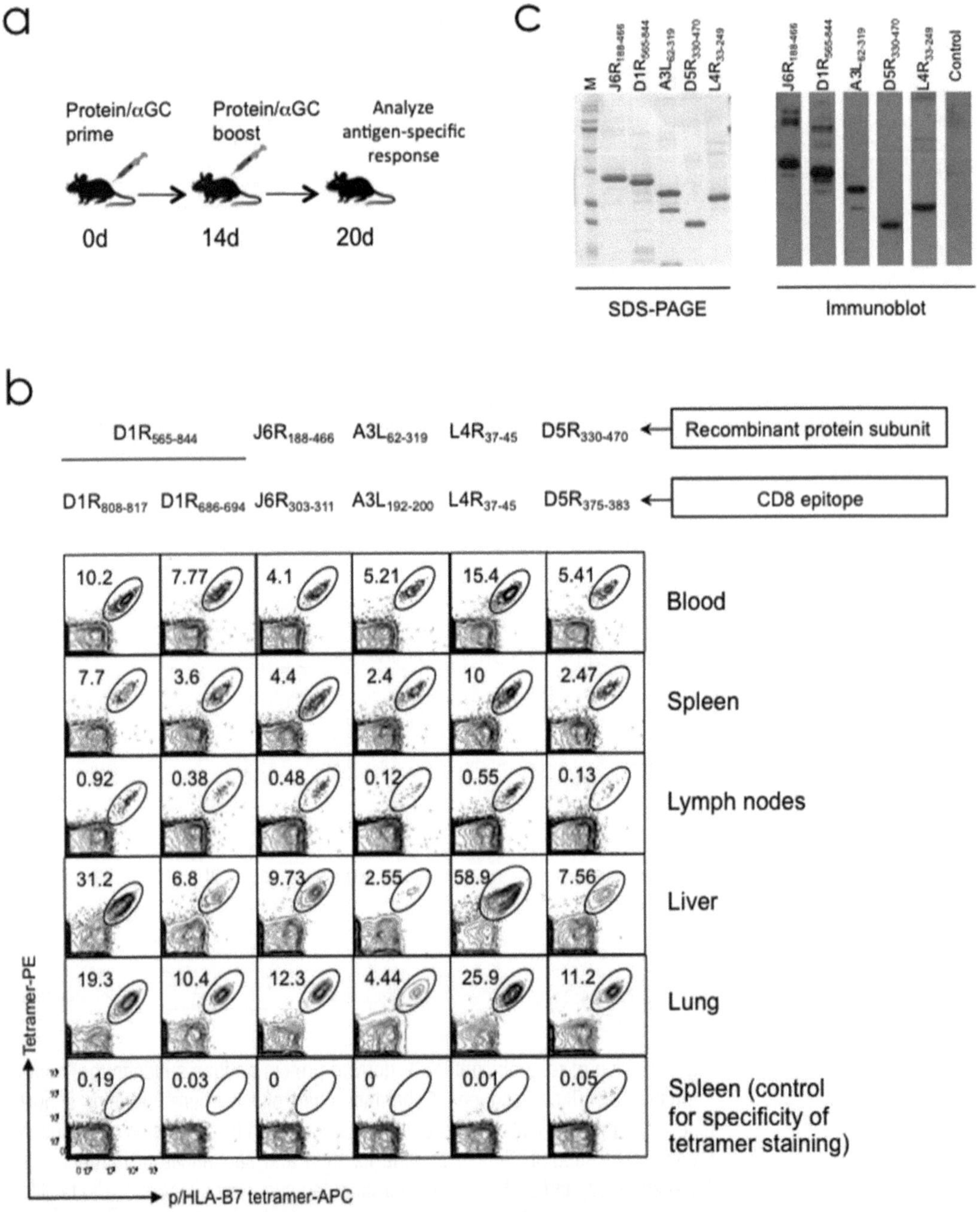

Fig. 3 Efficient stimulation of antigen-specific immune responses is achieved through prime and boost immunization with αGalCer-formulated protein antigens. (**a**) Experimental design. Purified protein antigen is formulated with αGalCer and administered to mice by intraperitoneal or intranasal route as indicated. Antigen-specific immune responses were assessed ~6 days after booster immunization. (**b**) Representative example showing that immunization with αGalCer-formulated VACV-derived recombinant protein subunits elicited a robust epitope-specific $CD8^+$ T cell response. Individual proteins containing HLA-B7.2 restricted $CD8^+$ epitopes (*see* Fig. 2) were formulated with αGalCer and administered to groups of $B7^{tg}$ mice IP as in shown in (**a**). On d6 after boost, various tissues and blood were harvested from each group of immunized mice and assessed with B7.2

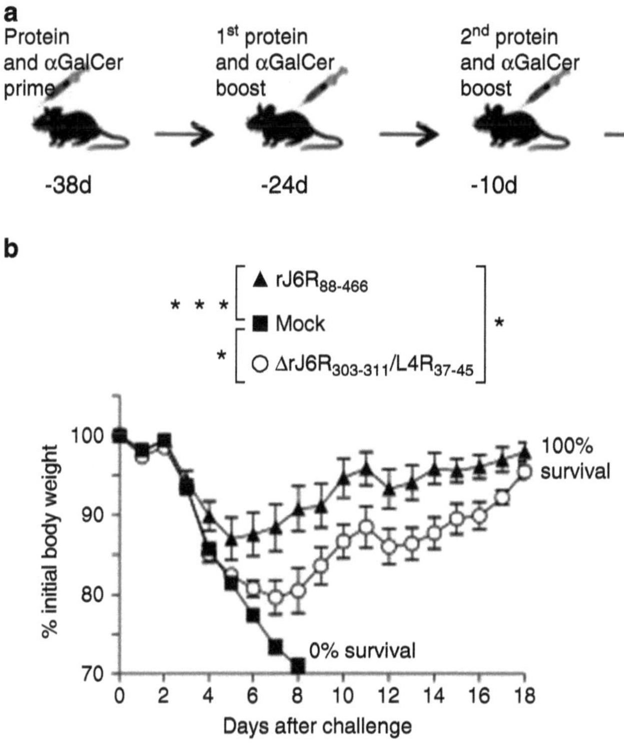

Fig. 4 Protection from lethal VACV infection upon vaccination with VACV-derived antigenic protein that contains CD8+ epitope. (**a**) Vaccination and challenge strategy. Three groups of mice ($n = 5$ mice per group) were immunized by IP route with αGalCer-formulated VACV-derived protein antigens rJ6R$_{88-466}$ (contains protective CD8+ epitope), or engineered ΔrJ6R$_{303-311}$/L4R$_{37-45}$ (contains non-protective CD8+ epitope), or mock-vaccinated as indicated. Vaccinated mice were challenged with VACV and observed during the ensuing 18 days for severity of disease. Elicitation of J6R$_{303-311}$ (protective epitope) or L4R$_{37-45}$ (non-protective epitope) epitope-specific CD8+ was confirmed with corresponding tetramers in blood of vaccinated mice on d 8 after second boost. (**b**) Protection of protein and αGalCer-vaccinated mice from lethal respiratory VACV challenge. All mock-vaccinated mice succumbed to the disease by d8 post-infection. Both protein and αGalCer-vaccinated groups were protected from severe weight loss and death. Replacing protective CD8+ epitope J6R$_{303-311}$ in rJ6R$_{88-466}$ with non-protective L4R$_{37-45}$ epitope showed that protection is mediated by J6R$_{303-311}$-specific CD8+ T cells with partial contribution from other immune responses against the protein antigen. ***$p < 0.001$; *$p < 0.05$ as compared to mock on d8 post challenge as defined by ANOVA with Dunnett's post-test; mean ± SEM. *Symbols* indicate proteins used for vaccination

Fig. 3 (continued) tetramer for epitope-specific CD8+ T cells. Epitope-specific CD8+ T cells were detected using a dual-fluorochrome labeling approach as described previously [28, 66]. Contour plots are gated on live CD8+ T lymphocytes; numbers indicate percent epitope-specific CD8+ T cells. Panel was reproduced from Ref. 28 with permission from the Journal of Clinical Investigation. (**c**) Representative example showing that immunization with αGalCer-formulated VACV-derived recombinant protein subunits elicited antigen-specific antibody responses. SDS-PAGE (*left*) and western blot (*right*) of purified VACV-derived subunits. Each lane was loaded with ~4 μg protein for SDS-PAGE and ~0.5 μg protein for immunoblot. Blots were probed with 1:500 sera dilution from mice primed and boosted with the indicated individual proteins, and developed with anti-mouse HRP-conjugated secondary antibodies. *M* molecular weight standards, from top to bottom: 250, 150, 100, 75, 50, 37, 25, 20, 15 kDa

2 Materials

Reagents and equipment described herein can be substituted with equivalent alternatives from other vendors.

2.1 Adjuvant Preparation

1. Fisherbrand™ class A clear glass threaded 6 ml vials with caps (Fisher Scientific).
2. αGalCer (Funakoshi, Japan); *see* Table 1 for structure. To dissolve αGalCer, use 5.6% sucrose, 0.75% l-histidine, and 0.5% Tween 20 in sterile water for injection (WFI) for cell culture with heating at 80 °C until dissolved (*see* **Note 1**). Make a 0.2 mg/ml stock solution and store at −20 °C.

2.2 Antigen Preparation

The immunization protocol reported herein was validated with the use of vaccinia virus (VACV)-derived recombinant proteins designed and produced in our laboratory [28] and with the model antigen ovalbumin. The following materials are required to obtain recombinant protein antigens for immunizing mice:

1. *E. coli* BL21-Gold(DE3) Competent Cells (Agilent Technologies) transformed with plasmid encoding desired protein antigen.
2. LB broth: To 800 ml H_2O add 10 g tryptone, 5 g yeast extract, and 10 g NaCl. Adjust pH to 7.5 with 0.5 M NaOH and bring the final volume to 1 L with dH_2O. Sterilize the solution by autoclaving.
3. Kanamycin (Km): Make 50 mg/ml stock solution in sterile dH_2O and store at −20 °C.
4. Glucose: Make 40% (w/v) stock solution and sterilize by autoclaving.
5. LB agar plates containing 50 μg/ml Km and 1% glucose.
6. Isopropyl β-d-thiogalactoside (IPTG): Make 1 mM stock in sterile dH_2O and store at −20 °C.
7. Sterile phosphate-buffered saline (PBS), 1×: 137 mM NaCl, 2.7 mM KCl, 10 mM Na_2HPO_4, 2 mM KH_2PO_4.
8. Ni-NTA agarose.
9. Cell lysis buffer A: 50 mM NaH_2PO_4, 300 mM NaCl, 5 mM imidazole (pH 8.0). Sterilize using Complete Filtration Unit with 0.2 μm filter (VWR) and store at room temperature (RT).
10. Lysozyme.
11. Wash buffer B: 50 mM NaH_2PO_4, 300 mM NaCl, 10 mM imidazole (pH 8.0). Filter sterilize (*see* Subheading 2.2, **item 9**) and store at room temperature (RT).

12. Elution buffer C: 50 mM NaH_2PO_4, 300 mM NaCl, 250 mM imidazole (pH 8.0). Filter sterilize (*see* Subheading 2.2, **item 9**) and store at RT.
13. Solubilization/wash buffer D: 20 mM Tris HCl, 300 mM NaCl, 8 M urea, 10 mM imidazole (pH 8.0) (*see* **Note 2**). Filter sterilize (*see* Subheading 2.2, **item 9**) and store at RT.
14. Elution buffer E: 20 mM Tris–HCl, 300 mM NaCl, 8 M urea, 100 mM imidazole (pH 8.0). Filter sterilize (*see* Subheading 2.2, **item 9**) and store at RT.
15. 10–12 % Sodium dodecyl sulfate (SDS)-polyacrylamide gel (*see* **Note 3**).
16. Sodium dodecyl sulfate-polyacrylamide gel electrophoresis (SDS-PAGE) running buffer: 0.025 M Tris–HCl (pH 8.3), 0.192 M glycine, 0.1 % SDS.
17. Loading dye solution (5×): 0.03 M Tris–HCl (pH 6.8), 10 % SDS, 25 % 2-mercaptoethanol, 0.1 % bromophenol blue, 45 % glycerol. Store at −20 °C.
18. Bovine serum albumin (BSA) lyophilized powder: Prepare 0.2 mg/ml stock in 1× loading dye solution. Store at −20 °C.
19. Spectra Multicolor Broad Range Protein Ladder (Thermo Fisher).
20. GelCode Blue Stain Reagent (Thermo Fisher).
21. Optional: Pierce High Capacity Endotoxin Removal Spin Columns, 0.25 ml (Thermo Fisher).
22. Slide-A-Lyzer Dialysis Cassette, 10 K MWCO, 3 ml (Thermo Fisher).
23. Pierce disposable polypropylene columns, 5 ml (Thermo Fisher).
24. Falcon disposable polypropylene centrifuge tubes, 50 ml (Corning).
25. Disposable Safe-Lock Tubes, 1.5 ml (Eppendorf).
26. Disposable centrifuge tubes, 250 ml (Corning).
27. Nalgene baffled shake flask, 2000 ml (Sigma).
28. Disposable syringes, 5 ml (BD Biosciences).
29. Disposable Millex-GV Syringe Filter Unit, 0.22 μm (EMD Millipore).
30. Disposable 28 mm syringe filter, 0.45 μm (Corning).
31. Nalgene Oak Ridge High-Speed PPCO Centrifuge Tubes, 50 ml (Thermo Scientific).
32. Orbital shaker incubator.
33. 550 Sonic Dismembrator (Fisher Scientific).

34. Precision Microprocessor-Controlled 280 Series Water Bath (Thermo Scientific).
35. Mini-PROTEAN 3 Mini Vertical electrophoresis system (Bio-Rad) with Power Station 300 plus power supply (Labnet International, Inc).
36. Eppendorf 5415D microcentrifuge.
37. Refrigerated Sorvall RT7 centrifuge with RTH-750 rotor.
38. Sorvall RC-5B refrigerated centrifuge with SS-34 rotor.
39. DU 530 UV/Vis Spectrophotometer (Beckman).

2.3 Immunizations

1. Mice: All mice used for immunization were 6–10-week-old males from the following strains: B6-*K0D0;B*07;02tg* (B7^{tg}) human leukocyte antigen (HLA) class I transgenic (tg) mice were bred in house. B7^{tg} mouse is described elsewhere [56]. C57BL/6 (B6) mice were purchased from Jackson Laboratories (Bar Harbor, ME). All animal procedures were approved by the Institutional Animal Care and Use Committee (IACUC) at Vanderbilt University.
2. Anesthesia: 10 mg/ml KETAVED (ketamine HCl injection, USP; Vedco) and 1 mg/ml xylazine HCl Injection (xylazine; Vanderbilt pharmacy) in sterile WFI. Ketamine/xylazine anesthesia should be approved by an IACUC at user institution.
3. Purified recombinant antigen or albumin from chicken egg white (ovalbumin, Ova) at 0.5–2 mg/ml in sterile PBS (*see* **Note 4**).
4. Sterile insulin syringes, 1 ml (BD Biosciences).
5. Sterile filter pipet tips, 1–200 μl (VWR).

2.4 Lymphocyte Isolation

1. SmartBox Auto CO_2 System for rodent euthanasia (Euthanex).
2. Refrigerated Sorvall RT7 centrifuge with RTH-750 rotor and plate adaptors.
3. Hausser Scientific Hemocytometer (Fisher Scientific).
4. Forceps.
5. Surgical scissors.
6. Falcon sterile disposable cell strainer, white, 70 μm (Fisher Scientific).
7. BD sterile disposable Slip Tip syringes, 5 ml (Fisher Scientific).
8. Sterile disposable Falcon polypropylene centrifuge tubes, 15 ml (Fisher Scientific).
9. Falcon sterile disposable 60 mm × 15 mm Petri dishes (Corning).
10. Optional: Capillary tubes, heparinized (Fisher Scientific) or plain (Fisher Scientific).

11. Dimethyl sulfoxide (DMSO).
12. Dasatinib (LC Laboratories): Dissolve to 1 mM in DMSO and store in 0.05 ml aliquots at −20 °C.
13. FACS buffer: PBS containing 2% heat-inactivated fetal bovine serum (FBS) and 50 nM dasatinib. Make and use fresh (*see* **Note 5**).
14. Collagenase (Sigma).
15. Complete RPMI medium (cRPMI): RPMI-1640 with l-glutamine and HEPES supplemented with 10% FBS, 1× penicillin/streptomycin solution and 1.75 μl of cell culture grade 2-mercaptoethanol.
16. Lung digestion medium: cRPMI (*see* Subheading 2.4, **item 15**) containing 2 mg/ml collagenase and 50 nM dasatinib.
17. Gibco ACK lysing buffer (Thermo Fisher).
18. Trypan blue solution, 0.4% in PBS (Fisher Scientific).

2.5 Tetramer Staining, Intracellular Cytokine Staining (ICCS), and Flow Cytometry

1. 10 mM Peptide epitope (purity ≥95%; Schufer-N, Denmark) dissolved in sterile DMSO.
2. Brefeldin A (Sigma). Prepare stock solution at 10 mg/ml in methanol.
3. BD GolgiStop Protein Transport Inhibitor (BD Biosciences).
4. Phorbol 12-myristate 13-acetate (PMA) (InvivoGen): Make 1 mg/ml stock solution in sterile WFI and store at −20 °C. Protect from light.
5. Ionomycin (Sigma): Dissolve in sterile DMSO to make 3 mM ionomycin solution and store at −20 °C.
6. cRPMI (*see* Subheading 2.4, **item 15**).
7. FACS buffer (*see* Subheading 2.4, **item 13**).
8. BD Cytofix/Cytoperm Fixation and Permeabilization Solution (BD Biosciences).
9. BD Perm/wash buffer, 10× solution (BD Biosciences).
10. Optional: AccuCheck counting beads (Thermo Fisher).
11. UltraComp eBeads (eBioscience).
12. Falcon 96 Well Round Bottom Cell Culture Plate (Corning).
13. Fisherbrand Polypropylene Microtiter Tubes, 1.2 ml (Fisher Scientific).
14. Refrigerated Sorvall RT7 centrifuge with RTH-750 rotor and plate adaptors.
15. LSR-II flow cytometer (BD Biosciences).
16. FlowJo flow cytometry software (Tree Star, Inc).
17. Tetramers, antibodies, and viability dyes: *See* Table 2.

Table 2
Flow cytometry reagents

Analysis[a]	Reagent	Antibody clone	Company[c]
Tet	$B8R_{70-79}$ (FPKNDFVSF)/B7.2-PE	–[b]	–
Tet	$L4R_{37-45}$ (FPRSMLSIF)/B7.2-PE	–	–
Tet	$A3L_{192-200}$ (SPSNHHILL)/B7.2-PE	–	–
Tet	$D1R_{686-694}$ (HPRHYATVM)/B7.2-PE	–	–
Tet	$D1R_{808-817}$ (RPSTRNFFEL)/B7.2-PE	–	–
Tet	$D5R_{375-383}$ (LPKEYSSEL)/B7.2-PE	–	–
Tet	$J6R_{303-311}$ (MPAYIRNTL)/B7.2-PE	–	–
Tet	$Ova_{257-264}$ (SIINFEKL)/H-2Kb-PE	–	–
Tet	Anti-CD8α-Pacific Blue	Clone 53–6.7	BD Biosciences
ICCS	Anti-CD8α-PerCP-Cy5.5	Clone 53–6.7	BD Biosciences
Tet	Anti-B220-FITC	Clone RA3-6B2	BD Biosciences
ICCS	Anti-B220-APC-Cy7	Clone RA3-6B2	BD Biosciences
Tet	Anti-CD11c-FITC	Clone N418	Tonbo Biosciences
ICCS	Anti-CD3ε-PE	Clone 145-2C11	BD Biosciences
Tet	Anti-CD4-FITC	Clone H129.19	BD Biosciences
Tet	Anti-CD11b-FITC	Clone M1/70	Tonbo Biosciences
ICCS	Anti-CD107a-FITC	Clone 1D4B	BD Biosciences
ICCS	Anti-IFN-γ-allophycocyanin (APC)	Clone XMG1.2	BD Biosciences
Tet	Propidium iodide	–	BD Biosciences
ICCS	Fixable Viability Dye eFluor 450	–	eBioscience

[a] *Tet* p/MHC class I tetramer used for staining, *ICCS* intracellular cytokine staining

[b] p/B7.2, $H2K^b$ monomers and tetramers were made in-house according to published methods ([28, 83], see also "Production protocols" at http://tetramer.yerkes.emory.edu/); all tetramers are labeled with phycoerythrin (PE) and stored as 50 μg/ml stock at +4 °C

[c] Representative vendors from which the reagents were purchased. These reagents are also available from the other vendors as well

3 Methods

Follow institutional biosafety and waste disposal regulations when working with chemicals and biologicals. Experimentation involving mice must comply with the experimenters' IACUC regulations. The procedures described here were approved by IACUC at Vanderbilt University.

3.1 Preparation of Antigen

This section describes the preparation of recombinant protein antigen that was used to immunize mice. The sample protocol described below includes the production, purification, and formulation of a VACV protein produced as a recombinant protein by biosynthesis in *Escherichia coli* (*E. coli*). This protocol was validated for ten different recombinant proteins, three of which were produced in soluble form, with the remaining seven proteins produced in insoluble form as inclusion bodies (IB). Isolated protein antigens proved to be suitable for in vivo immunogenicity and protection studies. Each investigator should optimize this protocol to ensure optimal yield, purity, and solubility of the protein of interest.

1. Plate bacteria transformed with the desired plasmid on freshly prepared LB agar plate containing 50 μg/ml Km and 1 % glucose; incubate overnight at +37 °C. Follow general rules of aseptic techniques when working with *E. coli*; that is, perform these procedures around the blue flame of a Bunsen burner.
2. Inoculate single colony into 2 ml of LB broth containing 50 μg/ml Km and 1 % glucose; incubate overnight at +37 °C (*see* **Note 6**).
3. Inoculate 250 ml LB broth containing 50 μg/ml Km (no glucose) with 1 ml of bacterial culture prepared as from Subheading 3.1, **step 2**, in 2000 ml Nalgene baffled shake flask; incubate at +37 °C with vigorous shaking (~150 rpm) to *A600 nm* = 0.8–1.0 (this level of growth takes ~4 h).
4. Induce expression of the recombinant gene by adding IPTG to 1 mM and continue incubation for an additional 4 h. Optional: Perform analysis of cellular fractions, i.e., total cell lysate as well as soluble and insoluble fractions, by 10–12 % SDS-PAGE to verify expression and solubility of the recombinant protein. Pause point: Bacterial culture can be stored overnight at +4 °C, or if the protein is produced as IB, cells can be harvested by centrifugation as in Subheading 3.1, **step 5**, and stored frozen at −80 °C, if necessary, for a long period of time.
5. Pellet cells by centrifugation at 3300 × *g* for 20 min at +4 °C. Discard the supernatant; carefully resuspend the pellet in 5 ml of cell lysis buffer A; then add 5 ml of the same buffer containing 4 mg/ml lysozyme; transfer to 50 ml polypropylene tube and incubate for 30 min on ice.
6. Sonicate with the 550 Sonic Dismembrator ten times for 10 s on ice using a setting of 5 on the Amplitude Control Knob, which is the highest setting for the micro-tip probe. Follow the manufacturer's instructions for the instrument in use.
7. Transfer the cell lysate into 50 ml Nalgene Oak Ridge High-Speed PPCO Centrifuge tube, and centrifuge at 7670 × *g* for 20 min at +4 °C. Harvest the pellet and proceed to **step 8** if protein is produced as IB; harvest supernatant and proceed to **step 9** if soluble protein is produced.

8. To purify IB, discard supernatant and resuspend the pellet in 10 ml cell lysis buffer A without lysozyme by sonication as in Subheading 3.1, **step 6**, followed by centrifugation as in **step 7**. To solubilize protein in the IB, resuspend pellet in 0.5 ml PBS by sonication as in Subheading 3.1, **step 6** first, then add 9.5 ml solubilization/wash buffer D (*see* **Note 7**).
9. Filter the supernatant through a 45 μm filter into a 15 ml polypropylene tube; add 2 ml Ni-NTA slurry, mix, and incubate with rotation for 2 h at +4 °C (*see* **Note 8**).
10. Pellet the resin at 300 × *g* for 5 min at +4 °C and carefully remove the supernatant (*see* **Note 8**). Resuspend resin in 14 ml of the appropriate wash buffer: for native protein purification, use wash buffer B; for solubilized denatured protein, use solubilization/wash buffer D. Centrifuge the solution at 300 × *g* for 5 min at +4 °C. Repeat this wash step.
11. Re-suspend the resin in 5 ml of the corresponding wash buffer as in Subheading 3.1, **step 10** and transfer to a disposable 5 ml polypropylene column. Wash the column four times with 5 ml wash buffer B (for native protein purification) or D (for solubilized denatured protein purification).
12. Elute with 3 ml elution buffer C (for native protein purification) or elution buffer E (for denatured protein purification). Sterilize the eluted protein by filtration through a Millex 0.22 μm filter and store at +4 °C on ice. Use for immunization within the next 2 days.
13. Assess purity of isolated protein using 10–12% SDS-PAGE. SDS-PAGE analysis has been described elsewhere [57] and, hence, is not described here. Quantify purified protein; one approach is to use a known amount of BSA protein that is separated by SDS-PAGE on the same gel as the recombinant proteins for quantification by densitometry. An average yield of purified recombinant VACV protein is ~1.5–6 mg, which corresponds to ~0.5–2 mg/ml in the eluted fraction.
14. Recommended: Follow vendor's protocol to further purify protein with the use of endotoxin removal spin column (Subheading 2.2, **item 21**) or, alternatively, using the recently published protocol (*see* **Note 9**). Otherwise, proceed to **step 15** (optional) or **step 16**.
15. Optional: Dialyze protein that was eluted under native conditions to exchange the elution buffer with PBS (*see* **Note 10**).
16. Remove urea from protein that was purified under denaturing conditions (*see* **Note 11**). Dialyze eluted protein against 500 ml PBS at RT; this will promote protein precipitation when urea is removed (*see* **Note 12**). Centrifuge at 10,000 × *g* for 5 min at RT, remove supernatant, and re-solubilize precipi-

tate in 300 μl of 1 % SDS. This should yield ~5–20 mg/ml of protein. Incubate at +37 °C until completely dissolved. Store at RT and use for immunization over the next 2 days. Note that SDS precipitates upon thawing SDS-solubilized protein stored at −20 °C, as will the protein stored with it.

3.2 Immunizing Mice

The most common routes for immunizing a mouse are intraperitoneal (IP), subcutaneous (SQ), intravenous (IV), and intranasal (IN). SQ is commonly used for tracking $CD8^+$ T cell responses in the draining lymph node [37]. Intramuscular (IM) administration is not generally recommended, as the muscle of the mouse is small. The route of immunization used determines trafficking properties of antigen-specific $CD8^+$ T cells and influences the anamnestic immune response at the initial site of pathogen invasion [58]. Hence, choice of immunization route will depend on the investigator's goal and infection model. Below, we describe protocols for IP and IN immunizations, which have been shown to elicit robust and protective $CD8^+$ T cell responses against lethal VACV infection in mice ([28] and unpublished data). IP immunization induces a robust systemic response, resulting in antigen-specific $CD8^+$ T cells circulating through the blood and secondary lymphoid organs, such as the spleen. IN immunization, in addition to eliciting a systemic response will stimulate a robust local mucosal immune response within the lungs [59]. Generating a robust antigen-specific $CD8^+$ T cell response generally requires two immunizations—prime and boost. Experimentation involving mice must comply with the investigator's IACUC regulations.

1. Thaw 0.2 mg/ml αGalCer stock solution at RT, and mix gently by pipetting (*see* **Note 13**).
2. Prepare appropriate volume of inoculum by mixing protein with αGalCer. For IN immunization, prepare 50 μl of mixture that contains 20–100 μg of protein (45 μl of 0.5–2 mg/ml solution) and 1 μg of αGalCer (5 μl of 0.2 mg/ml stock) per mouse. For IP immunization, prepare 200 μl of mixture that contains the same amount of protein and αGalCer per mouse as for IN immunization. If protein is insoluble and contains SDS, adjust SDS concentration with sterile PBS accordingly to final SDS concentration ≤ 0.05 % in the inoculum. For example, add 4 μl re-solubilized protein at 5–20 mg/ml in 1 % SDS from Subheading 3.1, **step 16**, and 5 μl of 0.2 mg/ml αGalCer stock to 191 μl of PBS (*see* **Note 14**). Proceed with **step 3** for IP immunization, or **step 4** for IN immunization.
3. For IP immunization, inject 200 μl of the inoculum IP into a $B7.2^{tg}$ mouse (*see* **Note 15**).
4. For IN immunization, anesthetize a $B7.2^{tg}$ mouse with 150 μl of ketamine-xylazine (*see* **Note 16**). After the mouse is deeply anesthetized (confirmed by the absence of foot reflexes in

response to a mild pinch), gradually release 50 μl of the inoculum into both nostrils at the same time with a micropipette. Adjust the rate of release so as to allow the mouse to inhale the inoculum without forming bubbles. This should cause a rapid increase in the breathing rate. Hold the mouse in an upside down position for another couple of minutes until its breathing gradually returns to normal. Observe mice until recovery from anesthesia (*see* **Note 17**).

5. Boost mice 14 days after primary immunization as follows: prepare mixture of protein and αGalCer as in **step 1** and inoculate mice as in **step 2** (*see* **Notes 18–20**).

3.3 Isolation of Lymphocytes and Flow Cytometry

Note that all experimentation involving mice must comply with the investigator's IACUC regulations. In addition, flow cytometry should be performed by trained personnel and in accordance with institutional regulations. Refer elsewhere for detailed overviews of flow cytometry acquisition and data analysis [60, 61].

1. Sacrifice mouse using SmartBox Auto CO_2 System.
2. For each mouse, prepare two 60 mm Petri dishes and place on ice. For IP-immunized mice, remove the spleen and put on top of a 70 μm cell strainer placed inside the Petri dish. For IN-immunized mice, remove the spleen and lungs and place inside separate Petri dishes, each with a 70 μm cell strainer. Harvest spleen or lungs from non-immunized mice as negative controls. Proceed with **step 3** to isolate splenic lymphocytes or **step 6** to isolate lung lymphocytes (*see* **Note 21**).
3. To each spleen, add 2.5 ml ACK lysis buffer at RT. Using the plunger end of a 5 ml syringe, mash the tissue over the cell strainer to disperse leukocytes. Pass the cell suspension one more time though the cell strainer and transfer into a 15 ml polypropylene centrifuge tube. Incubate for 2 min at RT to lyse red blood cells (RBCs). Add 10 ml cRPMI with dasatinib to dilute ACK lysis buffer.
4. Centrifuge the cell suspension at 300×*g* for 5 min at +4 °C. Decant supernatant.
5. Resuspend each splenocyte suspension by gentle pipetting in 5 ml FACS buffer and place on ice. To stain splenocytes with various fluorochrome-conjugated antibodies, proceed to **step 9** (*see* **Note 22**).
6. Rinse the harvested lungs with PBS to remove blood. Mince tissue with a scalpel; transfer the minced lung tissue into a 15 ml polypropylene centrifuge tube containing 2 ml cRPMI supplemented with dasatinib and 2 mg/ml collagenase and let digest for 1 h at +37 °C.

7. Pour the digested lung slices onto a 70 μm cell strainer placed inside a Petri dish. Using the plunger end of a 5 ml syringe, mash the tissue over the cell strainer to disperse leukocytes.
8. Follow Subheading 3.3, **steps 3–4**, to lyse RBCs, prepare single-cell suspension, then resuspend cells from each lung in 2 ml of FACS buffer, and place on ice (*see* **Note 22**).
9. Count viable cells with a hemocytometer or counting beads. The expected recovery is ~0.5–1 × 10^7 leukocytes per 1 ml of cell suspension from processed lungs or spleen (*see* **Note 23**).
10. Add 200 μl of cells from each sample, including control non-immunized mouse leukocytes, into a 96-well round-bottom plate. Optional: If absolute count of tetramer-positive $CD8^+$ T cells is required, we recommend using counting beads (*see* **Note 23**). Centrifuge plate at 828 × *g* for 2 min at +4 °C. Discard the supernatant.
11. Resuspend the cells in 100 μl of FACS buffer containing anti-B220-fluorescein isothiocyanate (FITC), -CD4-FITC, -CD11b-FITC, -CD11c-FITC (all at 1:200 dilution), -CD8α-Pacific Blue (1:100 dilution), and 1.5 μg/ml of corresponding R-phycoerythrin (PE)-labeled tetramer. Incubate for 1 to 2 h at +4 °C (*see* **Note 24**).
12. Dilute the staining reaction with 200 μl of FACS buffer and spin plate at 800 × *g* for 2 min at +4 °C to wash the cells. Discard the supernatant.
13. Resuspend the cells in 200–300 μl of FACS buffer containing 1:2000 dilution of 50 μg/ml propidium iodide stock solution, which incorporates into the nuclei of dead cells and, thereby, allowing differentiation between dead and viable cells in flow cytometry experiments. Transfer cells into 1.2 ml Microtiter Tubes; store on ice for up to 2 h before acquisition.
14. Prepare an acquisition template using FACSDiva software containing four fluorochromes to reflect the staining panel.
15. Set up compensation by using an unstained control and single stained compensation control samples.
16. Set up an acquisition layout containing the following plots: forward scatter (FSC)-A versus side scatter (SSC)-A. Create a gate for the lymphocyte population, and a FSC-W versus FSC-H followed by SSC-W versus SSC-H gate to discriminate singlet population. Create a histogram to display live/dead cells for propidium iodide with a gate to discriminate propidium iodide-negative live population; FITC ("dump" channel) versus CD8α-Pacific Blue to create $CD8^+$ T cell gate; CD8α versus tetramer to create $tetramer^+$ gate (Fig. 5).
17. Collect 5000–10,000 total $CD8\alpha^+$ events and export FCS files for the analysis in FlowJo software.

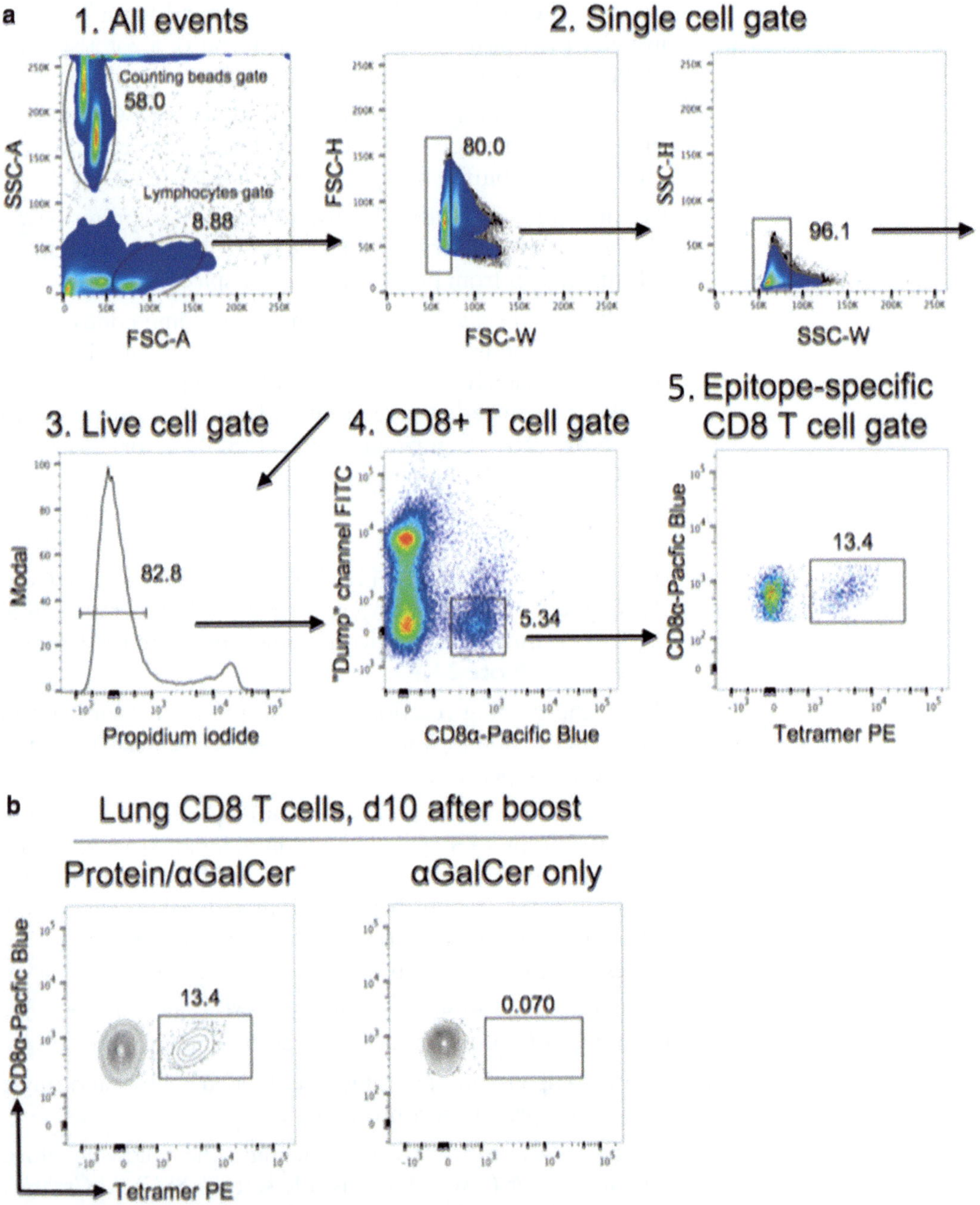

Fig. 5 Analysis of epitope-specific CD8⁺ T cells by tetramer staining. (**a**) Representative example showing gating strategy and identification of epitope-specific CD8⁺ T cells. Cells harvested from the lungs of rL4R/B8R$_{70-79}$ protein/αGalCer primed and boosted B7^{tg} mice (IN route) were analyzed by four-color flow cytometry following staining with B8R$_{70-79}$/B7.2 tetramer. (**b**) Representative flow cytometry contour plots showing specificity of B8R$_{70-79}$/B7.2 tetramer staining upon immunization with αGalCer-formulated protein antigen

18. In FlowJo, to determine the frequency of antigen-specific, i.e., tetramer$^+$, CD8$^+$ T cells, apply gates as in Subheading 3.3, **step 16**. To determine background from non-specific tetramer staining, create tetramer gate for "CD8α versus tetramer" subset for cells from non-immunized control mouse, then apply it to the cells from a mouse immunized with protein and adjuvant. To determine the frequency of tetramer$^+$ CD8$^+$ T cells, subtract the background from each experimental value. If using counting beads, refer to vendor's protocol to determine absolute number for the desired lymphocyte subset.
19. Optional: The remaining unstained cells can be cryopreserved at −80 °C in cRPMI containing 10% DMSO for CD8$^+$ T cell phenotyping in additional experiments if needed at a later time (*see* **Note 25**).

3.4 CD8 T Cell Re-stimulation and Staining for Intracellular Interferon-γ

Staining for intracellular interferon-γ (IFN-γ) can be optionally used as a complementary assay to validate the presence of functional antigen-specific CD8$^+$ T cells after immunization.

1. Harvest spleen and isolate lymphocytes as reviewed in Subheading 3.3, **steps 1–4**. Work under aseptic conditions using a laminar flow hood; do not use dasatinib in any medium during tissue processing and cell incubation. Include dasatinib in FACS buffer only during the staining procedure for flow cytometry.
2. Resuspend cells from each spleen in 5 ml of cRPMI. Add 200 μl of cell suspension containing ~2×10^6 lymphocytes and 50 μl of anti-CD107a-FITC antibody (optional, *see* **Note 26**) to each of three wells of 96-well round-bottom plate. To the first well, add 50 μl of cRPMI containing 50 μM antigenic peptide epitope to 10 μM final. Add 50 μl of cRPMI to the second well; this will serve as a negative control for CD8$^+$ T cell re-stimulation. Add 50 μl of cRPMI containing PMA and ionomycin to a final concentration of 50 ng/ml PMA plus 2 μg/ml ionomycin to the third well; this will serve as a positive control for CD8$^+$ T cell stimulation.
3. Incubate for 2 h at +37 °C in CO_2 incubator (5% CO_2), then add 50 μl cRPMI containing a combination of vesicular transport inhibitors, such as brefeldin A (10 μg/ml final) and GolgiStop (1:1500); incubate for an additional 4 h, for a total of 6 h. These inhibitors will allow for intracellular accumulation of secreted proteins including cytokines such as IFN-γ at levels that are readily detectable by flow cytometry.
4. Spin plate at 828 × *g* for 2 min at +4 °C. Discard the supernatant, resuspend in 250 μl of PBS, and spin again at 828 × *g* for 2 min at +4 °C to wash the cells. Discard the supernatant.

5. Resuspend the cells in 100 μl of PBS containing eFluor 450 amino-reactive viability dye (1:2000). Incubate 30 min at +4 °C.
6. Add 200 μl of FACS buffer and centrifuge plate at 828 × *g* for 2 min at +4 °C to wash the cells. Discard the supernatant.
7. Resuspend the cells in 100 μl of FACS buffer supplemented with dasatinib and containing anti-B220-APC-Cy7 (allophycocyanin-cyanine7 tandem dye) (1:100), -CD3ε-PE (1:100) and -CD8α-PerCP-Cy5.5 (peridinin chlorophyll-cyanine5.5 tandem dye) (1:200) antibodies (*see* **Note 27**). Incubate for 1 h at +4 °C.
8. Add 200 μl of FACS buffer and spin plate at 828 × *g* for 2 min at +4 °C to wash the cells. Discard the supernatant.
9. Resuspend the cells in 100 μl of BD Cytofix/Cytoperm and incubate for 10 min at +4 °C.
10. Wash the cells twice by adding 200 μl of 1× BD Perm/wash and centrifuging at 828 × *g* for 2 min at +4 °C. Discard the supernatant.
11. Resuspend the cells in 100 μl of 1× BD Perm/wash containing anti-IFN-γ-allophycocyanin (1:200) antibody. Incubate for 1 h at +4 °C.
12. Add 200 μl of 1× BD Perm/wash and centrifuge plate at 828 × *g* for 2 min at +4 °C to wash the cells. Discard the supernatant, resuspend in 200–300 μl of FACS buffer, and transfer cells into 1.5 ml microtubes. Stained cells can be stored on ice for up to 4 h before data acquisition. Alternatively, cells can be fixed as in Subheading 3.4, **step 9**, washed with FACS buffer as in **step 8**, resuspended in 200–300 μl of FACS buffer, and stored at +4 °C up to 16 h before data acquisition. Longer storage times have not been tested.
13. Prepare an acquisition template for six fluorochromes and set up compensation as detailed in Subheading 3.3, **steps 14–15**.
14. Set up an acquisition layout containing the following plots: forward scatter (FSC)-A versus side scatter (SSC)-A. Create a gate for the lymphocyte population and an SSC-W versus SSC-H gate to identify the singlet population. Create a histogram to display live/dead cells for eFluor450 with a gate to identify live cells; B220-APC-Cy7 versus CD3ε-PE to create T cell gate: CD8α-PerCP-Cy5.5 versus CD3ε-PE to create $CD8^+$ T cell gate; CD107a-FITC versus IFN-γ-allophycocyanin to create $CD107a^+IFN\text{-}\gamma^+$ $CD8^+$ T cell gate (Fig. 6).
15. Analyze sample as detailed in Subheading 3.3, **steps 17–18**. To determine frequency of $CD107a^+IFN\text{-}\gamma^+$ $CD8^+$ T cells, subtract the background from a well without antigenic peptide epitope from each experimental value.

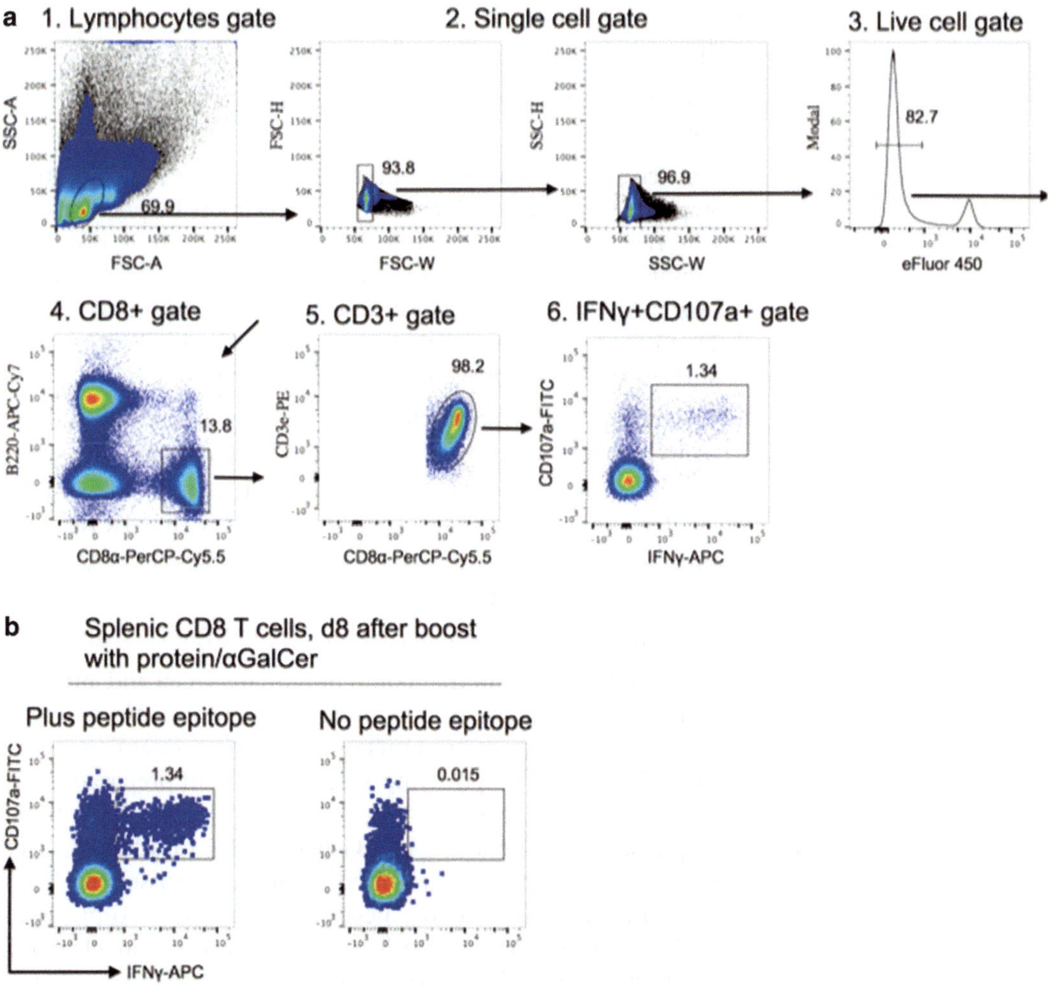

Fig. 6 Analysis of epitope-specific CD8⁺ T cells by intracellular cytokine staining (ICCS). (**a**) Representative example showing gating strategy and identification of epitope-specific CD8⁺ T cells. Cells harvested from the spleen of protein/αGalCer primed and boosted mice (IP route) were re-stimulated in vitro with the indicated antigenic peptide epitope, then stained with the indicated antibodies and analyzed by six-color flow cytometry. (**b**) Representative flow cytometry plots showing that IFN-γ was specifically induced by a subset of CD8⁺ T cells after peptide epitope re-stimulation

4 Notes

1. For preparation and storage of αGalCer, use only glass vials to minimize leaching of impurities out of a plastic container and adsorption of the lipid to plastic (*see* Subheading 2.1, **item 1**).
2. All urea-containing buffers should be made fresh. At physiological pH, urea produces cyanate that can cause carbamylation of proteins by reacting with amino, carboxyl, and sulfhydryl groups, which may alter their stability and function.

3. Refer to methods described elsewhere [57] for making protein electrophoresis gel and performing SDS-PAGE.
4. Proteins purified from IBs may contain up to 0.05 % SDS for solubility.
5. Low concentrations of dasatinib were reported to substantially improve CD8+ T cell detection with tetramers by preventing T cell receptor internalization [62]. Dasatinib is a reversible inhibitor that targets a wide variety of protein kinase C family enzymes [63]. Hence, we routinely use dasatinib in FACS buffer instead of sodium azide to maintain the TCR at the cell surface and for improved staining and cell viability.
6. Use freshly transformed bacterial colonies grown on plates; or alternatively, plate transformed bacteria from frozen glycerol stock.
7. Prior resuspension of IB in PBS through vigorous sonication facilitates further solubilization of proteins within IB by using urea-containing solubilization/wash buffer D. Centrifuge cells at 7670 × *g* for 20 min at +4 °C and harvest the supernatant.
8. Save an aliquot of the supernatant for SDS-PAGE analysis.
9. LPS is a TLR4 ligand that could potentiate T cell and antibody responses and, hence, we recommend its removal. Nonetheless, we did not find trace amounts of endotoxin contaminants and other impurities co-purifying with the protein preparations to contribute substantially to the elicitation of a CD8+ T cell response in the presence of αGalCer [28]. In addition, LPS removal in the past has resulted in dramatic losses of VACV protein. Should it become necessary to remove co-purifying endotoxins, use the recently described endotoxin clearance method by including a non-ionic detergent wash step during metal chelation affinity purification of the protein antigen [64].
10. This step is optional because components of elution buffer C do not affect the performance of the immunization protocol or antigen-specific immune responses.
11. Proteins purified under denaturing conditions contain a high concentration of urea, which is incompatible with the immunization protocol. Removal of urea by common laboratory approaches may result in protein aggregation. Stimulation of antigen-specific T cell responses in vivo does not require native conformation of protein antigen, but does require the protein to be in a reasonably soluble form. Although soluble urea-free protein can be obtained through in vitro refolding, such a procedure is laborious and requires optimization for each protein. We found that a low SDS concentration (0.01–0.05 %) is compatible with IP immunization protocol. This residual low concentration of SDS can promote protein solubility after the removal of urea by dialysis.

12. Some proteins can be refolded successfully and remain soluble after dialysis.
13. αGalCer solution should be clear; if appears cloudy, re-heat at +80 °C until dissolved. Repeated freeze and thaw does not affect the reagent's performance as long as the solution upon thawing remains clear and has not changed color.
14. Prepare mixture of protein with αGalCer right before immunization; usage of SDS-containing protein for IN immunization has not been validated.
15. For the first experiment, we recommend setting up a control wherein the mouse is inoculated IP with the same formulation but without protein antigen. Leukocytes harvested from this mouse after immunization will serve as a control to determine the background of the tetramer staining assay. An additional control for the performance of the reagents and immunization protocol that can be considered is the inclusion of a C57BL/6 mouse immunized by either the IP or IN route with 1 μg of αGalCer and 50 μg of ovalbumin (Ova) as detailed in the main protocol. Ova-specific $CD8^+$ should be readily detected with the readily available $H2K^b$/SIINFEKL tetramer (NIH Tetramer Core, Emory University, Atlanta, USA; http://tetramer.yerkes.emory.edu/) in the spleen on day 6–14 after boost.
16. Depending on the weight of the mouse, the amount of anesthesia can vary from 125 to 165 μl.
17. For the first experiment, we recommend setting up a control wherein the mouse is inoculated IN with the same formulation containing PBS and αGalCer but without protein antigen. Lymphocytes harvested from this mouse after immunization will serve as a control to determine the background of the tetramer staining assay.
18. Usually, antigen-specific $CD8^+$ T cells can be detected at low frequency on days 8–14 after primary immunization. At least one booster immunization substantially increases their frequency, which is more desirable for immunological and vaccination studies.
19. For the first time, before the mouse is sacrificed and leukocytes harvested, it may be necessary to confirm that immunization has induced antigen-specific $CD8^+$ T cells of detectable frequency. This can be accomplished by assessing mouse blood leukocytes. A robust antigen-specific $CD8^+$ T cell response should be readily detected systemically the blood on day 6–14 after boost.
20. Although it is not reviewed in the protocol here, protein antigen and αGalCer immunization also induces antigen-specific antibody responses that can be assessed in mouse serum (but *see* Fig. 3C).

21. Harvested organs can be left on ice while additional mice are being processed or reagents are being prepared for up to 24 h. Longer storage times have not been tested.
22. Cell suspensions can be left on ice for up to 8 h while additional tissues are being processed. Longer storage times have not been tested.
23. We found that precise counting of $CD8^+$ T cells in the lungs requires counting beads. Counting beads are added directly to staining solution to account for cell losses, assuming proportional bead and cell losses during washes. When working with counting beads, follow vendor's protocol at https://tools.thermofisher.com/content/sfs/manuals/PCB100_accucheck_beads_man.pdf.
24. The investigator should determine optimal staining conditions, such as concentration of tetramer, incubation temperature, and time; each of these parameters will differentially influence experimental outcome.
25. Cryopreservation does not affect staining performance but may affect viability. An expected lymphocyte viability after thawing is 80% or higher.
26. CD107a is a marker for degranulation activity of immune effector cells including $CD8^+$ T cells. Staining with anti-CD107a antibody is optional and performed during re-stimulation of cells.
27. Upon in vitro re-stimulation, epitope-specific $CD8^+$ T cells markedly down-regulate their T cell receptor from the cell surface and, hence, stain poorly with the complex of peptide/MHC tetramers.

Acknowledgements

Supported by Vanderbilt University Discovery Grant as well as VA Merit Award (BX001444) and NIH Contracts (AI040079), Research (AI042284, HL121139), Core (CA068485, DK058404), and Center (CA068485) grants.

References

1. Plotkin SA, Plotkin SL (2011) The development of vaccines: how the past led to the future. Nat Rev Microbiol 9:889–893
2. Zepp F (2010) Principles of vaccine design-lessons from nature. Vaccine 28(Suppl 3):C14–C24
3. Amanna IJ, Slifka MK (2009) Wanted, dead or alive: new viral vaccines. Antiviral Res 84:119–130
4. Bevan MJ (2011) Understand memory, design better vaccines. Nat Immunol 12:463–465
5. Pulendran B, Ahmed R (2011) Immunological mechanisms of vaccination. Nat Immunol 131:509–517
6. Koff WC, Gust ID, Plotkin SA (2014) Toward a human vaccines project. Nat Immunol 15:589–592
7. Amanna IJ, Slifka MK (2011) Contributions of humoral and cellular immunity to vaccine-induced protection in humans. Virology 411:206–215

8. Moss B (2011) Smallpox vaccines: targets of protective immunity. Immunol Rev 239:8–26
9. Rees AR (2015) The antibody molecule: from antitoxins to therapeutic antibodies, 1st edn. Oxford Medical Histories/Oxford University Press, Oxford, p 384
10. Jenner E (1809) Two cases of Small-Pox Infection communicated to the Foetus in Utero under peculiar circumstances, with additional remarks. Med Chir Trans 1:271–277
11. Adkins B, Leclerc C, Marshall-Clarke S (2004) Neonatal adaptive immunity comes of age. Nat Rev Immunol 4:553–564
12. Swamy GK, Wheeler SM (2014) Neonatal pertussis, cocooning and maternal immunization. Expert Rev Vaccines 13:1107–1114
13. Verhasselt V (2015) Is infant immunization by breastfeeding possible? Philos Trans R Soc Lond B Biol Sci. doi:10.1098/rstb.2014.0139
14. O'Connell CJ, Karzon DT, Barron AL, Plaut ME, Ali VM (1964) Progressive vaccinia with normal antibodies. A case possibly due to deficient cellular immunity. Ann Intern Med 60:282–289
15. Blum JS, Wearsch PA, Cresswell P (2013) Pathways of antigen processing. Annu Rev Immunol 31:443–473
16. Segura E, Amigorena S (2015) Cross-presentation in mouse and human dendritic cells. Adv Immunol 127:1–31
17. Thomas PG, Keating R, Hulse-Post DJ, Doherty PC (2006) Cell-mediated protection in influenza infection. Emerg Infect Dis 12:48–54
18. Brown LE, Kelso A (2009) Prospects for an influenza vaccine that induces cross-protective cytotoxic T lymphocytes. Immunol Cell Biol 87:300–308
19. Kohlmeier JE, Woodland DL (2009) Immunity to respiratory viruses. Annu Rev Immunol 27:61–82
20. Kremer M, Suezer Y, Volz A, Frenz T, Majzoub M, Hanschmann KM, Lehmann MH, Kalinke U, Sutter G (2012) Critical role of perforin-dependent $CD8^+$ T cell immunity for rapid protective vaccination in a murine model for human smallpox. PLoS Pathog 8:e1002557
21. Goulding J, Bogue R, Tahiliani V, Croft M, Salek-Ardakani S (2012) $CD8^+$ T cells are essential for recovery from a respiratory vaccinia virus infection. J Immunol 189:2432–2440
22. Gordon SN, Cecchinato V, Andresen V, Heraud JM, Hryniewicz A, Parks RW, Venzon D, Chung HK, Karpova T, McNally J, Silvera P, Reimann KA, Matsui H, Kanehara T, Shinmura Y, Yokote H, Franchini G (2011) Smallpox vaccine safety is dependent on T cells and not B cells. J Infect Dis 203:1043–1053
23. Li CR, Greenberg PD, Gilbert MJ, Goodrich JM, Riddell SR (1994) Recovery of Hla-restricted cytomegalovirus (Cmv)-specific T-cell responses after allogeneic bone-marrow transplant - correlation with Cmv disease and effect of ganciclovir prophylaxis. Blood 83:1971–1979
24. Goulder PJR, Watkins DI (2008) Impact of MHC class I diversity on immune control of immunodeficiency virus replication. Nat Rev Immunol 8:619–630
25. Schmidt NW, Butler NS, Badovinac VP, Harty JT (2010) Extreme $CD8^+$ T cell requirements for anti-malarial liver-stage immunity following immunization with radiation attenuated sporozoites. PLoS Pathog 6:e1000998
26. Epstein JE, Tewari K, Lyke KE, Sim BKL, Billingsley PF, Laurens MB, Gunasekera A, Chakravarty S, James ER, Sedegah M, Richman A, Velmurugan S, Reyes S, Li M, Tucker K, Ahumada A, Ruben AJ, Li T, Stafford R, Eappen AG, Tamminga C, Bennett JW, Ockenhouse CF, Murphy JR, Komisar J, Thomas N, Loyevsky M, Birkett A, Plowe CV, Loucq C et al (2011) Live attenuated malaria vaccine designed to protect through hepatic CD8(+) T cell immunity. Science 334:475–480
27. Woodworth JSM, Behar SM (2006) Mycobacterium tuberculosis-specific CD8(+) T cells and their role in immunity. Crit Rev Immunol 26:317–352
28. Gilchuk P, Spencer CT, Conant SB, Hill T, Gray JJ, Niu X, Zheng M, Erickson JJ, Boyd KL, McAfee KJ, Oseroff C, Hadrup SR, Bennink JR, Hildebrand W, Edwards KM, Crowe JE Jr, Williams JV, Buus S, Sette A, Schumacher TN, Link AJ, Joyce S (2013) Discovering naturally processed antigenic determinants that confer protective T cell immunity. J Clin Invest 123:1976–1987
29. Gerdts V, Littel-van den Hurk SV, Griebel PJ, Babiuk LA (2007) Use of animal models in the development of human vaccines. Future Microbiol 2:667–675
30. Gerdts V, Wilson HL, Meurens F, van Drunen Littel-van den Hurk S, Wilson D, Walker S, Wheler C, Townsend H, Potter AA (2015) Large animal models for vaccine development and testing. ILAR J 56:53–62
31. van Hall T, van der Burg SH (2012) Mechanisms of peptide vaccination in mouse models: tolerance, immunity, and hyperreactivity. Adv Immunol 114:51–76
32. Koup RA, Douek DC (2011) Vaccine design for $CD8^+$ T lymphocyte responses. Cold Spring Harb Perspect Med 1:a007252
33. Remakus S, Rubio D, Ma X, Sette A, Sigal LJ (2012) Memory $CD8^+$ T cells specific for a

single immunodominant or subdominant determinant induced by peptide-dendritic cell immunization protect from an acute lethal viral disease. J Virol 86:9748–9759
34. Coffman RL, Sher A, Seder RA (2010) Vaccine adjuvants: putting innate immunity to work. Immunity 33:492–503
35. Duthie MS, Windish HP, Fox CB, Reed SG (2011) Use of defined TLR ligands as adjuvants within human vaccines. Immunol Rev 239:178–196
36. Cho HI, Celis E (2009) Optimized peptide vaccines eliciting extensive $CD8^{+}$ T-cell responses with therapeutic antitumor effects. Cancer Res 69:9012–9019
37. Liu H, Moynihan KD, Zheng Y, Szeto GL, Li AV, Huang B, Van Egeren DS, Park C, Irvine DJ (2014) Structure-based programming of lymph-node targeting in molecular vaccines. Nature 507:519–522
38. Saroja C, Lakshmi P, Bhaskaran S (2011) Recent trends in vaccine delivery systems: a review. Int J Pharm Invest 1:64–74
39. Moon JJ, Huang B, Irvine DJ (2012) Engineering nano- and microparticles to tune immunity. Adv Mater 24:3724–3746
40. Hermans IF, Silk JD, Gileadi U, Salio M, Mathew B, Ritter G, Schmidt R, Harris AL, Old L, Cerundolo V (2003) NKT cells enhance CD4+ and $CD8^{+}$ T cell responses to soluble antigen in vivo through direct interaction with dendritic cells. J Immunol 171:5140–5147
41. Singh N, Hong S, Scherer DC, Serizawa I, Burdin N, Kronenberg M, Koezuka Y, Van Kaer L (1999) Activation of NK T cells by CD1d and alpha-galactosylceramide directs conventional T cells to the acquisition of a Th2 phenotype. J Immunol (Cutting Edge) 163:2373–2377
42. Semmling V, Lukacs-Kornek V, Thaiss CA, Quast T, Hochheiser K, Panzer U, Rossjohn J, Perlmutter P, Cao J, Godfrey DI, Savage PB, Knolle PA, Kolanus W, Forster I, Kurts C (2010) Alternative cross-priming through CCL17-CCR4-mediated attraction of CTLs toward NKT cell-licensed DCs. Nat Immunol 11:313–320
43. Oseroff C, Peters B, Pasquetto V, Moutaftsi M, Sidney J, Panchanathan V, Tscharke DC, Maillere B, Grey H, Sette A (2008) Dissociation between epitope hierarchy and immunoprevalence in $CD8^{+}$ responses to vaccinia virus western reserve. J Immunol 180:7193–7202
44. Gottschalk C, Mettke E, Kurts C (2015) The role of invariant natural killer T cells in dendritic cell licensing, cross-priming, and memory CD8(+) T cell generation. Front Immunol 6:379
45. Hill TM, Bezbradica JS, Van Kaer L, Joyce S (2016) CD1d-restricted natural killer T cells. Encyclopaedia Live Sci. doi:10.1002/9780470015902.a0020180.pub2
46. Fujii S, Shimizu K, Smith C, Bonifaz L, Steinman RM (2003) Activation of natural killer T cells by alpha-galactosylceramide rapidly induces the full maturation of dendritic cells in vivo and thereby acts as an adjuvant for combined CD4 and CD8 T cell immunity to a coadministered protein. J Exp Med 198:267–279
47. Galli G, Pittoni P, Tonti E, Malzone C, Uematsu Y, Tortoli M, Maione D, Volpini G, Finco O, Nuti S, Tavarini S, Dellabona P, Rappuoli R, Casorati G, Abrignani S (2007) Invariant NKT cells sustain specific B cell responses and memory. Proc Natl Acad Sci U S A 104:3984–3989
48. Kamijuku H, Nagata Y, Jiang X, Ichinohe T, Tashiro T, Mori K, Taniguchi M, Hase K, Ohno H, Shimaoka T, Yonehara S, Odagiri T, Tashiro M, Sata T, Hasegawa H, Seino KI (2008) Mechanism of NKT cell activation by intranasal coadministration of alpha-galactosylceramide, which can induce cross-protection against influenza viruses. Mucosal Immunol 1:208–218
49. Reilly EC, Thompson EA, Aspeslagh S, Wands JR, Elewaut D, Brossay L (2012) Activated iNKT cells promote memory $CD8^{+}$ T cell differentiation during viral infection. PLoS One 7, e37991
50. Carreno LJ, Kharkwal SS, Porcelli SA (2014) Optimizing NKT cell ligands as vaccine adjuvants. Immunotherapy 6:309–320
51. Ko SY, Ko HJ, Chang WS, Park SH, Kweon MN, Kang CY (2005) alpha-galactosylceramide can act as a nasal vaccine adjuvant inducing protective immune responses against viral infection and tumor. J Immunol 175:3309–3317
52. Courtney AN, Thapa P, Singh S, Wishahy AM, Zhou D, Sastry J (2011) Intranasal but not intravenous delivery of the adjuvant alpha-galactosylceramide permits repeated stimulation of natural killer T cells in the lung. Eur J Immunol 41:3312–3322
53. Nishimura T, Kitamura H, Iwakabe K, Yahata T, Ohta A, Sato M, Takeda K, Okumura K, Van Kaer L, Kawano T, Taniguchi M, Nakui M, Sekimoto M, Koda T (2000) The interface between innate and acquired immunity: glycolipid antigen presentation by CD1d-expressing dendritic cells to NKT cells induces the differentiation of antigen-specific cytotoxic T lymphocytes. Int Immunol 12:987–994

54. Guillonneau C, Mintern JD, Hubert FX, Hurt AC, Besra GS, Porcelli S, Barr IG, Doherty PC, Godfrey DI, Turner SJ (2009) Combined NKT cell activation and influenza virus vaccination boosts memory CTL generation and protective immunity. Proc Natl Acad Sci U S A 106:3330–3335
55. Duwaerts CC, Gregory SH (2011) Targeting the diverse immunological functions expressed by hepatic NKT cells. Expert Opin Ther Targets 15:973–988
56. Alexander J, Oseroff C, Sidney J, Sette A (2003) Derivation of HLA-B*0702 transgenic mice: functional CTL repertoire and recognition of human B*0702-restricted CTL epitopes. Hum Immunol 64:211–223
57. Green M, Sambrook J. (2012) Molecular cloning. A laboratory manual (Fourth Edition) (Cold Spring Harbor Laboratory Press), Vol 3, p Protocol 8
58. Belyakov IM, Ahlers JD (2009) What role does the route of immunization play in the generation of protective immunity against mucosal pathogens? J Immunol 183:6883–6892
59. Li AV, Moon JJ, Abraham W, Suh H, Elkhader J, Seidman MA, Yen M, Im EJ, Foley MH, Barouch DH, & Irvine DJ (2013) Generation of effector memory T cell-based mucosal and systemic immunity with pulmonary nanoparticle vaccination. Sci Transl Med 5: 204ra130
60. Sharrow SO (2002) Overview of flow cytometry. Curr Protoc Immunol Chapter 5: Unit 5 1
61. Roederer M (2002) Multiparameter FACS analysis. Curr Protoc Immunol Chapter 5: Unit 5 8
62. Lissina A, Ladell K, Skowera A, Clement M, Edwards E, Seggewiss R, van den Berg HA, Gostick E, Gallagher K, Jones E, Melenhorst JJ, Godkin AJ, Peakman M, Price DA, Sewell AK, Wooldridge L (2009) Protein kinase inhibitors substantially improve the physical detection of T-cells with peptide-MHC tetramers. J Immunol Methods 340:11–24
63. Montero JC, Seoane S, Ocana A, Pandiella A (2011) Inhibition of SRC family kinases and receptor tyrosine kinases by dasatinib: possible combinations in solid tumors. Clin Cancer Res 17:5546–5552
64. Zimmerman T, Petit Frere C, Satzger M, Raba M, Weisbach M, Dohn K, Popp A, Donzeau M (2006) Simultaneous metal chelate affinity purification and endotoxin clearance of recombinant antibody fragments. J Immunol Methods 314:67–73
65. Wagner CS, Grotzke JE, Cresswell P (2012) Intracellular events regulating cross-presentation. Front Immunol 3:138
66. Hadrup SR, Bakker AH, Shu CJ, Andersen RS, van Veluw J, Hombrink P, Castermans E, Thor Straten P, Blank C, Haanen JB, Heemskerk MH, Schumacher TN (2009) Parallel detection of antigen-specific T-cell responses by multidimensional encoding of MHC multimers. Nat Methods 6:520–526
67. Kain L, Webb B, Anderson BL, Deng S, Holt M, Costanzo A, Zhao M, Self K, Teyton A, Everett C, Kronenberg M, Zajonc DM, Bendelac A, Savage PB, Teyton L (2014) The identification of the endogenous ligands of natural killer T cells reveals the presence of mammalian alpha-linked glycosylceramides. Immunity 41:543–554
68. Morita M, Motoki K, Akimoto K, Natori T, Sakai T, Sawa E, Yamaji K, Koezuka Y, Kobayashi E, Fukushima H (1995) Structure-activity relationship of alpha-galactosylceramides against B16-bearing mice. J Med Chem 38:2176–2187
69. Natori T, Koezuka Y, Higa T (1993) Agelasphins, Novel a-galactosylceramides from the marine sponge *Agelas mauritianus*. Tetrahedron Lett 34:5591–5592
70. Kawano T, Cui J, Koezuka Y, Toura I, Kaneko Y, Motoki K, Ueno H, Nakagawa R, Sato H, Kondo E, Koseki H, Taniguchi M (1997) CD1d-restricted and TCR-mediated activation of valpha14 NKT cells by glycosylceramides. Science 278:1626–1629
71. Birkholz AM, Girardi E, Wingender G, Khurana A, Wang J, Zhao M, Zahner S, Illarionov PA, Wen X, Li M, Yuan W, Porcelli SA, Besra GS, Zajonc DM, Kronenberg M (2015) A novel glycolipid antigen for NKT cells that preferentially induces IFN-gamma production. J Immunol 195:924–933
72. Schmieg J, Yang G, Franck RW, Tsuji M (2003) Superior protection against malaria and melanoma metastases by a C-glycoside analogue of the natural killer T cell ligand alpha-Galactosylceramide. J Exp Med 198:1631–1641
73. Li X, Fujio M, Imamura M, Wu D, Vasan S, Wong CH, Ho DD, Tsuji M (2010) Design of a potent CD1d-binding NKT cell ligand as a vaccine adjuvant. Proc Natl Acad Sci U S A 107:13010–13015
74. Aspeslagh S, Li Y, Yu ED, Pauwels N, Trappeniers M, Girardi E, Decruy T, Van Beneden K, Venken K, Drennan M, Leybaert L, Wang J, Franck RW, Van Calenbergh S, Zajonc DM, Elewaut D (2011) Galactose-modified iNKT cell agonists stabilized by an induced fit of CD1d prevent tumour metastasis. EMBO J 30:2294–2305

75. Aspeslagh S, Nemcovic M, Pauwels N, Venken K, Wang J, Van Calenbergh S, Zajonc DM, Elewaut D (2013) Enhanced TCR footprint by a novel glycolipid increases NKT-dependent tumor protection. J Immunol 191:2916–2925
76. Tyznik AJ, Farber E, Girardi E, Birkholz A, Li Y, Chitale S, So R, Arora P, Khurana A, Wang J, Porcelli SA, Zajonc DM, Kronenberg M, Howell AR (2011) Glycolipids that elicit IFN-gamma-biased responses from natural killer T cells. Chem Biol 18:1620–1630
77. Miyamoto K, Miyake S, Yamamura T (2001) A synthetic glycolipid prevents autoimmune encephalomyelitis by inducing TH2 bias of natural killer T cells. Nature 413:531–534
78. Yu KO, Im JS, Molano A, Dutronc Y, Illarionov PA, Forestier C, Fujiwara N, Arias I, Miyake S, Yamamura T, Chang YT, Besra GS, Porcelli SA (2005) Modulation of CD1d-restricted NKT cell responses by using N-acyl variants of alpha-galactosylceramides. Proc Natl Acad Sci U S A 102:3383–3388
79. Kinjo Y, Wu D, Kim G, Xing GW, Poles MA, Ho DD, Tsuji M, Kawahara K, Wong CH, Kronenberg M (2005) Recognition of bacterial glycosphingolipids by natural killer T cells. Nature 434:520–525
80. Mattner J, Debord KL, Ismail N, Goff RD, Cantu C 3rd, Zhou D, Saint-Mezard P, Wang V, Gao Y, Yin N, Hoebe K, Schneewind O, Walker D, Beutler B, Teyton L, Savage PB, Bendelac A (2005) Exogenous and endogenous glycolipid antigens activate NKT cells during microbial infections. Nature 434:525–529
81. Albacker LA, Chaudhary V, Chang YJ, Kim HY, Chuang YT, Pichavant M, DeKruyff RH, Savage PB, Umetsu DT (2013) Invariant natural killer T cells recognize a fungal glycosphingolipid that can induce airway hyperreactivity. Nat Med 19:1297–1304
82. Joyce S, Girardi E, Zajonc DM (2011) NKT cell ligand recognition logic: molecular basis for a synaptic duet and transmission of inflammatory effectors. J Immunol 187:1081–1089
83. Rodenko B, Toebes M, Hadrup SR, van Esch WJ, Molenaar AM, Schumacher TN, Ovaa H (2006) Generation of peptide-MHC class I complexes through UV-mediated ligand exchange. Nat Protoc 1:1120–1132

Chapter 26

Molecular Methods and Bioinformatic Tools for Adjuvant Characterization by High-Throughput Sequencing

Steven R. Wiley and Vanitha S. Raman

Abstract

Adjuvants in vaccine formulations are designed to enhance immune responses against a target antigen or pathogen. The ability of these vaccines to induce activation and differentiation of mature naïve B cells to produce pathogen-specific antibodies (immunoglobulins; Ig) helps guarantee long-lived humoral immunity. This process involves clonal expansion of antigen-specific B cells, genomic rearrangement of Ig heavy (IgH) and light (IgL) loci, somatic hypermutation (SHM), and clonal selection for affinity-matured antibody, resulting in a vast but directed repertoire of B cells expressing highly specific antibody proteins. High-throughput sequencing of the IgH and IgL complementary determining regions (CDRs) derived from various B cell populations provides an unprecedented way to observe dynamic responses of the humoral immune repertoire in response to vaccination. However, applying high-throughput sequencing (HTS) methodologies to multi-armed in vivo experiments requires careful coordination of sample preparation with downstream bioinformatics, particularly with regard to issues of quantitation, sequence fidelity, bar-coding, and multiplexing strategies. Here, we overview strategies of high-throughput sequencing and analysis of the adaptive immune complex loci applied to multi-armed, multiplexed experiments.

Key words High-throughput DNA sequencing, Adaptive immune system, Adjuvant, Vaccine, Bioinformatics, Immunoglobulin, Antibody, B cell, IgH, IgL, Complementarity determining region

1 Introduction

The majority of vaccines in use today protect against pathogens by their ability to induce vaccine-specific antibodies by activating different B cell subsets. These include both anti-bacterial and anti-viral vaccines [1]. Studies now show that B cells activated in response to these vaccines come from a variety of subsets including the marginal zone (MZ) B cells and the recirculating follicular B cells [2, 3]. These findings were demonstrated using high-throughput sequencing (HTS) of antibody repertoires in response to both anti-viral and anti-bacterial vaccines. HTS studies with anti-bacterial vaccines containing predominantly polysaccharide antigens versus protein–polysaccharide conjugates showed conjugate

Christopher B. Fox (ed.), *Vaccine Adjuvants: Methods and Protocols*, Methods in Molecular Biology, vol. 1494,
DOI 10.1007/978-1-4939-6445-1_26, © Springer Science+Business Media New York 2017

vaccines to induce more mutated sequences as compared to the former. The observed difference is characteristic of a T-dependent B cell response, which allows for somatic hypermutation (SHM) of the immunoglobulin variable region of both the heavy and light chains [4, 5].

Human and rodent antibodies consist of a dimer of two heavy and light chain pairs, IgH and IgL, which are encoded by large, complex loci. During the process of B cell development, variable (V), diversity (D), and joining (J) gene segments within these loci are rearranged by a process known as VDJ recombination [6]. The VDJ region encodes the portion of the antibody that binds to its cognate antigen, also known as the variable region. Most points of contact between the antigen and antibody are in three CDRs within the variable region, the largest of which, CDR3, is the major determinant of antigen specificity [7, 8]. The VDJ region is 5′ of the constant region gene segments, which undergo genomic rearrangements after B cell activation by the process of class switch recombination (CSR) [6]. CSR helps determine effector function, by changing isotype of the Ig molecule while still retaining antigen-specificity (encoded by CDRs).

Activated B cells may also undergo somatic hypermutation (SHM), a key feature of adaptive humoral immunity. This process is crucial for producing affinity-matured antibodies to specific epitopes exhibited by pathogens and vaccines alike [5]. This process takes place predominantly in the dark zones of germinal center (GC), wherein newly activated antigen-specific B cells activate the enzyme, activation-induced deaminase (AID) while undergoing rapid clonal expansion. AID in conjunction with other enzymes such as Uracil-DNA-Glycosylase (UNG) and Single-Strand-Selective Monofunctional Uracil-DNA Glycosylase 1 (SMUG-1) and mismatch repair protein MSH2 and MSH6 introduces mutations in specific "hotspots" of the Ig variable (V) region gene, allowing for a diverse antibody repertoire while retaining genomic integrity [9–11]. The "hotspots" for these mutations are now known to be located within the CDRs, primarily CDR1 of the IgV gene [7, 12, 13]. B cell with mutated Ig are then selected in the light zones of the GC for both antigen specificity and affinity, with the aid of follicular T helper cells (TFH cell) and the follicular dendritic cells (FDC) [9]. During this process, the FDC and TFH also aid these B cells to differentiate into long-lived antibody-producing plasma cells and/ or memory B cells. Signaling through the Toll-like receptors (TLR) is well known to influence this process of differentiation in the GC [14, 15]. The use of adjuvants containing TLR agonists to induce diversification of the immune repertoire however is a relatively new concept to help against rapidly changing pathogens [16].

HTS has made it possible to study populations of B cells as they develop in response to different vaccine adjuvant formulations on a previously unattainable scale [16]. HTS refers to a family of technologies (MiSeq, HiSeq, 454, Ion Torrent) that utilize massive parallelism to generate large numbers of sequence reads. Initially the average read length available using these technologies was not large enough to completely span the CDRs of IgH and IgL chains, which are approximately 400 bases long. This shortcoming was quickly overcome as the technologies matured. However, as the read length increases, the sequencing run times increase, and the read throughput decreases, so ideally, the choice of sequencing mode is the minimal sequence length that can comfortably cover the CDRs in order to maximize the total number of reads. Some of these technologies also can perform paired-end reads, meaning that every molecule sequenced generates two reads, starting from each end, and depending on the length of the read and size of the DNA, may overlap at their 3′ ends. A good choice for sequencing Ig CDRs using paired-ends is the Illumina 2 × 250 base kit, which produces paired-end reads averaging around 250 bases each.

2 Materials

2.1 Adjuvants for Immunization

1. Freund's incomplete and complete adjuvant (Sigma-Aldrich, St. Louis, MO).
2. Alhydrogel (Brenntag North America, Reading, PA).
3. Squalene oil-in-water emulsion (Invivogen, San Diego, CA).
4. TLR agonist containing adjuvants (Invivogen, San Diego, CA).

2.2 Cell Sorting

1. MACS reagents: automated or manual separators, columns, and magnetic beads (Miltenyi Biotec, San Diego, CA).
2. FACS reagents: Antigen-specific antibodies and appropriate buffers (BD Biosciences, San Jose, CA; Biolegend, San Diego, CA; Affymetrix Ebiosciences, San Diego, CA).
3. FACS Instruments: Cell sorters like BD FACSAria II (BD Biosciences, San Jose, CA) or MoFlo cell sorter (Beckman Coulter, Brea, CA) can be used.

2.3 RNA Isolation and RT Kits

1. RNAeasy Plus mini kit (Qiagen, Hilden, Germany).
2. RNAsin plus RNAse inhibitor (Promega, Madison, WI).
3. SuperScrip IV Reverse Transcriptase (Invitrogen, Waltham, MA).
4. Dynabeads® Oligo (dT)25 (Thermo Fisher, Waltham, MA).

2.4 PCR and Sample Prep

1. Phusion Hot Start Flex 2× Master Mix (NEB, Ipswich, MA).
2. QIAamp DNA Mini Kit (Qiagen, Hilden, Germany).
3. Nanodrop (Thermo Fisher, Waltham MA).
4. Qubit fluorometer (Invitrogen, Waltham MA).

2.5 HTS

1. MiSeq, HiSeq systems, (Illumina, San Diego, USA).
2. GS Junior, Junior+, FLEX+ System (Roche 454 Life Sciences, Branford, CT, USA).
3. Library MID Adaptors Kit (Roche 454 Life Sciences, Branford, CT, USA).
4. Ion Torrent (Applied Biosystems, Foster City, CA, USA).

3 Methods

3.1 Adjuvant Formulation and Administration

1. All vaccine and/or adjuvant formulation(s) of choice need to be used at a dose and route in which it has previously been shown to be effective in the species of interest.
2. Commonly used adjuvants are Alhydrogel (or Alum), Freund's adjuvants, squalene emulsions, and TLR4 containing formulations (e.g., AS04 andGLA-SE).
3. Vaccination protocols usually follow a prime-boost regimen, spaced from months to years, depending on species.
4. Vaccine-specific B cells can be found in peripheral blood 5–15 days post-primary immunization but tend to disappear from circulation shortly after. Boosting of this response helps bring back these cells into circulation and keeps their levels elevated for up to 6 weeks [17, 18].
5. Vaccine-specific effector long-lived plasma cells can be found in bone marrow 21 days post-primary immunization and last for a lifetime [19, 20].

3.2 Cell Sorting

1. Any primary tissue sample containing B cells is a complex mixture of B cells in multiple stages of differentiation as well as other cell types. The complexity of the RNA and DNA in the sample will depend on the degree to which this population has been refined by positive or negative selection.
2. Cells can be sorted using either Magnetic-activated cell sorting (MACS), or Fluorescence activated cell sorting (FACS), or a combination of both. Selection can be positive or negative; positive selection targets markers specific to the cell subset of interest. Negative selection actively selects for unwanted populations to enrich for an "untouched" subset of interest. Subsets of interest include antigen-experienced memory B cells, plasma cells, and marginal zone (MZ) B cells.
3. Follicular (FO) and MZ B cells in mice can be isolated from secondary lymphoid organs negatively by depleting T cells and antigen-presenting cells (APC) using magnetic beads (MACS) coated with anti-CD3, anti-CD11c, and anti-CD11b antibodies. FO and MZ B cells can be isolated from this first (T cell and APC-depleted) fraction using anti-CD23-coated magnetic

beads. This will negatively select for MZ B cells and positively select for FO B cells. Antigen-experienced FO B cells can be negatively isolated from the second fraction (T cell and APC-depleted) using the naïve B cell marker, IgD. Plasma cells can be isolated from the third fraction (enriched for antigen-experienced B cells) using the plasma cell marker, CD138. Alternatively, cells can be labeled with these markers and sorted using FACS directly into 96-well plates (for single cell sorting; *see* **Note 1**) or tubes (for select subsets) [21, 22].

4. Isolation of these populations from human PBMC can be accomplished by enriching for B cells using the pan-B cell marker CD19 using MACS before sorting for specific population by FACS. Distinct subsets can be isolated from the enriched fraction after staining for presence of CD20, CD38, CD27, IgM, IgD, and IgG. This combination of markers will allow for separation of naive (CD27−, IgM+, IgD+), circulating MZ (CD27+, IgM+, IgD+), IgM (only) memory (CD27+, IgM+, IgD−) and switched IgG memory (CD27+, IgM−, IgD−) cells. Inclusion of additional markers for chemokine receptors such as CXCR4 and HLA-DR expression will further help identify newly generated plasmablasts as well [3, 23].

3.3 Sample Preparation

1. Regardless of the starting cell population, the sequences representing the Ig variable regions need to be amplified out of a vastly more complex nucleotide mixture then flanked by appropriate sequences as required by the high-throughput sequencing technology of choice.
2. HTS experiments usually sequence reverse transcribed RNA rather than genomic DNA for several reasons: (a) the fraction of V-gene sequences, particularly in plasma cells which express high levels of antibody, can be much greater in RNA than genomic DNA, (b) all intron sequences have been spliced out, making it possible to completely sequence the CDRs through to Ig constant regions using small read lengths and (c) RNA expression profiles more closely reflect functional responses at the protein level. However, for some applications, such as clinical diagnostic tests which are intended to measure the clonality of B and T cell populations, direct amplification of genomic DNA is preferred (*see* **Note 2**).

3.4 RNA Extraction

1. RNA extraction protocols should try to minimize the time from sample harvest to lysing cells in RNA extraction buffer in order to prevent message degradation due to cell stress.
2. RNA extraction kits such as RNAeasy are cost effective and reliable ways to extract total RNA from cells.
3. Message RNA can be refined from total RNA by use of oligo-dt-coated magnetic beads. While this results in a sample enriched for Ig sequences which makes PCR amplification easier, it adds an additional processing step.

4. Similarly, addition of RNAse inhibitors is highly recommended as soon as the RNA is extracted from the cell lysis buffer, and ideally the next processing step should be performed as soon as possible, since purified RNA is highly sensitive to degradation by ubiquitous environmental enzymes.

3.5 Reverse Transcription

1. Reverse-transcription (RT) can be done using standard techniques of oligo-dt or random hexamer priming, which will generate a cDNA sampling of all species of RNA.
2. Another approach is to use gene-specific priming, which can restrict cDNA production to specific Ig isotypes of interest, such as only IgG subtypes.
3. If specific RT primers are used, it is possible at this step to introduce a Unique Molecular Indicator (UMI), which consists of a number (usually six or more) of random nucleotides synthesized into the reverse primer downstream of the Ig complementary region [24]. By enumerating the total number of distinct UMI sequences attached to a species of transcript rather than total sequence counts, we can control for different efficiencies of PCR amplification in addition to all other downstream sequencing steps. The UMI in effect counts individual cDNA generation events. It can also be helpful in identifying cross-group contamination (*see* **Note 3**).
4. Use of engineered reverse transcriptase enzymes such as superscript will increase fidelity and yield of the RT step.

3.6 Barcoding/Multiplexing

1. The high cost of a single high-throughput sequencing run relative to the number of samples generated by a multi-armed controlled experiment, all but mandates use of a strategy for multiplexing the samples from different experimental groups into a single run using a bar-coding strategy.
2. This can be done with the vendor specified bar-code tags, introducing custom bar-code tags, or a combination of both.
3. Custom bar-code lengths need only be long enough to enumerate the total number of experimental groups. For example, if there are 16 groups, a two nucleotide bar code is the minimum required, which will be a small fraction of the total amplicon.
4. Bar-codes can be added to the 3′ end of the amplicon unit during the RT step if gene specific primers are used, or at either the 3′ or 5′ ends during PCR (*see* **Note 4**).

3.7 Amplification, Adaptoring

1. All major commercial high-throughput sequencing methods require that you place technology specific sequences at the ends of the amplicon. For example, in the case of Illumina, required sequences include a capture sequence and a read-primer sequence. These sequences can be added during the initial PCR amplification or afterwards by a secondary PCR or by ligating adaptors to the ends of the PCR product.

2. There is a variety of commercial adaptoring kits available which will incorporate vendor-specific bar-codes and required sequences. kits available which will incorporate vendor-specific bar-codes and required sequences-specific barend
3. Primer sets must be chosen carefully in order to prevent primer–dimer formation from overwhelming the PCR amplification. Primer–dimers form when the 3′ ends of the oligos are complementary to sequences within another primer, so the greater the complexity of primer mix, and the longer the primers, the greater potential for primer–dimer formation.
4. Using either a two-step PCR reaction or amplicon adaptoring has the advantage of minimizing primer–dimer formation by using shorter primers in the first reaction. Since these reactions are a mixture of many different amplicons, reverse transcriptase enzymes engineered for high fidelity and processivity, such as Flash Phusion are highly recommended, in order to reduce cross-over and miss incorporation events.
5. PCR cycling times will vary depending on the thermocyler hardware, but the extension times can be quite short due to the small target amplicon size of approximately 400 base pairs, especially if thin-walled PCR tubes are used.

3.8 Downstream Primers

1. Since there are so many different isotypes of Ig, studies usually focus on a subset such as IgG and IgM. The target isotypes determine the downstream reverse primer set, and are usually positioned close to the 5′ end of the CH1 domain.
2. If gene-specific primers are used in the RT reaction, the reverse primers' 3′ gene complementary region can be the same sequences as those of the RT primers. Due to the relatively small number of constant region genes, these can be covered by a small number of different oligonucleotides.
3. However, if a UMI sequence was incorporated during the RT step, the downstream PCR primers must match a designated region positioned at the 5' end of the RT primers in order for the UMI sequence to be incorporated in the amplicon.

3.9 Upstream Primers

1. In contrast to the relatively few downstream constant region genes, depending on the species from which the sample is derived, there can be around 100 potentially active VH genes, all of which must be primed upstream of the CDR1 region for complete variable region coverage.
2. The number of individual oligonucleotides required can be reduced, by using mixed-synthesis at single locations. Mixed-synthesis at multiple locations is also possible, however some oligonucleotides may be generated that are not completely complementary to any known gene (*see* **Note 5**).

3. One strategy is to break the VH primers into several separate reactions, which increases the amount of labor per sample, but reduces primer–dimer formation. Gel purification after PCR is often needed to separate the amplified V regions from smaller primer–dimer artifacts. Another approach is to use 5′ RACE in order to ligate an upstream target sequence at the upstream end, although it can be challenging to perform RACE efficiently.

3.10 Pooling and Quantifying

1. After final clean up using a method such QIAmp DNA mini-kit, all bar-coded samples must be pooled in equal amounts.
2. Quantification can be done either by UV spectroscopy with an instrument such as a Nanodrop, or using a dye-based method like that used by a Qubit fluorometer.
3. Final sample concentration is a critical parameter for most HTS technologies. In most cases, over or under loading the sequencing cell rapidly degrades performance.

3.11 Deconvoluting

1. The sequencing procedure varies depending on the technology, read length, and whether the reads are end-paired. Due to the expense and complexity of HTS, this is often done in dedicated labs on a free-for-service basis. These labs may also offer support for various preparation steps including ligation of sequencing adapters and sample quantitation. After the HTS run is performed, the vendor system will process all of the raw data into an easily accessible format such as FASTQ, in which vendor specific read/capture sequences have been trimmed and sequences are binned into files depending on vendor barcode [25]. At this point, initial sanity checks can be performed on the data.
2. Obviously sequences with missing or mispaired primers can be discarded, as well as sequences not having any expected custom bar-codes of UMI sequences at the right positions.
3. If the sequences are end-paired, then criteria such as a required minimum overlap length and quality scores within the overlap can be incorporated into the initial filter.
4. An overview of the bioinformatics process discussed in this chapter starting from this initial step is shown in Fig. 1.

3.12 Redundancy Reduction/Clustering

1. The massive amounts of sequence data produced by high-throughput methods generate a significant amount of redundant information. There can be thousands of individual reads derived from the same starting RNA if that message was present in sufficient abundance, which means that sequence reads should be clustered (grouped) using criteria loose enough to reduce redundancy, but sufficiently stringent so as to not group together distinct messages.

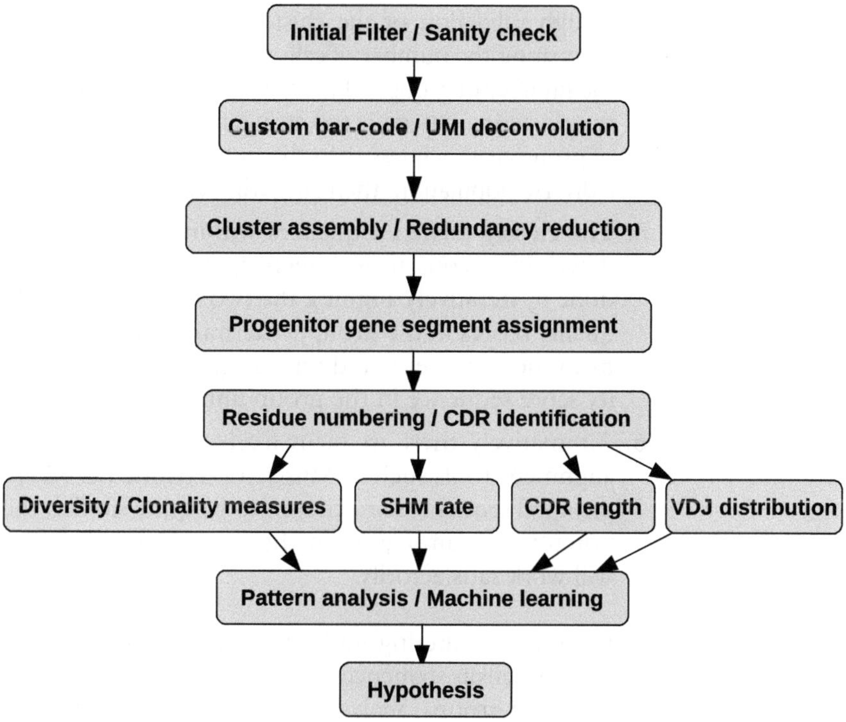

Fig. 1 Shown is a flowchart of a representative HTS Ig data analysis pipeline. After the initial steps are taken to filter, cluster, and identify the CDRs and closest genomic gene segments, a series of measurements can be assigned to each experimental group. These data can be analyzed for significant patterns or trends. If the experiment is sufficiently complex, machine learning techniques such as PCA may help in forming testable data-driven hypotheses

2. Initial grouping need only be performed on sets of sequences within a single experimental arm, as inter-arm comparison can be done later. Often grouping algorithms are iterative, building the largest cluster first, followed by the second largest, until no un-grouped sequences remain.
3. Clustering also requires criteria for inclusion or exclusion of a sequence into the group. Here is an example of an algorithm: (a) For each sequence in the set, calculate the set of all "neighbor" sequences by aligning it with every other sequence in the set using an insertion/deletion tolerant alignment method such as Smith-Waterman [26]. If the percent of matching nucleotides is above a cutoff value, the other sequence is added to the group. (b) Remove the largest group of sequences from unclustered set. (c) Repeat until no sequences remain in the unclustered group. If paired-end sequencing is being used, sequences which were initially excluded for not sufficiently overlapping can be added to clusters using the same criteria.

4. Rough validation of the clustering stringency can be done by comparing the number of cells present in the starting sample with the number of groups. If there are far more groups than cells then the clustering criteria is too stringent for the data. If the number of groups is much less than the number of input cells taken from a diverse population, then clustering criteria is too loose.
5. The closely related sequences within a group can be used to determine a consensus sequence, or group center. This can be done by iteratively aligning the two sequences with the highest quality scores in the group, determining a consensus sequence from the alignment, and repeating with the next highest quality score sequence in the group until all sequences are aligned.
6. Alternatively, there are many freely available multiple-sequence alignment tools such as Muscle or T-Coffe [27–29]. Since the grouped sequences are chosen to be quite similar, there is little potential for ambiguity in the consensus, and most methods will work satisfactorily.

3.13 Genomic and CDR Mapping

1. Once initial filtering and sanity checks have been performed, and consensus sequences have been derived from closely related sequence groups, analysis of the variable regions can begin.
2. Groups whose consensus sequences do not contain open reading frames in the amplicon can be eliminated at this point, since CDR location analysis depends on predicted protein sequence.
3. For the remaining groups, first steps in analysis of the sequences include (a) determining which are the most likely genomic progenitors of the V, D, J, and constant regions, and (b) mapping the predicted protein residues to the three CDRs.
4. Mapping the genomic genes can be done by taking a list of all the V, D, J, and C exon regions, and determining which has the best match to a group's consensus. Again, any insertion/deletion tolerant method of nucleotide alignment such as Smith-Waterman can be used for this purpose. One subtlety is that the D regions are so small that their sequences may not be unique to the site of D gene recombination, so the V and J region genes should be mapped first and the D regions matched only to the intervening sequences.
5. Antibody variable regions residues are labeled in a structurally consistent manner using either the Kabat or Chothia numbering schemes, which delineate CDR and framework regions. This is not a trivial task, and many different algorithms have been proposed to do this in the literature. One simple but effective method is to leverage a set of antibodies already mapped to the Chothia and Kabat schemes using 3D structural information (Dr. Andrew C.R. Martin's Group, http://www.bioinf.org.uk/), and use that as consensus sequence to which

```
                [  CDR1   ]              [ CDR2  ]                                       [ CDR 3 ]           [Const.]
glvrpsqslsltcsvtGYSITSGYYWNwirqfpgnklewmgYISYDGRNNynpslknrisitrdtfknqfflklnfvttedtatyycarEDYGSPFDYwghgttltvssatttapsv
   R             Y                             R  Y P        T   F         F   E     Y   ED   P     H
glvKpsqslsltcsvtgYsitsgyywnwirqfpgnklewmgyisydgSnnYnPslknrisiTrdtSknqfflklnSvttEdtatyYcar-Yygs-fdywgQgttltvssatttapsv
[                                             V3-6                                      ][ D1][     J2      ][  G3  ]
```

Fig. 2 Shown is the predicted translated protein sequence and CDR mapping of an example mouse IgH cluster compared to the nearest genomic gene segments. The cluster was assembled of 227 end-paired reads from a 2 × 250 Illumina HTS experiment, in which there were 90 different UMI sequences (data not shown). The *top sequence* is the translated cluster consensus annotated with the location of the CDRs and Ig constant domain. The *bottom sequence* shows alignments of nearest IgH loci gene segment translations. The *middle line* shows the location of nucleotide differences and the resulting predicted residue (which due to codon redundancy may not change the predicted amino acid at every location)

data sequences can be aligned using the hidden Markov model alignment program, Hmmer, which will align a single protein sequence to a multiple protein sequence alignment [30–32]. See Fig. 2 for an example of a mouse IgH HTS group consensus CDR mapping done by this method.

6. Thankfully, there is an online resource (IMGT/HighV-Quest, http://www.imgt.org) that will perform both the genomic mapping and residue numbering for many of the most commonly sequenced species. It accepts uploads of large numbers of sequences in fasta format, and performs CDR mapping that is considered to be state of the art. It will also classify the sequence as being productive or nonproductive. Unfortunately, if the species of interest is not available in HighV-Quest, it is up to the researcher to collect the set of V, D, J, and C Ig gene segments and perform the genomic mapping themselves (*see* **Note 6**). However, in many cases, CDR mapping performed by HighV-Quest using the most closely related species is likely to be sufficient.

3.14 Higher-Level Analysis

1. After grouping to eliminate sequence redundancy, performing basic variable region analysis to identify the most likely germline progenitor genes comprising the variable region, and mapping CDR and framework regions, a wide variety of higher-level statistics can be applied to the sequence data.
2. The length and percent mutation of the CDRs, particularly CDR3, correlates with affinity-maturation of the population. Methods originally devised to measure species diversity in ecological studies, such as the Simpson Diversity Index, methods based on Shannon entropy, and a variety of other measures can be applied to measure repertoire diversity and clonality in B and T cell populations [33, 34].
3. For many of these well-studied metrics, confidence scores can also be calculated using published formulas. However, applying diversity measures based on ecological concepts of species diversity relies on translating the concept of species in the

ecological sense to clustered consensus sequence variable regions generated by high-throughput sequencing. This can be done by applying criteria to judge whether or not two (group consensus) sequences represent the same clonal lineage as an analog to the concept of species. An easy method to do this is testing for identical CDR3 regions, since two antibodies with the identical CDR3 are highly likely to have related antigen specificity [3].

4. The distribution of V-gene families or V-D-J combinations can be assessed for differential expression between the different experimental arms. Until the advent of HTS, support for any hypothesis postulating a response biased towards a particular V gene family had to rely on a relatively low number of examples. However, using HTS, statements about V-gene distribution can be made with much greater confidence.
5. Presented with a large number of experimental groups, each with multiple of metrics, it can be difficult to identify the most significant trends. This job can be made easier by using automatic pattern recognition algorithms, such as, but by no means limited to, Principle Component Analysis (PCA) [35]. PCA reduces a large number of variables down to a smaller number that can optimally discriminate between groups and has proven useful in the analysis of HTS data.
6. Given the massive amount of sequence data produced by HTS experiments, automated methods to identify patterns in the data are likely to gain in popularity. Also, given the lack of standardization of Ig HTS protocols between different research groups, identification of robust higher-level trends by thorough methods such as PCA, offers the best chance of obtaining results that can be reproduced by multiple laboratories.
7. Although there is a growing set of software resources that can be leveraged to assist in analysis of Ig HTS data, in most cases a researcher will use multiple programs written in different languages to tailor the analysis to a specific experiment.
8. If a program is going to be repeatedly applied to the data such as a multiple sequence alignment program, which needs to be run over thousands of clusters it needs to be executed, or wrapped, by a master program that will feed it each group of sequences and handle the results.
9. While most programming languages can perform this task, the choice of language needs to take into account what software packages are available to assist in tasks like graphing, diversity calculation, and database storage and retrieval. Python (www.python.org) and Java (www.oracle.com/technetwork/java) are commonly employed for this purpose. Languages and programs that are designed for statistical and mathematical applications,

such as R (www.r-project.org) and Mathmatica (http://www.wolfram.com/mathematica), have many sophisticated features and packages that can be leveraged for HTS data analysis.

4 Notes

1. Bulk sequencing of IgH and IgL does not provide information as to which are paired together in naturally occurring antibodies. If the goal is to create functional antibodies, one approach is to sort single cells into multiwell plates, and then use a barcode strategy to keep track of the sequences derived from each well. This requires the technically difficult step of sequencing amplicons from single cells, and is inherently lower-throughput than bulk methods. Recently, it has come to light that for many antibodies, the light chain supports the heavy chain variable region structurally, but does not contact the antigen directly. In these cases, pairing a handful of diverse light chains with a given heavy chain is likely to produce a functional antibody. However, it has not been established whether antibodies made in this way are either higher-affinity or lower-affinity than naturally occurring heavy–light chain pairs.
2. There has been an effort to standardize clinical diagnostic applications which use HTS of Ig to diagnose a variety of human leukemias [36]. For clinical diagnostic applications, repeatable measurement of the diversity and clonality of the B cell and T cell repertoire is more important than analysis of the entire Ig variable region, so some of these tests use a set of standardized PCR primers, BIOMED-2 to amplify juncture regions between sites of genomic recombination (InVivoScribe, San Diego, CA, USA). Although this will not capture the entire antibody variable region, the benefit of using a standardized protocol could greatly increase reproducibility of vaccine adjuvant experiments in human subjects.
3. Given the extremely sensitive nature of PCR, there is always potential for cross-sample contamination. For example, if when comparing two samples from different organisms the most abundant sequences derived from one sample are present at a fractional abundance in the other--that is strong evidence of bleed-over between samples. This must be taken into account in any downstream analysis. If UMI tags were incorporated into the sequences, bleed-over can be confirmed, since virtually every individual UMI tagged sequence contaminating the second sample will also be present in the first.
4. A virtually unlimited number of bar-coded samples can be multiplexed in a single HTS run. However, the total number of reads from each sample will be reduced in proportion to the

total number of samples, so choosing how many samples to multiplex depends on the complexity of the samples, the desired degree of coverage per cell, and the total number of expected reads per run produced by the HTS technology of choice.

5. PCR primers using mixed synthesis reactions at more than one location run the risk of generating sequences that are not present in the target sequence set. For example, if in the same primer, a C-G-T mixed synthesis is used at one location and a T-A mixed synthesis is used at another position, six different types of primers will be generated, some of which may have no exact complementary sequences in the targeted gene segments.
6. If Ig loci of the experimental species is not well studied or annotated, as is the case for many nonhuman primates, it is incumbent on the researcher to identify the set of V, D, J, and C regions themselves. Also, the less studied a species is, the more likely it is that their genomic assemblies are incomplete, particularly in regions with large numbers of closely related genes, such as complex Ig loci. In this case, the researcher may have to search sequences of partially assembled genomic reads to identify a complete set of Ig gene segments.

References

1. Siegrist CA (2007) Vaccine immunology (general aspects of vaccination). Elsevier Vaccine Immunology Chapter 2:19
2. Jiang N, He J, Weinstein JA, Penland L, Sasaki S, He XS, Dekker CL, Zheng NY, Huang M, Sullivan M, Wilson PC, Greenberg HB, Davis MM, Fisher DS, Quake SR (2013) Lineage structure of the human antibody repertoire in response to influenza vaccination. Sci Transl Med 5(171):171ra119. doi:10.1126/scitranslmed.3004794
3. Galson JD, Clutterbuck EA, Truck J, Ramasamy MN, Munz M, Fowler A, Cerundolo V, Pollard AJ, Lunter G, Kelly DF (2015) BCR repertoire sequencing: different patterns of B-cell activation after two meningococcal vaccines. Immunol Cell Biol. doi:10.1038/icb.2015.57
4. Kelly DF, Snape MD, Clutterbuck EA, Green S, Snowden C, Diggle L, Yu LM, Borkowski A, Moxon ER, Pollard AJ (2006) CRM197-conjugated serogroup C meningococcal capsular polysaccharide, but not the native polysaccharide, induces persistent antigen-specific memory B cells. Blood 108(8):2642–2647. doi:10.1182/blood-2006-01-009282
5. Di Noia JM, Neuberger MS (2007) Molecular mechanisms of antibody somatic hypermutation. Annu Rev Biochem 76:1–22. doi:10.1146/annurev.biochem.76.061705.090740
6. Dudley DD, Chaudhuri J, Bassing CH, Alt FW (2005) Mechanism and control of V(D)J recombination versus class switch recombination: similarities and differences. Adv Immunol 86:43–112. doi:10.1016/S0065-2776(04)86002-4
7. Jolly CJ, Wagner SD, Rada C, Klix N, Milstein C, Neuberger MS (1996) The targeting of somatic hypermutation. Semin Immunol 8(3):159–168. doi:10.1006/smim.1996.0020
8. Xu JL, Davis MM (2000) Diversity in the CDR3 region of V(H) is sufficient for most antibody specificities. Immunity 13(1):37–45
9. Shlomchik MJ, Weisel F (2012) Germinal center selection and the development of memory B and plasma cells. Immunol Rev 247(1):52–63. doi:10.1111/j.1600-065X.2012.01124.x
10. Dingler FA, Kemmerich K, Neuberger MS, Rada C (2014) Uracil excision by endogenous SMUG1 glycosylase promotes efficient Ig class switching and impacts on A:T substitutions during somatic mutation. Eur J Immunol 44(7):1925–1935. doi:10.1002/eji.201444482
11. Maul RW, Gearhart PJ (2010) Controlling somatic hypermutation in immunoglobulin variable and switch regions. Immunol Res 47(1-3):113–122. doi:10.1007/s12026-009-8142-5

12. Cowell LG, Kim HJ, Humaljoki T, Berek C, Kepler TB (1999) Enhanced evolvability in immunoglobulin V genes under somatic hypermutation. J Mol Evol 49(1):23–26
13. Betz AG, Rada C, Pannell R, Milstein C, Neuberger MS (1993) Passenger transgenes reveal intrinsic specificity of the antibody hypermutation mechanism: clustering, polarity, and specific hot spots. Proc Natl Acad Sci U S A 90(6):2385–2388
14. Pasare C, Medzhitov R (2005) Control of B-cell responses by Toll-like receptors. Nature 438(7066):364–368. doi:10.1038/nature04267
15. Raman VS, Lind EF, Benson MJ, Noelle RJ (2007) Strategies for selective priming of memory B cells. Immunol Lett 109(2):93–100. doi:10.1016/j.imlet.2007.01.010
16. Wiley SR, Raman VS, Desbien A, Bailor HR, Bhardwaj R, Shakri AR, Reed SG, Chitnis CE, Carter D (2011) Targeting TLRs expands the antibody repertoire in response to a malaria vaccine. Sci Transl Med 3(93):93ra69. doi:10.1126/scitranslmed.3002135
17. Clutterbuck EA, Salt P, Oh S, Marchant A, Beverley P, Pollard AJ (2006) The kinetics and phenotype of the human B-cell response following immunization with a heptavalent pneumococcal-CRM conjugate vaccine. Immunology 119(3):328–337. doi:10.1111/j.1365-2567.2006.02436.x
18. Zhang X, Wang Q, Bi Y, Kou Z, Zhou J, Cui Y, Yan Y, Zhou L, Tan Y, Yang H, Du Z, Han Y, Song Y, Zhang P, Zhou D, Yang R, Wang X (2014) Kinetics of memory B cell and plasma cell responses in the mice immunized with plague vaccines. Scand J Immunol 79(3):157–162. doi:10.1111/sji.12146
19. Manz RA, Thiel A, Radbruch A (1997) Lifetime of plasma cells in the bone marrow. Nature 388(6638):133–134. doi:10.1038/40540
20. Slifka MK, Antia R, Whitmire JK, Ahmed R (1998) Humoral immunity due to long-lived plasma cells. Immunity 8(3):363–372
21. White HN, Meng QH (2012) Recruitment of a distinct but related set of VH sequences into the murine CD21hi/CD23- marginal zone B cell repertoire to that seen in the class-switched antibody response. J Immunol 188(1):287–293. doi:10.4049/jimmunol.1101264
22. McHeyzer-Williams LJ, Cool M, McHeyzer-Williams MG (2000) Antigen-specific B cell memory: expression and replenishment of a novel b220(-) memory b cell compartment. J Exp Med 191(7):1149–1166
23. Odendahl M, Mei H, Hoyer BF, Jacobi AM, Hansen A, Muehlinghaus G, Berek C, Hiepe F, Manz R, Radbruch A, Dorner T (2005) Generation of migratory antigen-specific plasma blasts and mobilization of resident plasma cells in a secondary immune response. Blood 105(4):1614–1621. doi:10.1182/blood-2004-07-2507
24. Kivioja T, Vaharautio A, Karlsson K, Bonke M, Enge M, Linnarsson S, Taipale J (2012) Counting absolute numbers of molecules using unique molecular identifiers. Nat Methods 9(1):72–74. doi:10.1038/nmeth.1778
25. Cock PJ, Fields CJ, Goto N, Heuer ML, Rice PM (2010) The Sanger FASTQ file format for sequences with quality scores, and the Solexa/Illumina FASTQ variants. Nucleic Acids Res 38(6):1767–1771. doi:10.1093/nar/gkp1137
26. Smith TF, Waterman MS (1981) Identification of common molecular subsequences. J Mol Biol 147(1):195–197
27. Edgar RC (2004) MUSCLE: multiple sequence alignment with high accuracy and high throughput. Nucleic Acids Res 32(5):1792–1797. doi:10.1093/nar/gkh340
28. Edgar RC (2004) MUSCLE: a multiple sequence alignment method with reduced time and space complexity. BMC Bioinformatics 5:113. doi:10.1186/1471-2105-5-113
29. Notredame C, Higgins DG, Heringa J (2000) T-Coffee: A novel method for fast and accurate multiple sequence alignment. J Mol Biol 302(1):205–217. doi:10.1006/jmbi.2000.4042
30. Eddy SR (2009) A new generation of homology search tools based on probabilistic inference. Genome Inform 23(1):205–211
31. Abhinandan KR, Martin AC (2008) Analysis and improvements to Kabat and structurally correct numbering of antibody variable domains. Mol Immunol 45(14):3832–3839. doi:10.1016/j.molimm.2008.05.022
32. Kabat EA, Wu TT (1991) Identical V region amino acid sequences and segments of sequences in antibodies of different specificities. Relative contributions of VH and VL genes, minigenes, and complementarity-determining regions to binding of antibody-combining sites. J Immunol 147(5):1709–1719
33. Simpson EH (1949) Measurement of diversity. Nature 163
34. Arnaud-Haond S, Duarte CM, Alberto F, Serrao EA (2007) Standardizing methods to address clonality in population studies. Mol Ecol 16(24):5115–5139. doi:10.1111/j.1365-294X.2007.03535.x
35. Pearson K (1901) On lines and planes of closest fit to systems of points in space. Philos Mag 2(11)
36. Langerak AW, Groenen PJ, Bruggemann M, Beldjord K, Bellan C, Bonello L, Boone E, Carter GI, Catherwood M, Davi F, Delfau

-Larue MH, Diss T, Evans PA, Gameiro P, Garcia Sanz R, Gonzalez D, Grand D, Hakansson A, Hummel M, Liu H, Lombardia L, Macintyre EA, Milner BJ, Montes-Moreno S, Schuuring E, Spaargaren M, Hodges E, van Dongen JJ (2012) EuroClonality/BIOMED-2 guidelines for interpretation and reporting of Ig/TCR clonality testing in suspected lymphoproliferations. Leukemia 26(10):2159–2171. doi:10.1038/leu.2012.246

INDEX

A

Adaptive immunity....202, 307
AF03....7, 8, 166–168, 171–173, 176, 178, 183
α-galactosylceramide....321–348
Alpha-tocopherol....4, 6, 177, 183
Aluminum salts
  AdjuPhos®....185, 192
  Alhydrogel®....185, 188, 254, 263–271
  aluminum hydroxyphosphate....181, 182, 185
  aluminum nanoparticles....189–190
  aluminum oxyhydroxide....181, 182, 185, 196, 254, 257
  antigen adsorption....186–187
  antigen characterization....184
  antigen desorption....187–188
Antibodies....2, 9, 10, 19, 20, 166, 307, 309, 315, 316, 321, 330–331, 335, 340, 344, 345, 353–357, 362, 364, 365
Antigen presenting cells (APCs)....2, 5, 6, 8, 16, 30, 128, 146, 201, 306, 311, 323, 356, 357
Antigen production....155
Anti-tumor immune responses....202
Aqueous extract....88–92
AS01....7, 9, 74
AS03....4, 6, 8, 9, 166, 167, 177, 183
AS04....3–5, 182, 183, 356
AS15....9

B

B cells....2, 16, 17, 306, 308–310, 323, 353, 354, 356, 357, 363, 365
Biodegradable....6, 8, 184, 201–212
Bioinformatics....353–366
Biosynthesis....96, 102, 175, 337
Block copolymer gels....154

C

CAF01....7
Cancer vaccine....6, 9, 201–212
Carbopol....156, 157, 161
C-C chemokine receptor type 1 (CCR1)....30
C-C chemokine receptor type 4 (CCR4)....108, 110–114, 116–120, 122, 123
CD1d....323
CD4 T cell....114, 115, 146, 323
CD8 T cell....7, 118, 119, 146, 310
CD69....307, 309, 310
CD80....306, 307, 309
CD86....306, 307, 309
CD154....314, 316
Cervarix®....3, 5, 202
Chemical synthesis....46, 88
Cholesterol....7, 74, 75, 81–82, 175
CIMAvax EGF®....6, 183
Complementary determining regions (CDRs)....354, 355, 357, 359, 361–364
Complete Freund's adjuvant (CFA)....5, 311
CpG-containing oligodeoxynucleotides (CpG-ODN)....16, 17, 19, 20, 24, 202–204
Cyclic di-GMP (cdGMP)....146, 147
Cyclic dinucleotides....145, 146
Cytokine signature....295–303, 313–320, 321–348
Cytometric bead array....319

D

Danger-associated molecule pattern (DAMP)....5
Delivery system....3, 4, 7, 127, 227, 323
Dendritic cells (DCs)....16, 17, 30, 108, 201, 308, 322, 327
Dimethyldioctadecylammonium (DDA)....7, 138–141
dmLT....156, 158, 159
DNA....5, 16, 24, 30, 97, 98, 120, 121, 136, 203, 204, 328, 354–357, 360
Dynamic light scattering (DLS)....76, 174, 237, 239–251

E

ELISpot....118, 119, 313–320
Emulsions
  association with antigen....6
  characterization....173–175
  high pressure homogenization/microfluidization....166, 169
  high shear mixing....131
  manufacturing....169, 171, 176
  phase inversion temperature method....166, 171–173, 184
Engerix-B®....20–24

Christopher B. Fox (ed.), *Vaccine Adjuvants: Methods and Protocols*, Methods in Molecular Biology, vol. 1494,
DOI 10.1007/978-1-4939-6445-1_26, © Springer Science+Business Media New York 2017

Enzyme-linked immunosorbent assay (ELISA)................21, 159, 285, 296, 297, 299, 300, 319
ERG-1 gene..96, 97, 101
Ergosterol..96, 97, 101, 102, 104

F

Fendrix®..5
Flagellin...16, 30
Flow cytometry........................ 109, 115, 117, 302, 306, 314, 315, 317, 319, 335–336, 340–343, 345
FluAd®..166
Fluorescence spectroscopy............... 208–209, 263–271, 286
Forced degradation.................................. 228, 230, 232, 234
Formulation................3–5, 7, 74, 82–83, 153–162, 166, 168, 174, 176, 181, 184, 188, 191, 192, 195, 203, 210, 211, 215–220, 227–251, 253, 263–267, 273, 285, 288, 290, 295–303, 306, 310, 354, 356
Fourier transform infrared (FTIR) spectroscopy.................................. 253, 254, 286
Freeze drying.. 78, 216, 224
Freeze-thawing.. 229, 232–234, 237

G

Genetic engineering..95
Glucopyranoside lipid adjuvant (GLA)............... 7, 255, 257, 258, 310
Glucopyranosyl lipid adjuvanted stable nanoemulsion (GLA-SE).........................7, 217, 221, 274, 276, 277, 280, 281, 286, 288, 290, 291
Glycosylation... 58, 59, 61–64, 264
GM-CSF..314
Granulocyte...6, 308

H

Helicobacter suis... 111, 119–121
Hepatitis B...5, 9, 16, 181, 182
HEPLISAV-B™.. 17, 18, 20–24
High-performance liquid chromatography (HPLC)....................... 46, 75, 76, 78, 79, 85, 88, 97–101, 104, 174, 211, 255
High-throughput DNA sequencing (HTS)............353–366
History...v, 15, 20, 254
Hydroxypropyl methylcellulose (HPMC).............. 156, 157, 161, 162

I

Ig heavy (IgH).. 354, 355, 363, 365
IgL..354, 355, 365
IL-2...110, 116, 117, 314, 316
IL-5..314–316
IL-12...30, 110
IL-17A..316
IL-18...30, 310
Imidazoquinoline...38, 145, 203
Imiquimod..202, 203
Immunogenicity.......................... 3, 6, 15, 18–20, 22, 24, 87, 108, 159, 162, 166, 182–184, 193, 197, 202, 228, 313–320, 322, 323, 328, 337
Immunoglobulin G (IgG)............................... 160, 357–359
Immunostimulating complexes (ISCOMs)....................7, 82
Inactivated vaccine...2, 3
Incomplete Freund's adjuvant (IFA)................................5, 6
Inflammasome...5, 310
Innate immunity..203, 296
In silico...107–123
Interferon alpha (IFN-α)..16, 17
Interferon gamma (IFN-γ)........................16, 110, 116, 121, 122, 296, 297, 299, 301–303, 309, 310, 314–316
Intracellular cytokine staining (ICS)........ 313–320, 335–336
ISCOMATRIX®...7

J

Janeway, Charles..v, 2, 202
Jenner, Edward..1, 2, 322

L

Lipid extraction...99, 101
Lipopolysaccharide (LPS)........................5, 16, 30, 118, 183, 202, 211, 346
Liposomes
- association with antigen...137
- characterization..74
- extrusion.. 81, 131, 148
- high shear mixing...131, 132
- homogenization..130
- inkjet...132
- lipid film hydration................. 81, 85, 129, 139, 141, 142
- manufacturing.................................... 129–132, 139–141
- microfluidics..133–136
- solvent injection..132
- sonication.. 131, 139–140
- supercritical fluid..132

Liquid chromatography (LC).......................... 74–78, 88–91
Live attenuated vaccine..2, 321
Luminex®...297, 319
Lymph node...................................6, 19, 117, 145–151, 239, 305–311, 314, 339
Lymphocytes.....................314, 315, 330–331, 340–343, 347
Lyophilization.......................................67, 68, 211, 215–220

M

Malaria...45, 74, 88
Manufacturing of adjuvants......127–142 , 165–178, 181–197
Mass spectrometry (MS)....................18, 67, 174 , 165–178, 181–197
Matrix M-2...9
Mechanical stress...228, 230–232
Mechanism of action.............. 3, 5, 6, 8, 16, 24, 74, 273, 296

Metabolic engineering........96
MF59®........3, 4, 6, 8, 165–167, 170, 176, 177, 183, 306
MHCI........309
MHCII........309
Mineral oil........5, 49, 57, 184
Monocytes........6, 19, 30, 309
Monophosphoryl lipid A (MPLA)........4–7, 147–149, 151, 183, 202–204, 207, 208, 211
Montanide® ISA 51........6, 184
Mucosal........24, 153–155, 159, 160, 165, 177, 339
Multivariate modeling........258–259

N

NALP3........5
Nanoparticles........8, 135, 136, 140, 146, 186, 189, 193, 204–205, 240, 248
Nanoparticle tracking analysis (NTA)........175, 239–251
Narcolepsy........9, 10
Native PAGE........286–287, 290–292
Natural killer (NK) cells........16
Natural killer T (NKT) cells........323, 327, 328
Natural product........46
Neutrophils........6, 296, 306, 308
NOD-like receptors (NLRs)........30
Nucleotide oligomerization domai (NOD)........42

O

O-phthalaldehyde (OPA) assay........263–271, 286

P

Pandemrix®........183
Partial least squares modeling........253–259
Particle shape........205, 208
Particle size........85, 86, 104, 129, 166, 170, 174, 189, 203, 205–207, 228, 232, 237, 239–241, 248–250
Pathogen-associated molecular patterns (PAMPs)........2, 3, 16, 202
Pattern recognition receptors (PRRs)........2, 16, 145, 202
Peripheral blood mononuclear cells (PBMC)........34, 114, 115, 296, 302, 357
Phospholipid........7, 104, 139, 146, 177
Photostability........229, 230, 233–235, 237, 238
Poloxamer........154, 161, 222
Poly(I:C)........323
Poly(lactic-co-glycolic) acid (PLGA)
  adjuvant loading........205
  adjuvant release........205, 211
  characterization........204–205
Polymeric microparticles........8
Polyoxyethylene(12)-ceto-stearylether........172
Polysorbate 80........4
Purification........34, 47, 51–65, 70, 97, 103, 104, 118, 146, 149, 328, 329, 337, 338, 346, 360

Q

QB-90........88, 90–92
QS-21
  formulation
  synthesis........46
Quil-A®........73–75, 77, 85, 88, 89
Quillaja brasiliensis........88
Quillaja saponaria (QS)........6, 45, 73, 74, 88

R

Raw material source........176
Recombinant vaccine........2, 107
Regulatory T cell........108–110, 114–115, 117
Resiquimod........145, 203–205, 207, 209
Respiratory syncytial virus
Ribi, Edgar........183
RIG-I and RIG-I ligands........145
RNA........30, 120, 121, 136, 145, 202, 355–358, 360

S

Saccharomyces cerevisiae........95, 96
Safety........2–5, 9, 15, 18, 19, 23–25, 29, 38, 42, 70, 108, 175, 176, 184, 189, 202, 297, 321
Saponin
  formulation........73, 74
  purification........65
  synthesis........47, 65–68
Scalability........131, 133, 136
Site of injection (SOI)........2, 5, 6
Size-exclusion chromatography........150
Small molecule........9, 108, 113, 145, 146
Smallpox........322
Sodium dodecyl sulfate-polyacrylamide gel electrophoresis (SDS-PAGE)
  Coomassie stain........186, 193, 197, 274–280 , 287–293, 331–346
  gold stain........274, 275, 279
  PVDF membrane........274–275, 278–279
  silver stain........274, 275, 279, 282
Solid phase extraction (SPF)........97, 100
Somatic hypermutation (SHM)........354
Sorbitan monooleate........170, 178
Sorbitan trioleate........4
Squalene........4, 6–8, 101, 102, 165–171, 173, 175–178, 183, 237, 287, 310, 355, 356
Squalene monooxygenase........96, 97, 101
Stability........3, 5, 8, 24, 46, 129, 155, 165, 173, 174, 176, 177, 202, 210, 227–239, 273, 280, 285, 296, 301, 345
Stable emulsion (SE)........8, 166, 167, 177
STING........146
Stressed stability........227–238
Sublingual........119, 153–162
Subunit vaccine........3, 15, 29, 45, 107, 127, 136–138, 322

T

T cells 2, 117–119, 296, 300–303, 306, 308–310, 314, 322, 323, 327, 328, 330–331, 339, 341–345, 347, 348, 356, 357, 363, 365
TDB. *See* Trehalose dibehenate (TDB)
Th1 .... 5, 7, 16, 18, 29, 30, 108, 202, 203
Th2 .... 5, 16, 29, 109–110, 115–116
Th17 314
T helper (Tfh) 354
T helper type 2 (Th2) 183
Thermoresponsive 153–162
Thermostable 215–220
Thin-layer chromatography (TLC) 40, 50, 51, 53, 75, 77, 78, 89, 91–92, 97, 98, 100, 101, 103, 104
Toll-like receptors (TLRs)
  biological activity 87
  characterization 16, 322–323
  formulation 322–323
  synthesis 177
Trehalose dibehenate (TDB) 7, 138–141
Triterpene 46, 47, 52–54, 63, 69, 70
Tumor necrosis factor (TNF) 19, 314, 316

U

Ultracentrifugation 150, 286–288

V

Vaccinia virus 322, 332, 339
Variable, diversity, and joining (VDJ) region 354
Varicella zoster virus (shingles) .... v, 45, 88
Venezuelan Equine Encephalitis 2
Virosomes 4, 183, 184

W

WEC50 7
Whole-blood assay 297, 299

Y

Yeast 18, 176, 332

Z

Zeta potential 173, 175, 204, 208, 210, 237, 241

MIX
Papier aus verantwortungsvollen Quellen
Paper from responsible sources
FSC® C105338

If you have any concerns about our products,
you can contact us on
ProductSafety@springernature.com

In case Publisher is established outside the EU,
the EU authorized representative is:
Springer Nature Customer Service Center GmbH
Europaplatz 3, 69115 Heidelberg, Germany

Printed by Libri Plureos GmbH
in Hamburg, Germany